# MicroLED Devices and Systems

For a complete listing of titles in the
*Artech House Applied Photonics Library,*
turn to the back of this book.

# MicroLED Devices and Systems

Khaled Ahmed

ARTECH
HOUSE
BOSTON | LONDON
artechhouse.com

**Library of Congress Cataloging-in-Publication Data**
A catalog record for this book is available from the U.S. Library of Congress.

**British Library Cataloguing in Publication Data**
A catalogue record for this book is available from the British Library.

**Cover design by Joi Garron**

ISBN 13: 978-1-68569-049-6


**685 Canton Street**
**Norwood, MA 02062**



10 9 8 7 6 5 4 3 2 1

*To Leila*

# Contents

# Foreword

I first met Khaled Ahmed in April 2021 through colleagues at Intel Corporation who spoke highly of his reputation and expertise in microLED technology. As an Intel Fellow in the Office of the Chief Technology Officer (CTO), driving advanced research and development (R&D) programs, I felt the need to explore alternative technological directions beyond what my team had in-hand and working. Although our experimental technology showed all the hallmarks of viability and potential, I was concerned that we might be missing a superior solution.

At that time, the world was reeling from the COVID-19 pandemic with record-breaking rates of infection, political tensions were heating up to levels not seen in decades, climate heating was exacerbated by activities like bitcoin mining, and educational institutions faced unprecedented challenges. Amid these crises, science and technology continued to achieve remarkable feats: a helicopter flew on Mars for the first time thanks to the scientists behind NASA's programs, a house was 3D printed from clay for the first time, and numerous brilliant minds were addressing critical future problems.

By the time I started looking for an expert in microLED technology, I was the principal investigator of a program partly funded by the Defense Advanced Research Projects Agency (DARPA) Hierarchy Identify Verify Exploit (HIVE) to develop a first demonstration of an at-scale computing architecture that had optical networks directly attached for breakthrough scalability and energy efficiency. High-speed networks had been optical for many years, but traditionally required complex protocol conversions and electrical drivers, consuming significant what computers want to operate on—wide, parallel electric input/output (I/O)—and converted into.

In the DARPA HIVE program, which led to Intel's Programmable Integrated Unified Memory Architecture (PIUMA) technology, we integrated optical I/O with compute silicon, achieving substantial improvements in energy efficiency and latency by eliminating unnecessary conversion processes. We exposed the wide parallel electrical I/O directly to the optical transceivers, and allowed experimental optical chiplets to do direct conversion to the native speed and encoding for optical transmission. Putting these units into the same package gave us significant advantages in energy and orders of magnitude improvement in latency. We also used a global shared address space construct that allowed us to radically expand upon a high-radix network construct to make low-diameter networks, effectively reducing the end-to-end latency of operations that would be critical to the future of petabyte-scale problems in analytics, artificial intelligence (AI), and high-performance computing (HPC) domains. That resulting PIUMA design was eventually revealed at HotChips 2023.

While my team continued to innovate with direct copackaged optical I/O, I grew increasingly concerned about the challenges posed by laser-based photonic data communications. Modern interfaces face numerous obstacles, such as data links requiring training and firmware, microcontrollers to enable and tune devices during operation, design for test and resiliency with an ever-increasing complexity, and other facets of standard designs. When combining these day-to-day problems with novel challenges of precise temperature control to keep optical links stable, susceptibility to noise in supply voltages, and an order-of-magnitude increase in the complexity of tuning and retaining stable links, I became concerned about the hurdles to realizing economic viability of this technology for high-volume manufacturing. It's a different scale of problem to make 10 thousand units in a year versus the scale at which Intel builds products in the 1 billion units-per-year basis.

Through my research and industry discussions, I learned that microLED technology, adapted from visual displays to data communications, could potentially address many of these issues. That technology was an adaptation of microLEDs from visual displays (lightbulbs) to data communications (focused flashlights). From that initial concept, I was introduced to Khaled, a senior principal engineer in the Technology Manufacturing Group with extensive experience in microLEDs for displays.

Khaled's profound knowledge of microLEDs and his efforts to make mass manufacturing of display-oriented microLEDs both ubiquitous and affordable were impressive. I was particularly interested in their potential for wide parallel digital I/O, given their mature fabrication processes and cost-effectiveness.

Khaled proved to be an exceptional partner. He patiently explained what I needed to understand about the intricacies of microLED devices and their development for display technologies. He also understood the risks associated with laser-based photonics and that I was looking for a technology that could be adapted to support the unique properties of data communications and the technical challenges (requirements) for viable products in the 2030 and beyond timeframe. was eager to explore innovative ideas. Khaled was a willing partner in exploring ideas and trying out things that others would think ridiculous, because he could see the payoff if the ideas were successful in changing how the entire industry operates.

Over the three years following our first contact, Khaled demonstrated his problem-solving ability, economic foresight, and thorough approach to addressing technical challenges, profoundly influencing my thinking about problems and solutions. While I would like to think that I had some small part to play in expanding Khaled's vision and direction, I believe the opposite is far truer in that Khaled has changed how I think about problems and their solutions.

Data communication fundamentally involves transmitting information from point A to point B with minimal energy, latency, and cost, without loss of information. Optimizing these parameters involves complex trade-offs as you explore real-world implementation choices. Every transmission medium is noisy and introduces errors; every technical approach for data transmission has a direct cost and then many indirect costs in connectors, cables, and aging effects; and latency is determined by factors greater than the raw transmission of information, typically through protocols, error recovery, and software stacks.

MicroLED technology presents a promising solution but requires addressing numerous technical problems beyond photon generation. Early on, Khaled partnered with Intel Labs to measure the optical transmission properties of display-optimized microLEDs for data communications. While bulk display devices could be modulated at very high speed, their radiance of light in a hemispherical manner was very problematic—too many photons are lost to make a nice visual display, which means very poor energy efficiency in getting the photons from point A to point B. This required Khaled to understand the inherent challenges of going from a lightbulb, to a lightbulb with a focusing lens, to fabricating devices that are intrinsically prefocused and have little side emission of photons. And one of the most compelling aspects to this technology, other than the relatively inexpensive nature of the mature processes for fabrication, is that it is far less temperature sensitive than current laser-based photonic approaches for data communications.

Further challenges included integrating light into waveguides for longer transmissions and ensuring reliable, easy-to-service products. This raised questions for what kinds of materials could be used for waveguides, how they can be carefully aligned, and how they can be converted to use pluggable adaptors on the sides of packages to enable highly reliable and easy-to-service products. Khaled explored these challenges intrinsic in dealing with the photodetectors when noncoherent light from microLEDs coming from point A will cover the surface of the destination point B in an uneven pattern.

Through each challenge and concept, Khaled was a fantastic partner to explore the art of the possible. Once a problem was well understood and defined, Khaled would go back to first principles and model the device physics to understand the limits of what could be achieved. Armed with detailed simulations, Khaled would then move into the more practical aspects of designing a solution and not an ingredient that stood alone. I appreciate the effort that Khaled has spent chasing this vision of future with me, and his patience as we have had classical ups-and-downs in getting this work to move forward. It is my hope that we are standing at the precipice of the next major advance in networking by using microLED devices or their adjacent peers, and that this text will help entice more people to working in this area.

*Josh Fryman, PhD*
*Intel Fellow, Office of the CTO*
*July 2024*

# Preface

Microscale light-emitting diodes (microLEDs) were first proposed two decades ago and have been the subject of intense research for the past decade by academia and industry. They can solve at least three problems: (1) power consumption in mobile displays (as in smartphones, smartwatches, and laptops), (2) high brightness in TV displays and augmented reality displays, and (3) parallel optical interconnect (data communication) in data centers and artificial intelligence compute systems.

The mobile display industry revenue surpassed approximately 50 billion dollars in 2020 and is projected to represent approximately 75% of the 180+ billion-dollar display market in 2026. Samsung introduced the first microLED TV in 2019. Apple has been reported to work on microLED displays for watches since 2014. However, in March 2024, it was reported that Apple decided to cancel their microLED program for watches due to manufacturing problems related to transferring microLEDs with high yield. The display industry has spent approximately 7 billion dollars in research and development over the past decade. On the other hand, there is a growing interest in microLEDs as emitters for data communication between semiconductor chips. Such a solution will solve several problems including energy consumption, high data rate, latency, and cost.

The data communication applications will leverage a decade's worth of academic research on visible light communication using microLEDs.

The microLED body of literature addresses several aspects of the technology, and the number of research papers is growing exponentially with time. Since each research group focuses on one application or the other, and the papers report empirical results for a diverse set of applications, there is a growing need for a theoretical framework that can be used to benchmark and understand the results from various research groups and various applications. Without such a framework, the efficiency of the industry reaching a solution that is production-worthy will be very poor. The idea of using a solid theoretical framework to advance a technology is not new. This has been tested in the semiconductor industry for more than 50 years now. Since microLEDs are optoelectronic devices, they need theoretical frameworks for both electronic and optical device behavior, as well as for how the devices work in a system (be it a display or a data communication system).

In this book, a theoretical framework (validated by experiments) is introduced in the form of a number of white-box analytic or semianalytic mathematical models that are based on physics. These models will provide intuition needed by device engineers, display engineers, manufacturing engineers, and metrology engineers working in the fields of displays and data communication, which will help them design and manufacture optimal devices for each application.

The book also provides models for a display system and data communication system to help system engineers understand and assess the gaps of commercially available microLEDs versus what is needed for a specific system. Again, instead of using black-box numerical models, the book uses the same theme used for device modeling: white-box and analytic or semianalytic system models. In doing so, the trade-offs between the system key performance indicators can be understood and properly addressed.

This book is designed for engineers who want to start with physics-based intuition to design microLED-based systems within about 80% accuracy, then follow with running experiments and more sophisticated models to capture the top 20% of design accuracy. This 80-20 approach is proven to work in many fields including the semiconductor industry.

Gordon Moore once said, "What can be done, can be outdone," as mentioned by Intel CEO Pat Gelsinger in a LinkedIn post in 2023. This is the essence of innovation. At this phase in the lifecycle of microLEDs, there is a need to predict what can be done and what can be outdone with microLEDs.

This book provides an innovation framework for microLED devices and systems. An innovation framework is a foundational set of practices and tools that helps organizations or individuals generate ideas, evaluate those ideas, and turn the best ideas into a value-add for the business. It arranges the general steps of the innovation process into clear stages that help leaders decide whether to pivot course, pause, or continue funding the work. Innovation is not a straight path—it's iterative, with an unknown destination. Each step along the way provides an opportunity to learn, pivot, and work toward the best possible outcome.

An innovation frame work is built on three pillars or phases. Each phase of the innovation framework has a distinct goal:

1. *Conception:* The goal of the first phase of the framework is to identify problem-solution fit. This means proving that your customers (or segments of your customers) have a problem worth solving—and your proposed solution could solve their problem. You know you are ready to move on to the next phase when you can craft a concept pitch. Your concept pitch should demonstrate what you have learned, justify the need to put a product into customers' hands for further learning, and detail the level of support you need (be it funding or headcount) to move on to the next phase. To achieve the goals of this phase, both physics-based mathematical models and mental models for how devices and systems operate are required.
2. *Validation:* In the second phase of the framework, you're identifying product-market fit. Your goal in the validation phase is to prove that your solution not only solves your customer's problem but also has a growth market opportunity. Before moving on to the final phase, you will create a validation pitch to share with stakeholders. The validation pitch should show findings from experiments, demonstrate the product-market fit, and detail the support needed to move into the final phase. Again, to achieve the goals of this phase, both physics-based mathematical models and mental models, for how devices and systems operate, are required.
3. *Growth:* In the growth phase, you focus on determining how you will bring your new product or service to the broader market. This phase includes a wide set of scaling techniques to help you enable all the necessary moving parts.

While there are stages and steps to follow, there is also backward motion built into the framework to allow for learning and iteration. Feel free to repeat phases, jump back in the process, and customize the framework as you need.

The purpose of this book is to address many of the recent and current developments and to offer technical insights into the present and the foreseeable future of microLED devices and systems. In spite of the overwhelming complexity of the field, the following pages will provide information and mathematical models so that interested students and professionals may make qualified evaluations of existing and soon-to-appear microLED systems. We also present some innovative ideas of our own that we hope will stimulate further research and development.

This book will discuss the following constructive topics: fundamentals of operating principles of microLED devices, principles of microLED displays, compact mathematical models for the current-voltage characteristics of microLEDs, emissive power consumption in microLED displays, luminance-current characteristics of microLEDs, modulation frequency of a microLED, and coupling efficiency from microLEDs to optical fiber in an optical communication system, and energy consumption in digital optical communication systems based on microLEDs. The book concludes with a discussion of possible systems based on microLED devices.

# 1

# MicroLED Overview

## 1.1 Introduction

In the late 1800s, Thomas Edison invented the lightbulb. The conventional lightbulb, commonly called the Edison bulb, has been used for over one hundred years for a variety of applications including lighting and displays. The conventional lightbulb uses a tungsten filament enclosed in a glass bulb sealed in a base, which is screwed into a socket. The socket is coupled to an AC power or DC power source. The conventional lightbulb can be found commonly in houses, buildings, outdoor lighting, and other areas requiring light or displays. Unfortunately, drawbacks exist with the conventional lightbulb:

- It dissipates more than 90% of the energy used as thermal energy;
- It routinely fails due to thermal expansion and contraction of the filament element;
- It emits light over a broad spectrum, much of which is not perceived by the human eye;
- It emits in all directions, which is undesirable for applications requiring strong directionality or focus (e.g., projection displays, and optical data storage).

To overcome some of the drawbacks of the conventional lightbulb, several alternatives have been developed including fluorescent lamps, mercury vapor lamps, sodium vapor lamps, and gas discharge lamps such as neon lamps. These lamp technologies in general suffer from similar problems to Edison lamps as well as having their own unique drawbacks. For example, fluorescent lamps require high voltages to start, which can be in the range of a thousand volts for large lamps, and also emit highly nonideal spectra that are dominated by spectral lines.

In the past two decades or so, solid-state lighting has become more important due to several key advantages it has over conventional lighting technology. Solid-state lighting is lighting derived from semiconductor devices such as diodes that are designed and optimized to emit photons. Due to the high efficiency, long lifetimes, low cost, and nontoxicity offered by solid-state lighting technology, light emitting diodes (LEDs) have rapidly emerged as the illumination technology of choice. An LED is a two-lead light source typically based on a p-i-n junction diode, which emits electromagnetic radiation when activated. The emission from an LED is typically in a Lambertian radiation pattern. When a suitable voltage is applied to the leads, electrons and holes recombine within the device releasing energy in the form of photons. This effect is called electroluminescence, and the color of the light is determined by the energy bandgap of the semiconductor. Appearing as practical electronic components in 1962 [1] the earliest LEDs emitted low-intensity infrared light. Infrared LEDs are still frequently used as transmitting elements in remote-control circuits, such as those in remote controls for a wide variety of consumer electronics. The first visible-light LEDs were also of low intensity and limited to red. Modern LEDs are available across the ultraviolet and infrared wavelengths, with very high brightness.

The earliest blue and violet gallium nitride (GaN)-based LEDs were fabricated using a metal-insulator-semiconductor structure due to a lack of p-type GaN. The first p-n junction GaN LED was demonstrated by Amano et al. [2] using the low-energy electron beam irradiation (LEEBI) treatment to obtain p-type GaN in 1989. They obtained the current-voltage (I-V) curve and electroluminescence of the LEDs but did not record the output power or the efficiency of the LEDs. Nakamura et al. [3] demonstrated a p-n junction GaN LED using a low-temperature GaN buffer and the LEEBI treatment in 1991 with an output power of 42 $\mu$W at 20 mA. The first p-GaN/n-InGaN/n-GaN double heterostructure (DH) blue LEDs were demonstrated by Nakamura et al. in 1993 [4]. The LED showed a strong band-edge emission of InGaN in a blue wavelength regime with an emission wavelength of 440 nm under a forward-biased condition. The output power and the external quantum efficiency (EQE) were 125 $\mu$W and 0.22%, respectively, at a forward current of 20 mA. In 1994, Nakamura et al. [5] demonstrated commercially available blue LEDs with an output power of 1.5 mW, an EQE of 2.7%, and the emission wavelength of 450 nm. On October 7, 2014, the Nobel Prize in Physics was awarded to Isamu Akasaki, Hiroshi Amano, and Shuji Nakamura for "the invention of efficient blue light-emitting diodes which has enabled bright and energy-saving white light sources" [6] or, less formally, LED lamps.

By combining GaN-based LEDs with wavelength-converting materials such as phosphors, solid-state white light sources were realized. This technology utilizing GaN-based LEDs and phosphor materials to produce white light is now illuminating the world around us as a result of the many advantages over incandescent light sources including lower energy consumption, longer lifetime, improved physical robustness, smaller size, and faster switching. LEDs are now used in applications as diverse as aviation lighting, automotive headlamps, advertising, general lighting, traffic signals, and camera flashes. LEDs have allowed new text, video displays, and sensors to be developed, while their high switching rates can be very useful in communications technology. LEDs, however, are not the only solid-state light source and may not be preferable light sources for certain lighting applications. Alternative solid-state light sources utilizing stimulated emission, such as laser diodes (LDs) or superluminescent light-emitting diodes (SLEDs), provide many unique features advantageously over LEDs.

In 1960, the laser was demonstrated by Theodore H. Maiman at Hughes Research Laboratories in Malibu. This laser utilized a solid-state flash lamp-pumped synthetic ruby crystal to produce red laser light at 694 nm. Early visible laser technology comprised lamp-pumped infrared solid-state lasers with the output wavelength converted to the visible spectrum using specialty crystals with nonlinear optical properties. For example, a green lamp-pumped solid-state laser had three stages: (1) electricity powers lamp, (2) lamp excites gain crystal, which lases at 1064 nm, and (3) 1064 nm goes into frequency conversion crystal that converts to visible 532 nm. The resulting green and blue lasers were called lamped-pumped solid-state lasers with second harmonic generation (LPSS with SHG) that had a wall plug efficiency of ~1% and were more efficient than argon (Ar)-ion gas lasers, but were still too inefficient, large, expensive, and fragile for broad deployment outside of specialty scientific and medical applications. To improve the efficiency of these visible lasers, high-power diode (or semiconductor) lasers were utilized. These diode-pumped solid-state lasers with SHG (DPSS with SHG) had three stages: (1) electricity powers 808-nm diode laser, (2) 808 nm excites gain crystal, which lases at 1064 nm, and 1064 nm goes into frequency conversion crystal that converts to visible 532 nm. As high-power laser diodes evolved and new specialty SHG crystals were developed, it became possible to directly convert the output of the infrared diode laser to produce blue and green laser light output. These directly doubled or SHG diode lasers had two stages: (1) electricity powers 1064-nm semiconductor laser, and (2) 1064 nm goes into frequency conversion crystal that converts to visible 532-nm green light. These laser designs are meant to improve the efficiency, cost, and size compared to DPSS-SHG lasers, but the specialty diodes and crystals required make this challenging today.

Solid-state laser light sources, due to the narrowness of their spectra—which enables efficient spectral filtering, high modulation rates, short carrier lifetimes, a smaller size, and far greater surface brightness compared to LEDs—can be more preferable as visible light sources as a means of transmitting information with high bandwidth in many applications including lighting fixtures, lighting systems, displays, and projectors. Advancements of new GaN-based blue laser technology based on improved processes have substantially reduced manufacture cost and opened opportunities for utilizing the modulated laser signal and the light spot directly to measure and or interact with the surrounding environment, transmit data to other electronic systems, and respond dynamically to inputs from various sensors. Such applications are often referred to as smart lighting applications.

While LED-based light sources offer great advantages over incandescent based sources, there are still challenges and limitations associated with LED device physics. The first limitation is the droop phenomenon that plagues GaN-based LEDs. The droop effect leads to power rollover with increased current density, which forces LEDs to hit peak external quantum efficiency at very low current densities in the 1- to 100-A/cm$^2$ range.

## 1.2 What is a MicroLED?

A microscale LED (microLED) is an LED that has a surface-emitting diameter of less than 10 or 20 $\mu$m. The suggestion of using microLED structures for improving light extraction efficiency may be credited to Thibeault and DenBaars [7]. The first suggestion of using microLEDs in microdisplays may be credited to Jiang et al. from Kansas State University in 2001 [8]. Dawson's group was the first to suggest using blue microLEDs for visible light communication in 2010 [9]. In 2014 Apple acquired a start-up company, LuxVue, which had proposed techniques for manufacturing small displays for smartwatch applications (e.g., diameter ~1–2") by transferring microLEDs from growth wafers to a glass backplane. LuxVue suggested the use of electrostatic force to pick microLEDs from growth substrate (e.g., sapphire wafers) and place them onto a glass or complementary metal-oxide-semiconductor (CMOS) substrate, forming a two-dimensional display array. Since 2014, dozens of start-ups received funding to address one aspect or another of making microLED displays for mobile devices. In Figure 1.1, the industry research and development (R&D) spending on microLED devices and systems is compared to R&D spending on comparably complex technologies such as CMOS technology nodes. The R&D spending per year on microLED technology is far less than similar complex

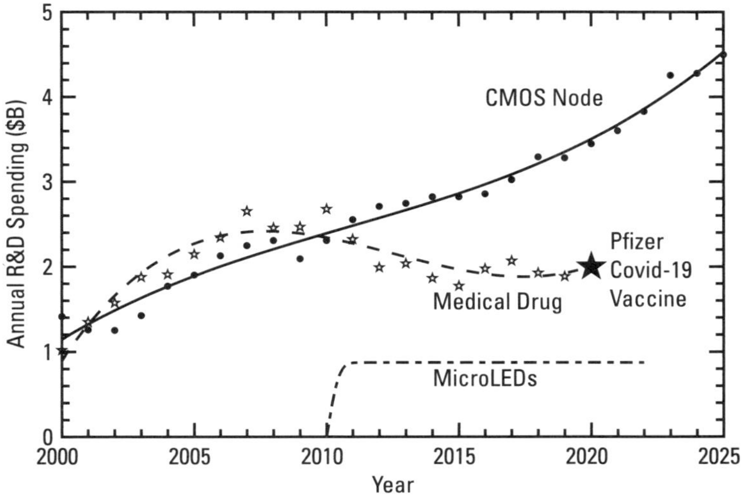


**Figure 1.1** R&D spend per year on various significant technologies including CMOS technology nodes and drugs. The microLED spend is averaged over 8 years (data for each year is not readily available) and drug development [10].

technologies. It is posited here that for microLED-based devices to find their way to the marketplace as products used by a large number of humans, more spending may be necessary.

The simplest microLED structure includes a stack of semiconductor layers that form a p-i-n diode, with "p" being the semiconductor region doped with p-type dopant, "n" the semiconductor region doped with n-type dopant, and "i" the semiconductor region that is not intentionally doped. The "i" region is a quantum well. The quantum well comprises two undoped semiconductors of the same material as the p or n regions that sandwich a thin semiconductor layer that has a bandgap smaller than the bandgap of the two undoped semiconductor barriers surrounding it. The structure is schematically shown in Figure 1.2.

The wavelength of the emitted light in nanometers equals, to a first order, to $1240/E_g$, where $E_g$ is the energy gap of the quantum well semiconductor material. In operation, an electric current is passed into the microLED. The electric current comprises electrons injected from the n-type semiconductor toward the quantum well and holes injected from the p-type semiconductor towards the quantum well. If the quantum well is designed properly, most of the electrons and holes are confined in the well. The spatial confinement of electrons and holes results in recombination of the electrons and holes, involving electrons losing energy equaling that of the energy gap of the quantum well semiconductor material, to a first order. The loss of energy results in emission of light, according to the electroluminescence theory [11]. A perfectly efficient

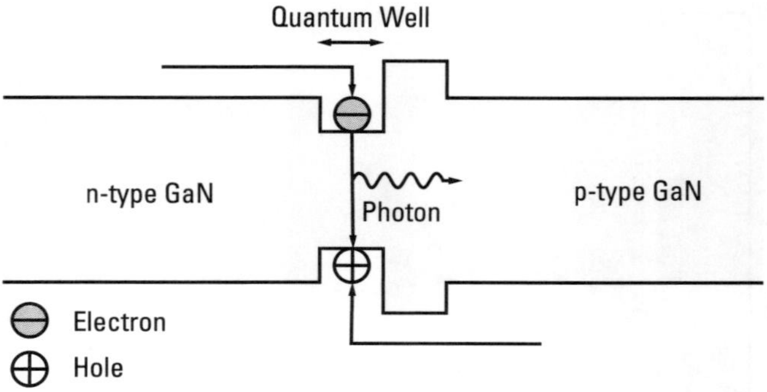


**Figure 1.2** Schematic of the energy band diagram of a typical LED structure. A thin active layer is sandwiched between a p-type and an n-type semiconductor with wider bandgap, forming a quantum well. Electrons injected from the n-type semiconductor recombine with the holes injected from the p-type semiconductor to produce a photon. In this example, the quantum well is made of indium gallium nitride (InGaN) and the n-type and p-type semiconductors are gallium nitride. To prevent electrons from leaking to the p-GaN, an electron barrier layer (EBL) is used next to the p-type GaN side.

microLED produces a photon for every electron injected into at the terminals of the device. In practice, however, some of the electrons do not get confined in the quantum well (they leak into the p-type semiconductor region) and do not produce emission. Also, some of the electrons recombine with holes by an energy transition assisted by a trap in the energy gap of the quantum well semiconductor, leading to nonradiative recombination (see Figure 1.3). The ratio of emitted photons divided by the injected electrons is defined as internal quantum efficiency (IQE).

The emitted light, an electromagnetic wave, will travel though the p-type (or n-type) semiconductor trying to leave the quantum well where they have been generated. Some of the energy carried by this light wave is absorbed by the p-type (or n-type) regions. Since the refractive index of the n-type or p-type semiconductor regions is greater than that of air (where an observer's eyes reside), some of the energy carried by the light wave will be reflected at the semiconductor/air interface and trapped inside the semiconductor regions, and only a small fraction will exit to the observer's eyes (e.g., 5%). The fraction of light exiting the device is called light extraction efficiency (LEE). For large LEDs, roughening the surface where light exits the device results in improving LEE to around 25% (e.g., see [13]). In microLEDs, sidewall reflections of light results in even larger LEE (e.g., 35%) (see Figure 1.4). This improvement in LEE was the original motivation for using microLEDs for lighting application [7].

Ever since microLEDs were suggested for display applications [8], it became obvious that microLEDs will present an economic advantage since on a given semiconductor wafer many more microLED emitters can be made to form a display that demands millions of emitters. In Figure 1.5, the estimated

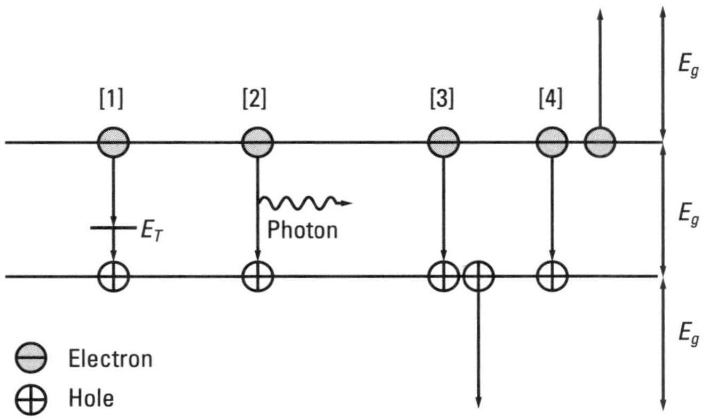


**Figure 1.3** Schematic illustrating various recombination mechanisms [12]: (1) nonradiative recombination via a trap located in the bandgap of the material, (2) band-to-band radiative recombination, (3), and nonradiative electron-electron Auger recombination (4).

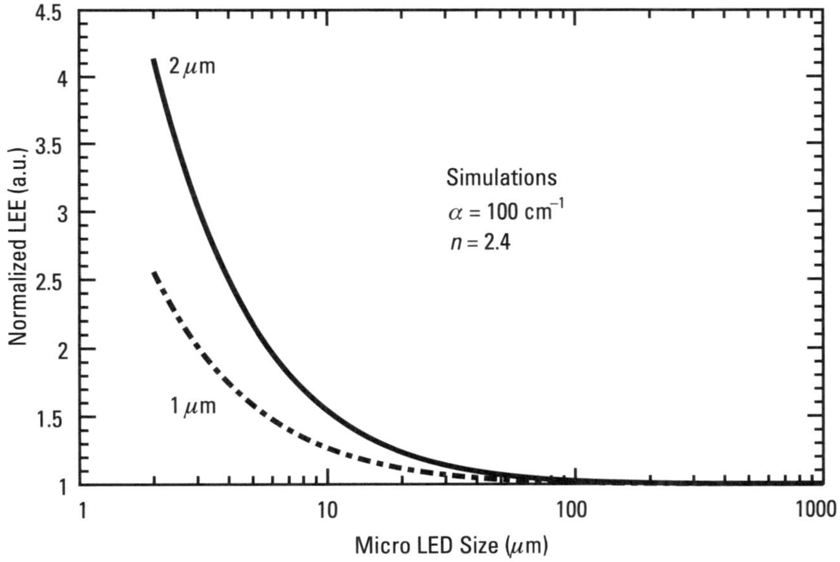


**Figure 1.4** Simulated improvement in light extraction efficiency (LEE) with reduction of LED size using the model described in [14] for two values of the microLED thickness of 1 and 2 $\mu$m. The improvement in LEE is due to increased light reflections on the sidewalls of the microLEDs that result in higher light exiting the device.

cost of producing a 14" microLED display is plotted as a function of microLED size for two different growth wafer sizes of 8" and 12" diameters. A smaller microLED size results in smaller production cost for a given wafer size. For a

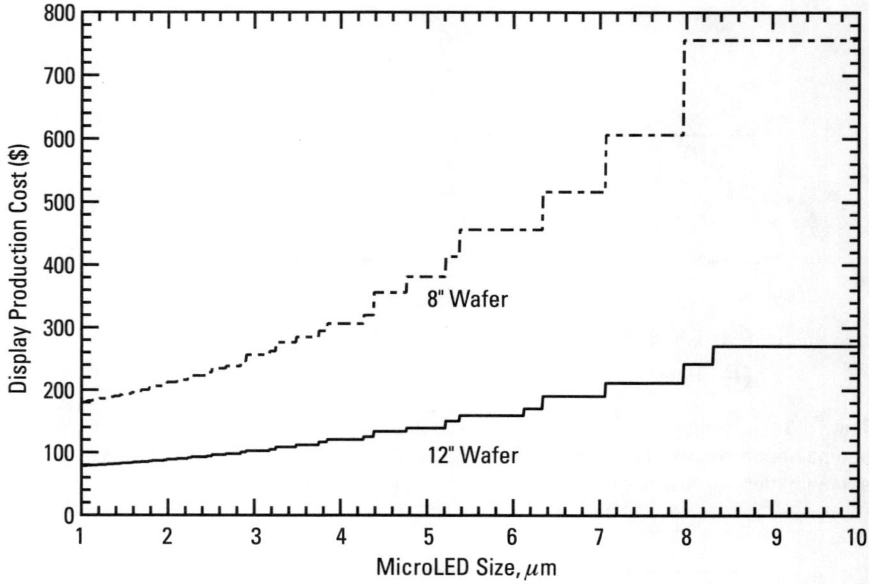


**Figure 1.5** Estimated display production cost for 14″ diagonal microLED display using a truly massive transfer technology for 12″ and 8″ wafers. It is assumed that monolithic red, green, and blue (RGB) is achievable and two redundant microLEDs per color per pixel are possible. The cost of production decreases as the microLED diameter decreases for a given wafer size.

given microLED size, the production cost is much lower when a larger growth wafer diameter is used.

Compared to organic LEDs (OLEDs), inorganic microLEDs made of high-quality crystalline semiconductors promise much higher luminance (by its ability to carry much higher current) without compromising its lifetime. Simulated current-voltage characteristics for an OLED and a microLED is shown in Figure 1.6. At a given voltage, much higher current can be injected in a microLED compared to an OLED. This means that microLEDs can be made to be much brighter than OLEDs.

MicroLEDs have been considered for high-speed digital communication applications owing to their much smaller device capacitance compared to conventional large LEDs [9]. The calculated modulation frequency of microLEDs as a function of switching energy is shown in Figure 1.7. It is clear that as the size scales down the target bandwidth and switching energy are met.

## 1.3 Visible Light MicroLEDs

The first blue LED was fabricated by Nakamura in 1993 [15]. GaN was used as p- and n-type semiconductor regions, and InGaN was used for the quantum

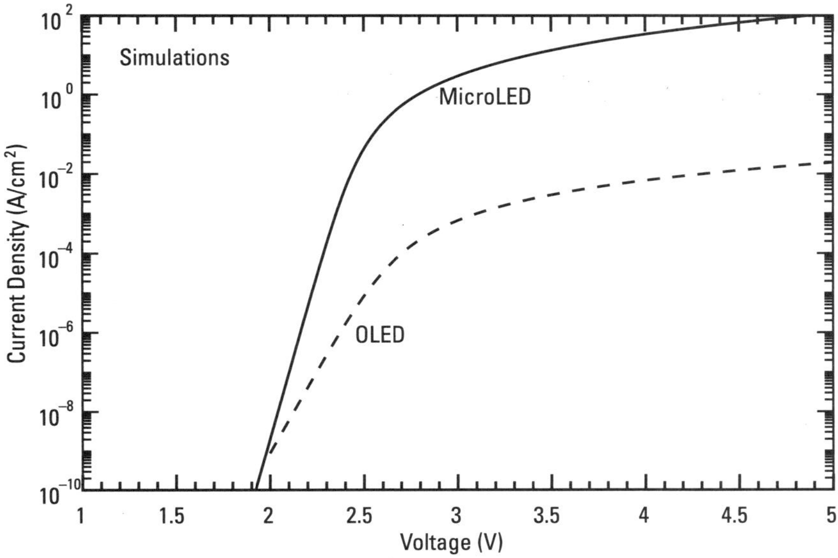


**Figure 1.6** Exemplary current-voltage curves for blue-emitting OLED and microLED. MicroLEDs have much higher (e.g., >1,000 times) drive current compared to OLEDs. Higher drive current is necessary for brighter emission. The difference is due to fundamental difference in device and material properties between inorganic and organic light-emitting diodes.

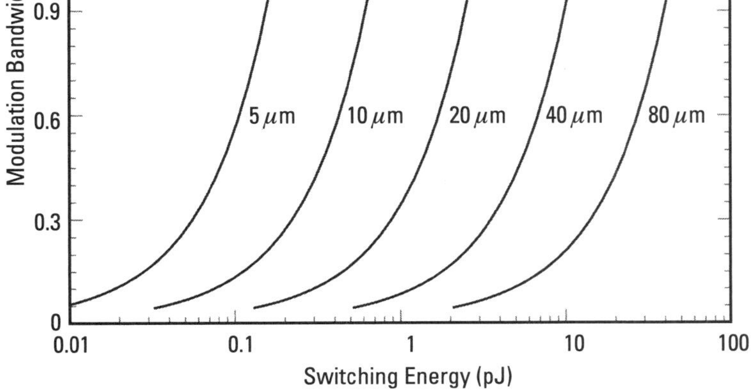


**Figure 1.7** Calculated electro-optical modulation bandwidth versus energy per bit for small- and large-size microLEDs. For a given microLED size, the current density is varied from 1 A/cm$^2$ to 1,000 A/cm$^2$.

well semiconductor layer. Later on, green LEDs were demonstrated using the same material system with InGaN quantum wells containing higher indium mole fraction (20% for blue and 32% for green) [16]. High-efficiency red InGaN-based LEDs has been elusive [17–22]. However, efficient red LEDs have been demonstrated using AlGaInP material for the quantum well layer [18–20].

The experimental EQE is plotted versus peak emission wavelength for the InGaN and the aluminum gallium indium phosphide (AlGaInP) material systems in Figure 1.8. The data points were obtained from published papers and books [18, 19]. Two envelope curves emerge for the two material systems. Indeed, the InGaN material system has been optimal for large-size green and blue LEDs, while AlGaInP has been optimal for large-size red LEDs. When the devices are scaled down to sub-10-$\mu$m range, the relatively large surface recombination velocity for AlGaInP results in fast degradation of red efficiency as the microLED shoreline size decreases. Envelope efficiency curves for semiconductor light emitting diodes (InGaN and AlGaInP) and organic light emitting diodes (OLEDs) are shown in Figure 1.9.

## 1.4 Types of MicroLED Structures

There are four significant types of microLED structures that have received the most attention: (1) planar [26–28], (2) core-shell nanowire [29–32], (3) axial

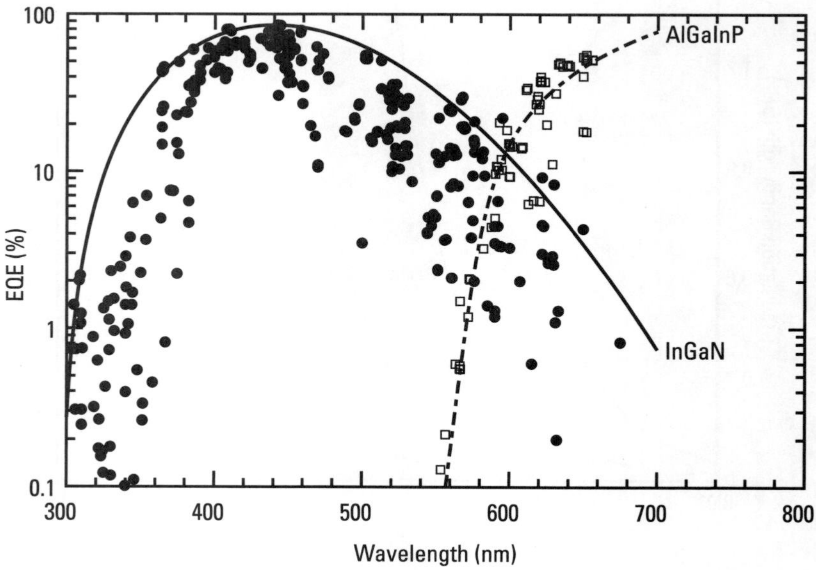


**Figure 1.8** Experimental EQE versus wavelength for InGaN- and AlGaInP-based LEDs with various sizes (20 $\mu$m to 1 mm in diameter). Data points were obtained from [17, 18, 20, 22–25].

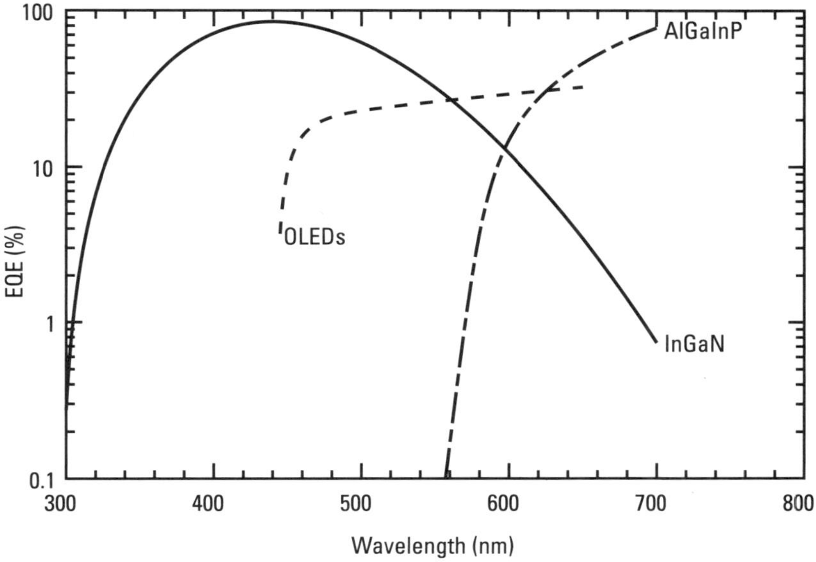


**Figure 1.9** Envelope curves for the EQE of InGaN-based LEDs (based on Figure 1.8), AlGaInP-based LEDs (based on Figure 1.8), and OLEDs (based on [17]). InGaN-based LEDs outperform both AlGaInP and OLEDs for the blue and green emission. OLEDs and AlGaInP LEDs outperform InGaN-based LEDs for red emission.

nanowire [22, 23, 33–35], and (4) nanopyramid [36–41]. Schematics for the above structures are shown in Figure 1.10.

Planar microLEDs have a stack of layers in a pancake manner. Starting from a sapphire wafer, a buffer layer made of aluminum nitride (AlN) is grown, followed by the growth of an n-type GaN layer (~1,000 nm). An undoped GaN layer (e.g., 12 nm in thickness) is then grown followed by the growth of a thin (e.g., 4 nm in thickness) quantum well (QW) layer made of InGaN. The mole fraction in the InGaN is adjusted to target a specific peak emission wavelength. For example, if the indium mole fraction is approximately 20% the microLED will emit light with peak wavelength at ~460 nm. The growth of the InGaN QW is followed by the growth of a barrier layer made of undoped GaN with thickness of ~12 nm. An aluminum gallium nitride layer (AlGaN), also known as electron barrier layer, is grown, followed by the growth of a p-type GaN layer. The stack of pancake layers is patterned into squares or circles, for example, with a diameter less than ~20 $\mu$m. The patterning step involves etching along sidewalls that inadvertently produces active traps that have been shown to degrade the quantum efficiency of the microLEDs, with larger degradation observed for smaller diameters [24–28, 43–45].

Core-shell nanowires can be grown on sapphire or silicon wafers using either metal-organic chemical vapor deposition (MOCVD) or molecular beam epitaxy (MBE) epitaxy. Starting from a sapphire wafer, for example, a thin (e.g.,

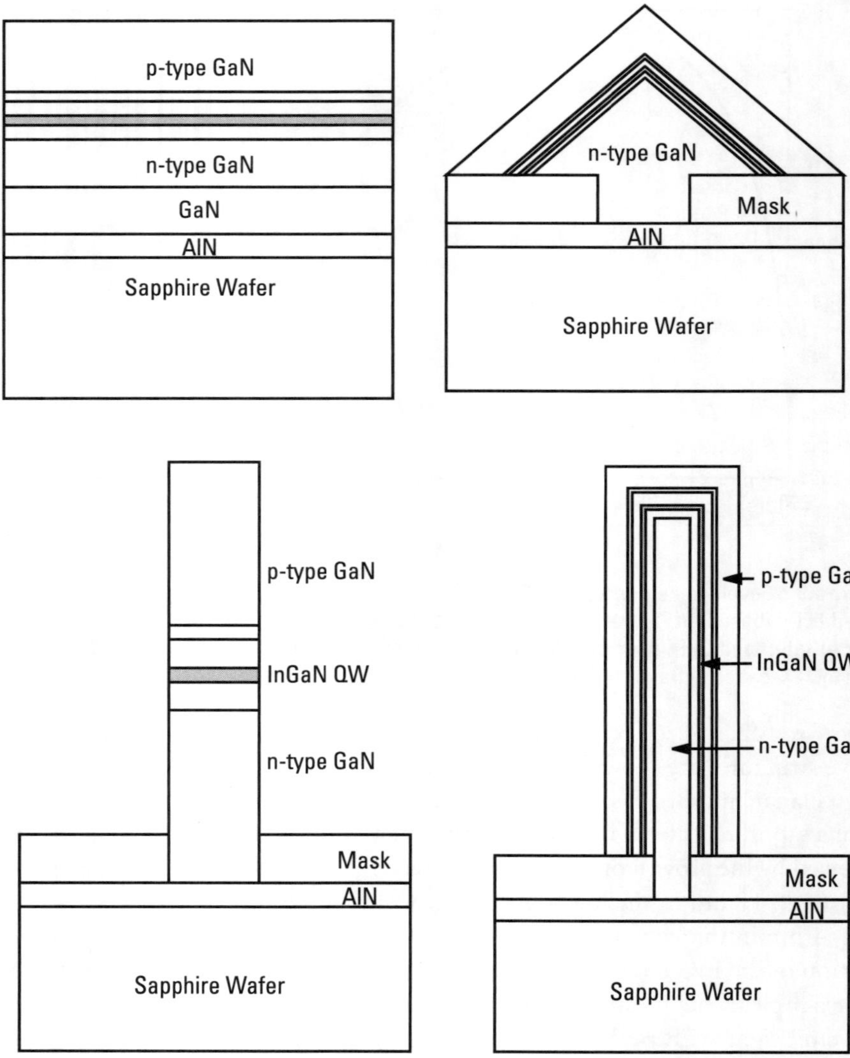


**Figure 1.10** Schematics of four different microLED structures. Top left is the planar structure, top right is the pyramid structure, bottom left is the axial nanowire structure, and bottom right is the core-shell nanowire structure.

50 nm) AlN layer is grown by MOCVD, followed by the growth of a thick (1–3 $\mu$m) of undoped GaN buffer. Then a silicon nitride (or other material) layer of ~100 nm is deposited and patterned into holes with diameter sizes of ~300 nm. After the surface of the undoped GaN at the bottom of the patterned trenches is cleaned, selective area epitaxy is done using MOCVD or MBE of n-type GaN core nanowire. After the n-type GaN nanowire cores are erected off of the substrate, an undoped GaN barrier shell is grown, followed by the growth

**Table 1.1**
Pros and Cons of Various MicroLED Structures

| | Planar | Core-Shell Nanowire | Axial Nanowire | Nanopyramid |
|---|---|---|---|---|
| **Material System** | InGaN/GaN | | | |
| **Demonstrated Substrates** | Sapphire | Sapphire, silicon | Sapphire, silicon | Sapphire, silicon |
| **Monolithic RGB Risk** | Very high | High | Medium | Low |
| **Risk of Scaling Substrate to Silicon 300 mm size** | Very high | Low | Low | Low |
| **Risk of Manufacturing** | Low | High | High | Medium |
| **Efficient Blue Demo** | Yes | Yes | Yes | No |
| **Efficient Green Demo** | Yes | No | No | No |
| **Efficient Red Demo** | No | No | No | No |
| **Growth Technology** | MBE, MOCVD | MOCVD, MBE | MBE | MOCVD |

of a quantum well shell made of InGaN, followed by the growth of another undoped GaN shell and an AlGaN electron barrier layer. Finally, a p-type GaN shell is grown.

Table 1.1 illustrates a benchmark of different microLED structure from the manufacturability perspective.

## References

[1] Holonyak, N., and S. Bevacqua, "Coherent (Visible) Light Emission from Ga (As1-xPx) Junctions," *Applied Physics Letters*, Vol. 1, No. 4, 1962, pp. 82–83.

[2] Amano, H., M. Kito, K. Hiramatsu, and I. Akasaki, "P-Type Conduction in Mg-Doped GaN Treated with Low-Energy Electron Beam Irradiation (LEEBI)," *Japanese Journal of Applied Physics*, Vol. 28, No. 12A, 1989, p. L2112.

[3] Nakamura, S., N. Iwasa, M. S. M. Senoh, and T. M. T. Mukai, "Hole Compensation Mechanism of p-type GaN Films," *Japanese Journal of Applied Physics*, Vol. 31, No. 5R, 1992, p. 1258.

[4] Nakamura, S., M. Senoh, and T. Mukai, "High-Power InGaN/GaN Double-Heterostructure Violet Light Emitting Diodes," *Applied Physics Letters*, Vol. 62, No. 19, 1993, pp. 2390–2392.

[5] Nakamura, S., "High-Power InGaN/AlGaN Double-Heterostructure Blue-Light-Emitting Diodes," in *Proceedings of 1994 IEEE International Electron Devices Meeting, IEEE*, December 1994, pp. 567–570.

[6] Heber, J., "Nobel Prize 2014: Akasaki, Amano & Nakamura," *Nature Physics*, Vol. 10, No. 11, 2014, pp. 791–791.

[7] Thibeault, B., and S. DenBaars, "Enhanced Light Extraction Through the Use of Micro-LED Arrays," US Patent US6410942B1, 2000.

[8] Jiang, H., S. Jin, J. Li, J. Shakya, and J. Lin, "III-Nitride Blue Microdisplays," *Applied Physics Letters*, Vol. 78, No. 9, 2001, pp. 1303–1305.

[9] McKendry, J., R. Green, A. Kelly, Z. Gong, et al., "High-Speed Visible Light Communications Using Individual Pixels in a Micro Light-Emitting Diode Array," *IEEE Photonics Technology Letters*, Vol. 22, No. 18, 2010, pp. 1346–1348.

[10] US Government Congressional Budget Office, https://www.cbo.gov/publication/57126.

[11] Piper, W., and F. Williams, "Theory of Electroluminescence," *Physical Review*, Vol. 98, No. 6, 1955, p. 1809.

[12] David, A., N. Young, C. Lund, and M. Craven, "The Physics of Recombinations in III-Nitride Emitters," *ECS Journal of Solid State Science and Technology*, Vol. 9, No. 1, 2019, p. 016021.

[13] Kim, J., " Improved Light Extraction Efficiency in GaN-Based Light Emitting Diodes," in *GaN and ZnO-based Materials and Devices* (S. Pearton, ed.), Berlin: Springer, 2011, pp. 153–164.

[14] Ahmed, K., "Model for Light Extraction Efficiency of MicroLEDs," TechRxiv, preprint, https://doi.org/10.36227/techrxiv.21944900.v1, 2023.

[15] Nakamura, S., T. Mukai, and M. Senoh, "High-Power GaN PN Junction Blue-Light-Emitting Diodes," *Japanese Journal of Applied Physics*, Vol. 30, No. 12A, 1991, p. L1998.

[16] Nakamura, S., M. Senoh, N. Iwasa, and S.-I. Nagahama, "High-Brightness InGaN Blue, Green and Yellow Light-Emitting Diodes with Quantum Well Structures," *Japanese Journal of Applied Physics*, Vol. 34, 1995, p. L797–L799.

[17] Ahmed, K., "Heuristics of OLED and Micro LED Efficiencies," *SID Symposium Digest of Technical Papers*, Vol. 52, No. 1, 2021, pp. 864–867.

[18] Hwang, J., R. Hashimoto, and S. Saito, "Green, Yellow, and Red LEDs," in *III-Nitride Based Light Emitting Diodes and Applications,* Second Edition (T.-Y. Seong, J. Han, H. Amano, and H. Morkoç, eds.), Vol. 2, Singapore: Springer Nature Singapore, 2017, pp. 239–266.

[19] Shchekin, O., and M. G. Craford, "History of Solid-State Light Sources," in *Handbook of Advanced Lighting Technology,* Vol. 1 (R. Karlicek, C.-C. Sun, G. Zissis, and R. Ma, eds.), Springer, 2017, pp. 41–70.

[20] Wang, G., X. Yi, T. Zhan, and Y. Huang, "The AlGaInP/AlGaAs Material System and Red/Yellow LED," in *Light-Emitting Diodes: Materials, Processes, Devices and Applications* (J. Li and G. Q. Zhang, eds.), Springer, 2019, pp. 171–202.

[21] P. Li, H. Li, H. Zhang, et al., "Red InGaN Micro-Light-Emitting Diodes (>620 nm) with a Peak External Quantum Efficiency of 4.5% Using an Epitaxial Tunnel Junction Contact," *Applied Physics Letters*, Vol. 120, No. 12, 2022, p. 121102.

[22] Pandey, A., Y. Xiao, M. Reddeppa, et al., "A Red-Emitting Micrometer Scale LED with External Quantum Efficiency >8%," *Applied Physics Letters*, Vol. 122, No. 15, 2023, p. 151103.

[23] Pandey, A., and Z. Mi, "III-Nitride Nanostructures for High Efficiency Micro-LEDs and Ultraviolet Optoelectronics," *IEEE Journal of Quantum Electronics*, Vol. 58, No. 4, 2022, pp. 1–13.

[24] Wong, M., J. Kearns, C. Lee, et al., "Improved Performance of AlGaInP Red Micro-Light-Emitting Diodes with Sidewall Treatments," *Optics Express*, Vol. 28, No. 4, 2020, p. 5.

[25] Wong, M., S. Nakamura, and S. DenBaars, "High External Quantum Efficiency III-Nitride Micro-Light-Emitting Diodes," in *Semiconductors and Semimetals, Volume 106: MicroLEDS* (H. Jiang and J. Lin, eds.), Elsevier, 2021, pp. 95–121.

[26] Bour, D. P., K. McGroddy, D. A. Haeger, et al., "LED Structures for Reduced Non-Radiative Sidewall Recombination," US Patent US9865772B2, 2017.

[27] Perkins, J. M., "Diffusion Revealed Blocking Junction," US Patent US10396241B1, 2017.

[28] McGroddy, K., H.-H. Hu, A. Bibl, C. K. T. Chan, and D. A. Haeger, "LED with Internally Confined Current Injection Area," US Patent US11101405B2, 2013.

[29] Ahmed, K., S. Dasgupta, and I.- C. Robin, "Nanowire Light Emitting Diodes with High Extraction Efficiency for Micro LED Displays," US Patent US16/147,748, 2018.

[30] Ahmed, K., "High Performance Light Emitting Diode and Monolithic Multi-color Pixel," US Patent US10957818B2, 2016.

[31] Ahmed, K., K. Parikh, and P. L. Chang, "Micro-LED Displays," US Patent US10177195B2, 2016.

[32] Monemar, B., B. Ohlsson, N. Gardner, and L. Samuelson, "Nanowire-Based Visible Light Emitters, Present Status and Outlook," in *Semiconductors and Semimetals, Volume 94, Semiconductor Nanowires II: Properties and Applications* (S. A. Dayeh, A. Fontcuberta i Morral, and C. Jagadish, eds.), 2016, pp. 227–271.

[33] Nami, M., and D. Feezell, "Optical Properties of Ag-Coated GaN/InGaN Axial and Core–Shell Nanowire Light-Emitting Diodes," *Journal of Optics*, Vol. 17, No. 2, 2015, p. 025004.

[34] Mi, Z., S. Zhao, and R. Wang, "High Efficiency Visible and Ultraviolet Nanowire Emitters," US Patent US10892379B2, 2019.

[35] Nguyen, H., S. Zhang, K. Cui, X. Han, and Z. Mi, "Molecular Beam Epitaxial Growth, Fabrication, and Characterization of High Efficiency InGaN/GaN Dot-in-a-Wire White Light Emitting Diodes on Si (111)," *ECS Transactions*, Vol. 35, No. 6, 2011, p. 41.

[36] Ahmed, K., A. Pancholi, S. Dasgupta, and C. Mair, "Micro Light-Emitting Diode Display Fabrication and Assembly," US Patent US15/988,656, 2018.

[37] Dasgupta, S., K. Ahmed, and A. Pancholi, "Micro-LED Structures for Full Color Displays and Methods of Manufacturing the Same," US Patent US11245053B2, 2019.

[38] Ahmed, K., and S. Dasgupta, "Micro Light-Emitting Diode Display Having Truncated Nanopyramid Structures," US Patent US16/435,312, 2019.

[39] Ahmed, K., "Display with Nano-Pyramid Light Emitting Diodes," US Patent US17/132,525, 2020.

[40] Ahmed, K., "Micro-LED Structures with Improved Internal Quantum Efficiency," US Patent US16/946,224, 2020.

[41] West, P., and K. Ahmed, "Micro LED Laser Release from Silicon Wafer," US Patent US17/485,398, 2021.

[42] Ahmed, K., A. M. Prakash, R. C. Woodbeck, and S. Pabba, "Structures for Micro LED Laser Release," US Patent US17/402,313, 2021.

[43] Olivier, F., S. Tirano, L. Dupré, B. Aventurier, C. Largeron and F. Templier, "Influence of Size-Reduction on the Performances of GaN-based Micro-LEDs for Display Application," *Journal of Luminescence*, Vol. 191, 2017, pp. 112–116.

[44] Wong, M., C. Lee, D. Myers, et al., "Size-Independent Peak Efficiency of III-Nitride Micro-Light-Emitting-Diodes Using Chemical Treatment and Sidewall Passivation," *Applied Physics Express*, Vol. 12, No. 9, 2019, p. 097004.

[45] Smith, J., R. Ley, M. Wong, et al., "Comparison of Size-Dependent Characteristics of Blue and Green InGaN MicroLEDs Down to 1 $\mu$m in Diameter," *Applied Physics Letters*, Vol. 116, No. 7, 2020, p. 071102.

# 2

# MicroLED Design: Physics and Technology

## 2.1 Introduction

A microLED operates according to the electroluminescence theory, which describes a mechanism by which electrical energy is transformed into light energy. The primary goal for increasing electroluminescence (EL) efficiency is to determine how to capture all or most of the electrogenerated excitons for emission. The EL efficiency is proportional to the radiative recombination rate.

GaN-based microLEDs have the potential to realize all visible emissions with the same material system. InGaN can offer emission across the entire visible range corresponding to a bandgap energy of 0.67–3.42 eV by tuning the alloy composition [1, 2]. This is shown in Figure 2.1. The GaN material system has been demonstrated to enable monolithic RGB LEDs on the same substrate [3–6]. If monolithic RGB on the same substrate can be realized, then it is possible to transfer the three colors in one step to a display backplane for manufacturing microLED displays, thus reducing production cost relative to conventional methods relying on transferring the three colors from three different wafers. Moreover, if monolithic RGB can be realized on the same wafer, augmented reality microdisplays would be possible at much reduced cost and much improved performance.

Despite the heavy development of these devices in the blue emission regime, which has led to extremely high-efficiency devices, emission at longer wavelengths such as green, yellow, amber, and red typically experiences much

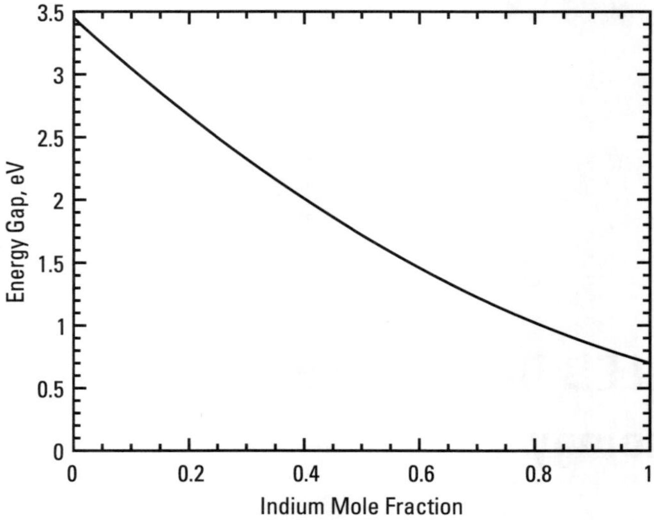


**Figure 2.1** Energy gap of InGaN versus indium mole fraction. Higher indium mole fraction results in a smaller energy gap, which is suitable for long wavelength emission.

lower quantum efficiencies, worsening with longer wavelengths, as shown in Figure 2.2.

Understanding the physical (and technological) challenges toward realizing efficient red, green, and blue emissions is the focus of this chapter. Before mathematical models are presented to calculate the radiative recombination coefficient and the emission wavelength as a function of applied electric current, a review of important concepts and technological aspects are necessary. In Section 2.2 a brief description of the microLED structure is given. In Section 2.3 the physical origin of lower-than-ideal microLED efficiency (quantum confinement Stark effect (QCSE)) is discussed. Mitigation strategies for the QCSE are discussed in Section 2.4. A physics-based analytical modeling framework is discussed in Section 2.5 to provide tools to quantify benefits from various mitigation strategies of the QCSE.

## 2.2 MicroLED Structure and Operation

Figure 2.3 shows the structure of the conventional nitride semiconductor microLED. The conventional nitride semiconductor microLED comprises an n-type semiconductor, a multiple quantum well (MQW) structure and a p-type semiconductor layer. In order to raise the lighting efficiency of the nitride semiconductor microLED, the MQW structure of the nitride semiconductor microLED comprises the barrier layers and the well layers to form the traps to capture the electrons and holes to increase the combination efficiency there-

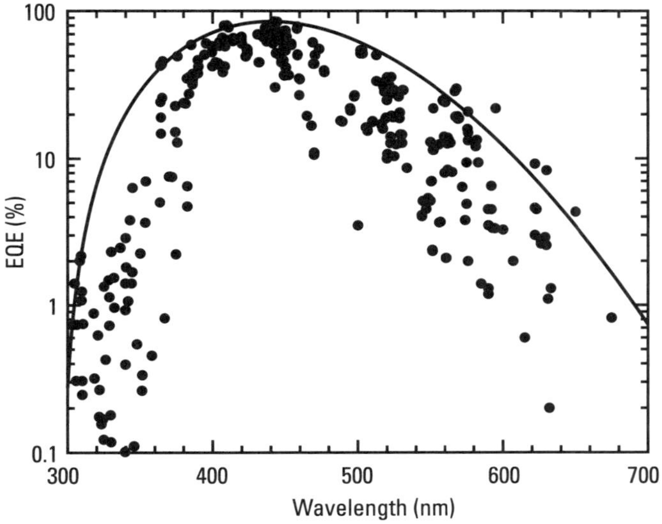


**Figure 2.2** Envelope of GaN LEDs EQE versus peak wavelength illustrating the sharp roll-off of efficiency below and above blue emission.

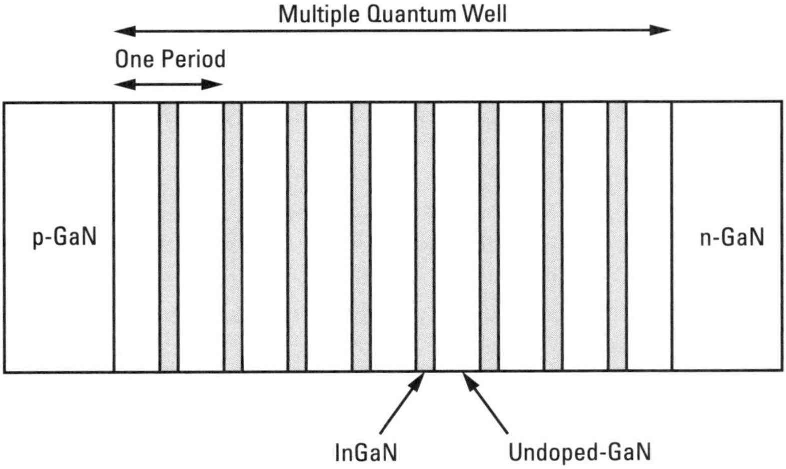


**Figure 2.3** Structure of a GaN microLED. Multiple quantum wells are sandwiched between two doped regions of opposite polarity (n-type and p-type). The QW is formed by a relatively narrow bandgap material such as InGaN sandwiched between two relatively large band gap materials such as GaN.

of. Generally, the MQW structure of the nitride semiconductor microLED is formed by multiple GaN layers and multiple InGaN layers stacked alternately. In an undoped, unpolarized QW the conduction and valence bands are flat (no built-in fields) as shown in Figure 2.4. The electron and hole wavefunctions are

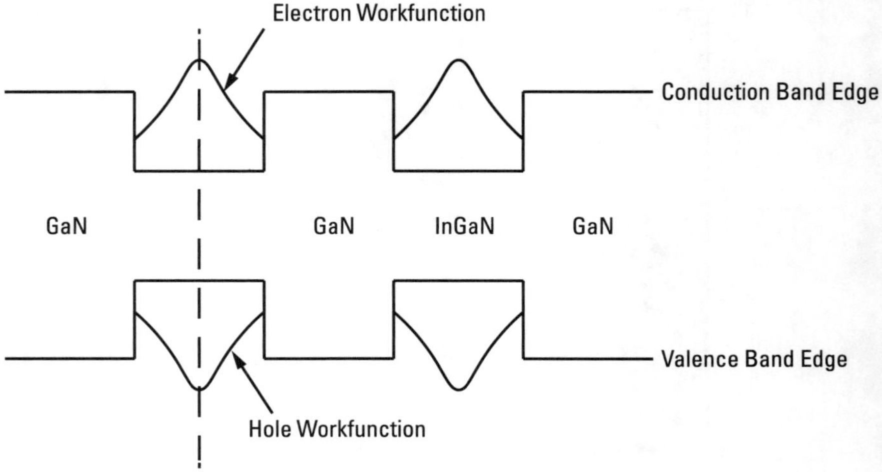


**Figure 2.4** Energy band diagram of two QWs with no built-in or applied external fields. The electron and hole wavefunctions are centered within the QW and overlap perfectly, thereby providing the largest oscillator (transition) strength.

centered within the QW and overlap perfectly, thereby providing the largest transition strength.

## 2.3 Quantum Confined Stark Effect: Wavefunction Polarization

The majority of GaN microLEDs used with existing display technologies are grown on the polar (0001) c-plane of wurtzite GaN. Nonbasal planes of GaN however, afford distinct advantages and different optical properties to the traditional c-plane GaN. Undesirably, due to the polarization-related electric fields inside the MQWs for c-plane GaN, the QCSE causes a lower energy recombination transition and a characteristic blue shift in the peak emission wavelength is observed as current density is increased [7]. Nevertheless, the lattice constant of the GaN layer does not match the lattice constant of the InGaN layer and the piezoelectric polarization in the MQW structure exists and the bottom of the well is tilted as shown in Figure 2.5. The distorted energy band structure ($E_c$ and $E_v$) causes the electron wave function and the hole wave function to be separated so that the peak of the electron wave function does not align with the peak of the hole wave function. When the electron wave function and the hole wave function are separated, the recombination efficiency of the electrons and the holes decreases and the light emitting efficiency is reduced. The situation that a distorted energy band structure ($E_c$ and $E_v$) makes the wave functions of electron and hole separated is named as QCSE. QCSE was first reported by

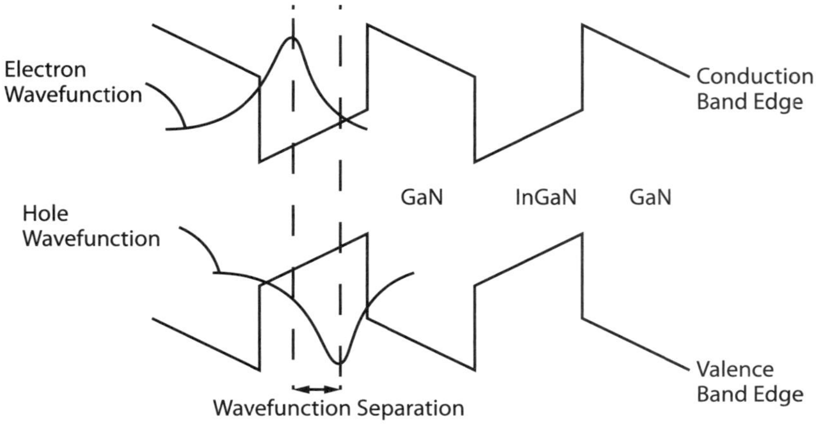


**Figure 2.5** Schematic illustration of the energy band diagrams for the effect of polarization field on electron and hole wavefunction separation, which is the QCSE.

Miller et al. in the context of GaAs-AlGaAs QW structures with electric field applied perpendicular to the layers [8].

Avoiding QCSE in InGaN microLEDs has been considered as an important milestone to realize the ultimate solid-state light sources for general illumination [9].

When a current is injected into the microLED structure, the band distortion due to polarization fields results in electron overflow, resulting in further reduction of the internal quantum efficiency.

The origin of the polarization field is spontaneous and piezoelectric polarization. A brief discussion of these two types is given here.

### 2.3.1 Spontaneous Polarization

Due to the small ionic radius of nitrogen compared to gallium and indium, GaN and InN are considered to be extremely polar [10]. N has a higher electronegativity than Ga, thus N atoms are able to attract more electrons than Ga atoms due to this difference in electronegativity. Hence, a polarization occurs that is referred to as spontaneous polarization ($P_{sp}$) (i.e., polarization at zero strain). This is schematically shown in Figure 2.6. This results in a permanent dipole moment. The intrinsic dipole moment is neutralized by free electric charge that builds up on the surface by internal conduction or from the ambient atmosphere. For GaN and InN, the spontaneous polarization coefficients are almost equal [10, 11]. The spontaneous polarization coefficient of $In_xGa_{1-x}N$ deviates from linearity (i.e., Vegard's law) and is interpolated by the following second-order polynomial of the alloy composition [12, 13].

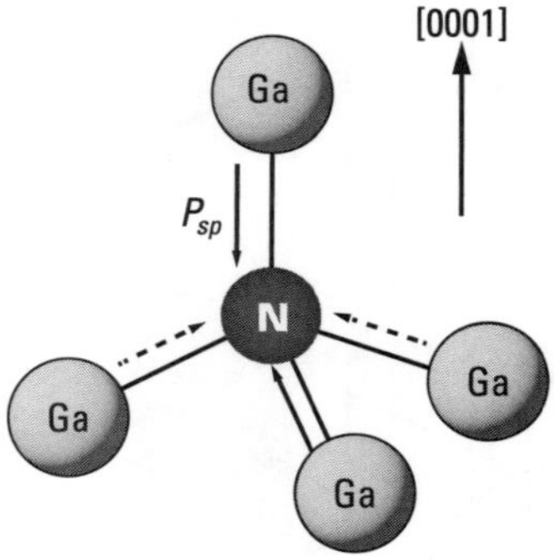


**Figure 2.6** Schematic illustration of the development of spontaneous polarization due to difference in electronegativity of nitrogen and gallium in GaN.

### 2.3.2 Piezoelectric Polarization

If a thin layer of a different lattice constant is grown on a bulk, it grows with a relatively low defect density; however, it gets biaxially strained as shown in Figure 2.7. Since $a_{\mathrm{InN}} > a_{\mathrm{GaN}}$ , therefore the InGaN QW is compressively strained. Strain can be used for altering and optimizing the electronic and optical properties of QWs by varying both the energy levels and the spatial extent of the wavefunctions. Due to this asymmetric deformation, charge redistribution occurs, which causes piezoelectric fields. The piezoelectricity gives rise to an electric field pointing from the substrate side (N face) to the surface side (Ga face). The electric field is dependent on the indium concentration $x$ such that $E_{pz} \sim 10 \cdot x\,\mathrm{MV/cm}$ [7].

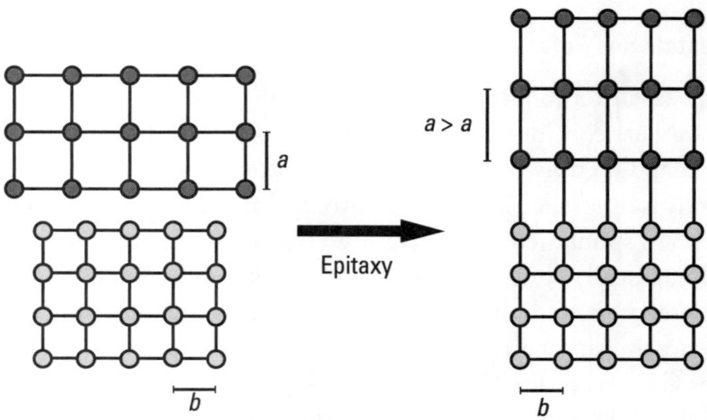


**Figure 2.7** Schematic illustration of the development of strain during epitaxy of a large lattice constant material A (e.g., InGaN) on a small lattice constant material B (e.g., GaN). Strain results in $a > a_0$ and development of a piezoelectric field.

The total polarization in a strained material ($P_{total}$) is considered to be the sum of both the spontaneous and piezoelectric polarizations. However, since $P_{pz} >> P_{sp}$, the spontaneous polarization is typically neglected [14].

## 2.4 Mitigation of QCSE

### 2.4.1 Nonpolar Devices

One approach to eliminating the spontaneous and piezoelectric polarization effects in GaN optoelectronic devices is to grow the devices on nonpolar planes of the crystal [15]. Such planes contain equal numbers of Ga and N atoms and are charge neutral. Furthermore, subsequent nonpolar layers are crystallographically equivalent to one another so the crystal will not be polarized along the growth direction.

Non-c-plane orientations, including nonpolar and semipolar orientations, exhibit reduced or eliminated internal electric fields in quantum well devices. Different planes in GaN crystals are shown in Figure 2.8. The reduction or elimination of this field in nonpolar and semipolar crystal orientations can result in improved device performance. However, the lack of native bulk substrates has limited the application of these crystal orientations. Unfortunately, nonpolar InGaN growth has proven challenging [15]. The lack of successful nonpolar InGaN growth can be attributed to several factors. First, the large lattice mismatches between InGaN and available substrates severely complicate InGaN heteroepitaxy. Second, InGaN must generally be grown at comparatively lower temperatures than GaN due to the propensity for indium to desorb from the growth surface at higher temperatures. Unfortunately, nonpolar nitrides are typically grown above 900°C and more often above 1050°C,

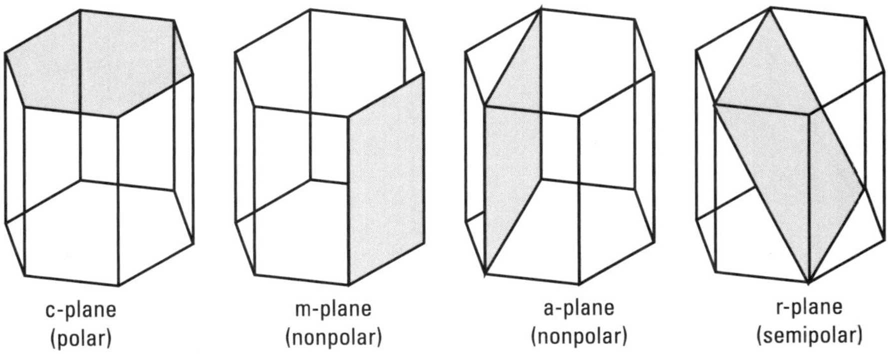


**Figure 2.8** Crystallography and orientation of group III-nitride layers growth along different planes.

temperatures at which indium readily desorbs from the surface. Third, high-quality nonpolar nitrides are typically grown at decreased pressures (<100 Torr) in order to stabilize the *a*- and *m*-planes relative to inclined facets. However, it has been previously widely reported that c-plane InGaN should be grown at atmospheric pressure in order to enhance indium incorporation and decrease carbon incorporation.

### 2.4.2 Core-Shell Nanostructures MicroLEDs

One method to alleviate the problems with planar device fabrication is to use GaN nanowires or microrods [16–20]. Such structures, shown in Figure 2.9, can be fabricated at high temperature with the appropriate shell structures to form a p-QW-n LED that is harvested from the growth substrate. The divergence from planar should provide a higher efficiency for light extraction. The diameter of the microrods and nanowires is typically small enough that the threading dislocation density is significantly reduced, increasing the IQE and lifetime. By controlling the crystallographic orientation of the GaN $\mu$-rods nonpolar or semipolar planes can be used for device fabrication, thereby reducing the effect of the QCSE, which, in turn, can also lead to improvements in the IQE [21].

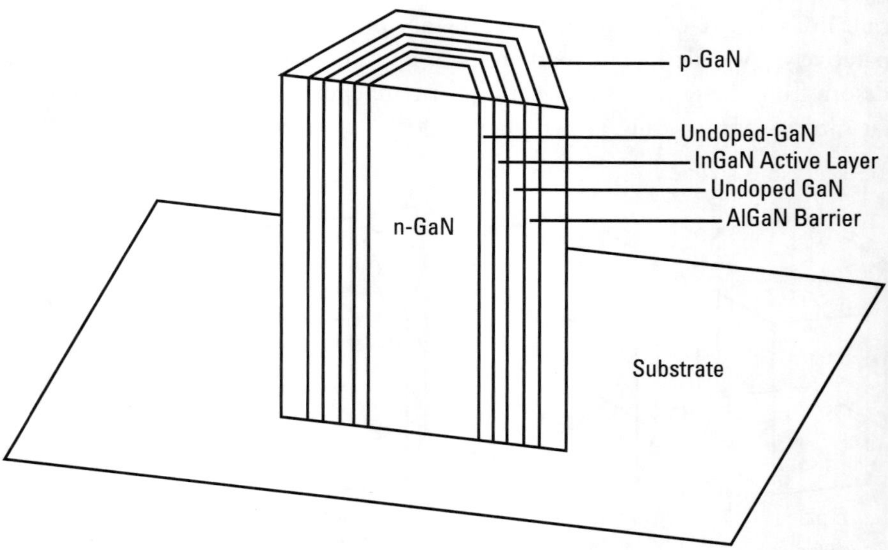


**Figure 2.9** Schematic illustration of a cross section of a core-shell nanowire with emission from the m-plane (sidewalls).

### 2.4.3 Graded Indium in InGaN

Adjusting the shape of the band gap of the QW layer has been proposed to minimize the influence of the polarization field by spreading the polarization-induced sheet charge into a quasi-volume space charge [22–24]. Two examples of bandgap profile are shown in Figure 2.10. However, convincing experimental data has not been provided.

### 2.4.4 Cubic GaN

GaN and alloys including AlGaN and InGaN exhibit both hexagonal (wurtzite) and cubic (e.g., zinc-blende) phases with crystal structures shown in Figure 2.11. For GaN and InGaN the hexagonal (h-GaN) phase is energetically preferred and with a few exceptions, all device applications including high-power transistors, LEDs, and laser diodes have been developed with h-GaN material. The wurtzite structure is described by two (or three) equivalent basal plane axes that are rotated 120° with respect to each other (the a-axes), all of which are perpendicular to a unique c-axis. Group III and nitrogen atoms occupy alternating c-planes along the crystal's c-axis. The symmetry elements included in the wurtzite structure dictate that III-nitrides possess a bulk spontaneous polarization along this c-axis. Furthermore, as the wurtzite crystal structure is noncentrosymmetric, wurtzite nitrides can and do additionally exhibit piezoelectric polarization also along the crystal's c-axis.

There are potential advantages to cubic (c-GaN) material and its alloys. One advantage is that the <001> direction (i.e., the direction of growth on the {001} crystal face) is not only free of spontaneous polarization, but also free of piezoelectric polarization. The bandgap of the cubic nitrides is slightly smaller than that of the wurtzite polytypes, and therefore the band-edge emission in bulk crystals of cubic InGaN has longer wavelength than in wurtzite crystals

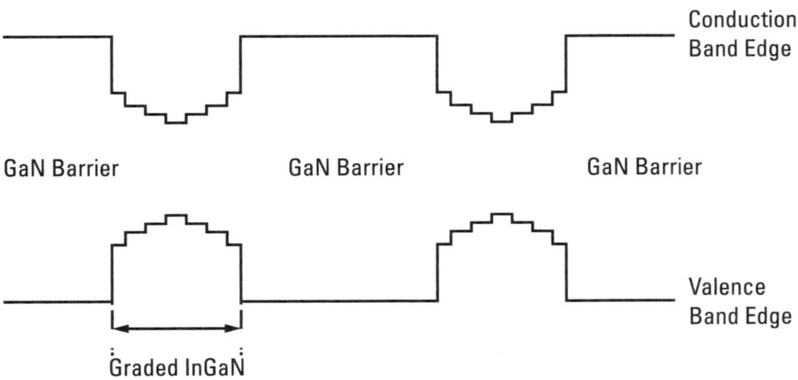


**Figure 2.10** Schematic illustration of graded indium InGaN QWs.

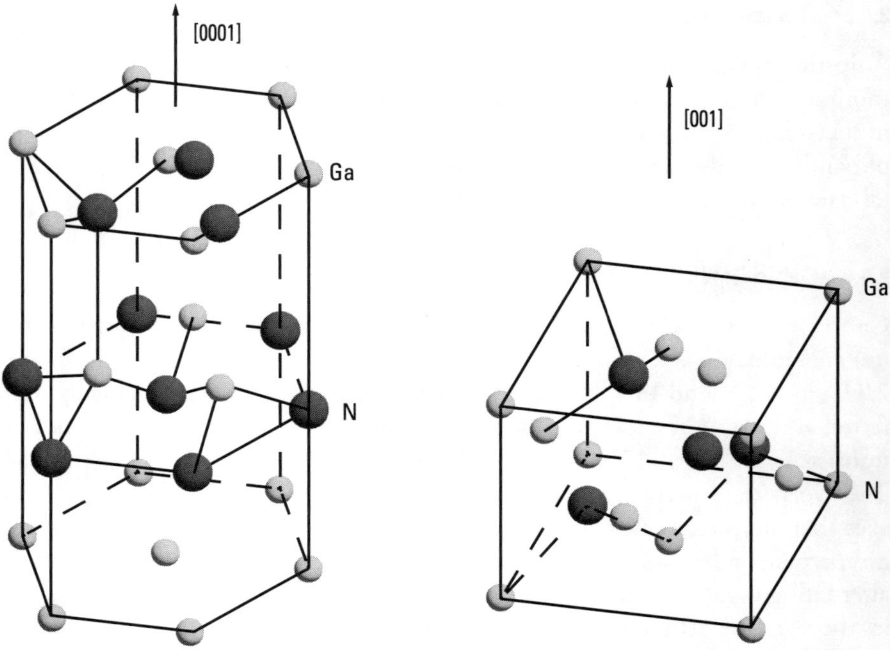


**Figure 2.11** Schematic illustration of the crystal structure of (left) hexagonal (wurtzite) and (right) cubic (zincblende) GaN. Unlike zincblende GaN, the wurtzite crystal structure is noncentrosymmetric.

with the same indium concentration. The general absence of internal electric fields in c-GaN LEDs can eliminate the blueshift associated with the QCSE [25–27]. However, approaches to avoid the preferential [0001] wurtzite crystal growth are challenging as they often produce a reduced crystal quality frequently combined with comparably lower deposition rates [28–30].

### 2.4.5 N-Polar Orientation

The Ga-polar orientation is the most common choice for nitride microLEDs. However, the N-polar orientation, which has demonstrated high performance in electronic applications, may be a promising option for longer wavelength InGaN microLEDs due to its higher indium uptake. The N-polar is demonstrated in Figure 2.12. Due to the direction of the polarization field against the forward bias, a larger forward bias decreases the polarization field in N-polar InGaN/GaN MQWs, resulting in a flat-band and reduced QCSE [31–36]. The energy band diagrams for Ga-polar and N-polar are shown in Figures 2.13 and 2.14, respectively.

Despite intensive research, the growth of micrometer-thick high-quality N-polar GaN based materials remains challenging [37–41]. For example,

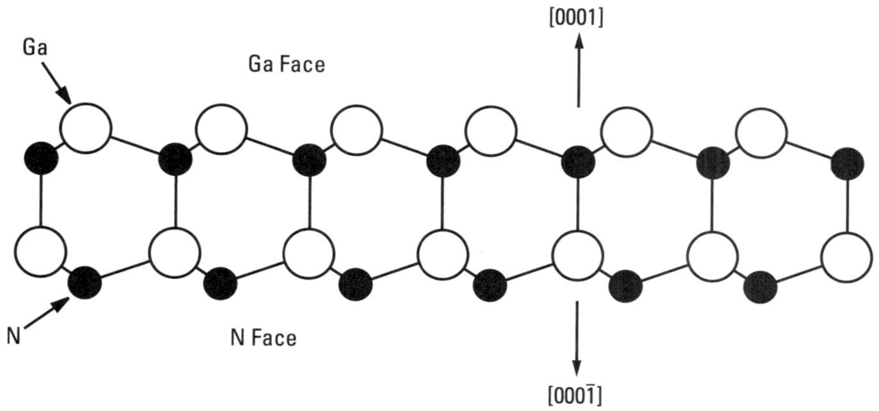


**Figure 2.12** Cross-sectional view of a wurtzite GaN crystal in a (11$\bar{2}$0) projection, indicating the inequivalent (0001) and (000$\bar{1}$) directions. GaN exhibits strong ionic character due to strong charge transfer between the highly electronegative nitrogen atom and the less electronegative III-metal gallium atom, which leads to polarization in the (0001) direction that is opposite to that in the (000$\bar{1}$) direction.

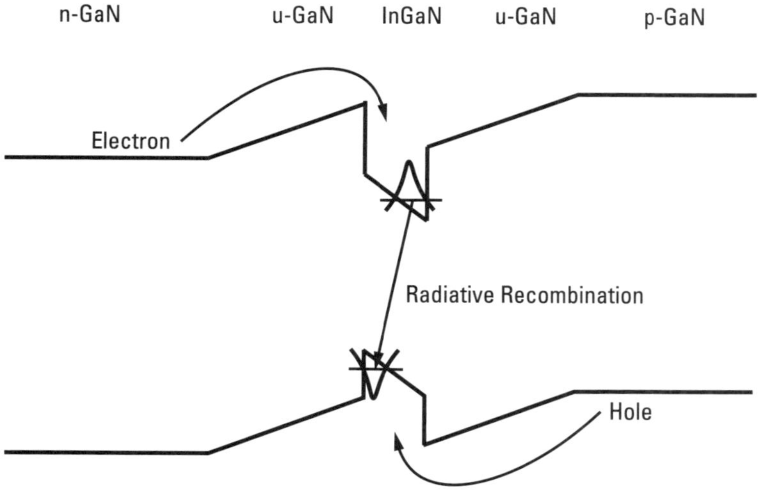


**Figure 2.13** Schematic illustration of the energy band diagrams for a gallium-polar InGaN/GaN microLED stack under forward bias. The polarization field is in the same direction as the applied field, resulting in more electron and hole wavefunction separation, and reduction of internal quantum efficiency.

growth with smooth surface morphology is relatively harder for the N-polar surface. It is also known that under a fixed growth condition, the N-polar growth exhibits higher O incorporation and much lower Mg incorporation, by

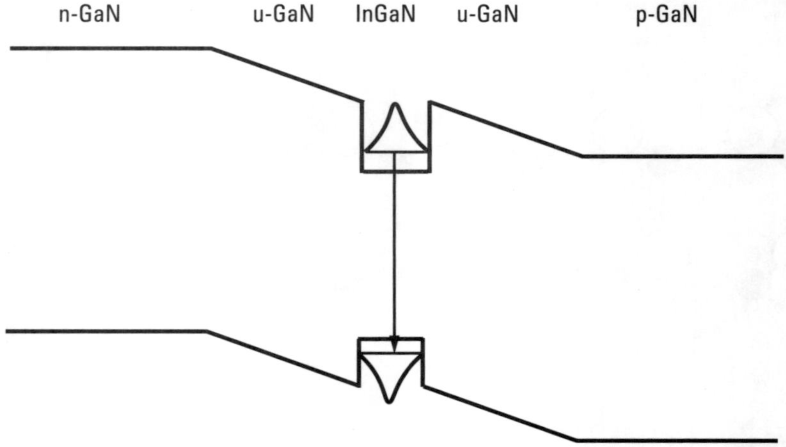


**Figure 2.14** Schematic illustration of the energy band diagrams for the nitrogen-polar InGaN/GaN microLED stack under forward bias. Since the polarization field is opposite to the applied field, internal field is compensated at some forward voltage resulting in improved electron and hole wavefunction overlap.

almost an order of magnitude, compared to metal-polar surface growth, which can make p-doping of N-polar GaN difficult.

### 2.4.6 Doped Barriers

Theoretical and experimental efforts have shown that it is possible to reduce the internal electric fields in the c-plane InGaN/GaN QWs through the use of doped barriers [42–47]. Placing heavily doped p- and n-type GaN barriers close to the QW leads to an increase in the p–n junction electric field, which counteracts the opposite polarization-induced electric field in the QW, resulting in a smaller net internal electric field, thereby improving the electron–hole wavefunction overlap on the microLEDs. The technique has been employed in thick and thin c-plane single QW microLEDs, and improved efficiency droop has been observed.

### 2.4.7 Axial Nanowire/Disk-in-Wire Architecture

A much reduced polarization field has been predicted by theory and realized by experiments using axial nanowire architecture [48–53]. A schematic of an axial nanowire is shown in Figure 2.15. Here, a nanowire with flat-top forming an n-GaN c-plane growth template is grown out of a silicon (Si) or sapphire wafer using selective area epitaxial growth. Then MBE is used to grow the barrier and QW structure, and finally the p-GaN contact layer. When the diameter of the

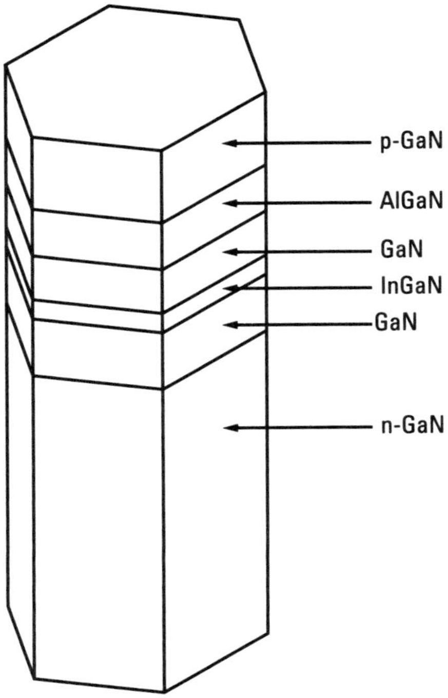


**Figure 2.15** Schematic illustration of axial nanowire.

nanowire is less than a critical value, strain is relaxed, which is the root cause for the piezoelectric field in conventional c-plane light-emitting diode structures.

## 2.5 Elementary Modeling Framework for MicroLED Operation

The objective of this section is to calculate the transition energy and radiative recombination coefficient versus indium mole fraction and QW width.

The simplest QW microLED to be dealt with consists of a single layer of material *A* embedded between two thick (thickness being much greater than the penetration length of the confined wave function) layers of material B, where *B* has a bandgap larger than *A* and where the band discontinuities are such that both types of carriers are confined in the *A* material (Figure 2.16).

Electroluminance theory states that emission wavelength is determined by the energy gap plus the quantum energy states for electrons and holes, and can be expressed by [54–56]

$$E_t \equiv E_{g,w} + \varepsilon_{1,n} + \varepsilon_{1,p} - E_b \tag{2.1}$$

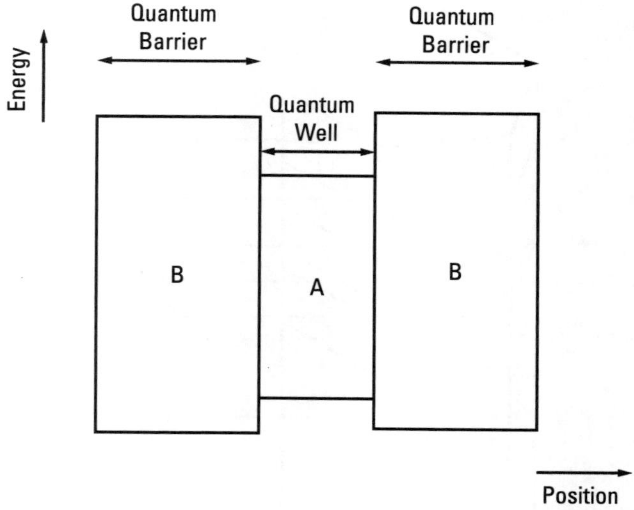


**Figure 2.16** Schematic illustration of a QW system where a QW material is sandwiched by two barrier materials. The barrier material has a wider bandgap compared to the QW material. The QW width is *d*.

where $E_{g,w}$ is the energy gap of the well material, $\varepsilon_{1,n}$ is the first confined state for electrons in the conduction band well, $\varepsilon_{1,p}$ is the first confined state for holes in the valence band well, and $E_b$ is the exciton binding energy.

GaN-based microLEDs feature a large free exciton binding energy (20 meV in bulk GaN), which makes excitons potentially stable at room temperature [57, 58]. The exciton binding energy was estimated to be 50 meV for 2 nm QW width including random alloy disorder [59]. The binding energy decreases with increased QW width due to the field-induced separation of electrons and holes: The binding energy was estimated to be ~30 meV for 3-nm wide QW. An increased indium composition causes competing effects: larger indium fluctuations, which lead to stronger localization and hence more Coulomb interaction, and stronger polarization fields, which separate electrons and hole, reducing their interaction. This leads to a slight reduction of the binding energy with increasing the indium mole fraction for any given QW width (binding energy decreases from ~50 to ~40 meV when indium mole fraction increases from 5% to 25% for 2-nm quantum well) [59]. Simple expressions for the confined exciton binding energy will be provided below.

It is therefore useful to review the calculations of first confined energy states in various QW configurations to understand the operation of a microLED. This can be done by solving the Schrodinger equation. The wavefunction can be described by the Schrodinger equation where $V(z)$ is the potential energy, $z$ is the distance along the confinement axis, $\varepsilon_n$ is the quantized energy states that result from the solution of (2.2), $m^*$ is the effective mass along the confinement axis, and $\hbar$ is Planck's constant:

$$\left(-\frac{\hbar^2}{2m^*(z)}\frac{\partial^2 y}{\partial z^2}+V(z)\right)\psi_n(z)=\varepsilon_n\psi_n(z) \tag{2.2}$$

### 2.5.1 Confined States in Various Quantum Well Configurations

#### 2.5.1.1 Infinitely Deep Square Quantum Well

In the infinitely deep well approximation, the solution to (2.2) is very simple, as the wave function must be zero in the confining layer B, and therefore also at the interface because of the continuity equations. Taking the $x$ abscissa origin at one interface (Figure 2.16), the solution of (2.2) can evidently only be ~ $\sin(n\pi z/d)$, $n$ being an odd or even integer. The confining energy $\varepsilon_1$ is then simply

$$\varepsilon_1=\frac{\pi^2\hbar^2}{2m^*d^2} \tag{2.3}$$

#### 2.5.1.2 Finite Square Quantum Well

The Schrodinger equation (2.2) in the finite-well case must satisfy the continuity of $\psi_n(z)$ and $(1/m^*)\partial\psi_n/\partial z$ at $z=-d/2$ and $z=d/2$.

Equation (2.2) can be exactly solved to yield the wave functions and energies from solving the following transcendental equation:

$$\tan(k_w\bullet d)=2\frac{m_w}{m_b}\frac{k_b}{k_w}\left[1-\left(\frac{m_w}{m_b}\bullet\frac{k_b}{k_w}\right)^2\right]^{-1} \tag{2.4}$$

where $k_b$ and $k_w$ are given by

$$k_w=\left(\frac{2m_w}{\hbar^2}\varepsilon_1\right)^{1/2} \tag{2.5}$$

$$k_b=\left(\frac{2m_b}{\hbar^2}(V_0-\varepsilon_1)\right)^{1/2} \tag{2.6}$$

with $m_w$ the effective mass in the well, $m_b$ the effective mass in the barrier, $V_0$ is the QW height, and $d$ is the QW width.

Approximate solution is given by considering the condition $k_w d << 1$. In this case $\tan(k_w d) \approx k_w d$. A simple approximate condition can be found for $\varepsilon_1$ as follows:

$$\varepsilon_1 \approx \frac{\pi^2 \hbar^2}{2m_w d^2}\left(1-\frac{2}{\sqrt{\sigma}+2}\right)^2 \quad (2.7)$$

$$\sigma = \left(\frac{m_w}{m_b}\right)^2 \frac{2m_b V_0}{\hbar^2} d^2 \quad (2.8)$$

where $\sigma$ is a dimensionless parameter that indicates the deviation from infinite QW approximation.

#### 2.5.1.3 Infinite Quantum Well with Applied Field

In real operating conditions, an external field is applied on the QW. It is therefore required to estimate the first confined state under such conditions. The first simple configuration involves infinite barrier height. In this case, the variational approach was used to estimate the first confined state by minimizing the following equation in terms of $\beta$ [60]:

$$\varepsilon_1(\beta) = \frac{\pi^2 \hbar^2}{2m^* d^2}\left[\left(1+\frac{\beta^2}{\pi^2}\right)+\xi\left(\frac{1}{2\beta}+\frac{\beta}{\beta^2+\pi^2}-\frac{1}{2}\coth\beta\right)\right] \quad (2.9)$$

where the parameter $\xi = qEd/(\pi^2\hbar^2/2m^* d^2)$ is the normalized electric field.

In the low field limit ($\xi << 1$) we find

$$\varepsilon_1 = \frac{\pi^2 \hbar^2}{2m^* d^2} - \frac{1}{8}\left(\frac{1}{3}-\frac{2}{\pi^2}\right)^2 \frac{m_w q^2 E^2 d^4}{\hbar^2} \quad (2.10)$$

In the high field limit ($\xi<<1$) we find

$$\varepsilon_1 = \frac{\pi^2 \hbar^2}{2m^* d^2} - \frac{1}{2} qEd + \left(\frac{3}{2}\right)^{5/3} \left(\frac{q^2 E^2 \hbar^2}{m_w}\right)^{1/3} \quad (2.11)$$

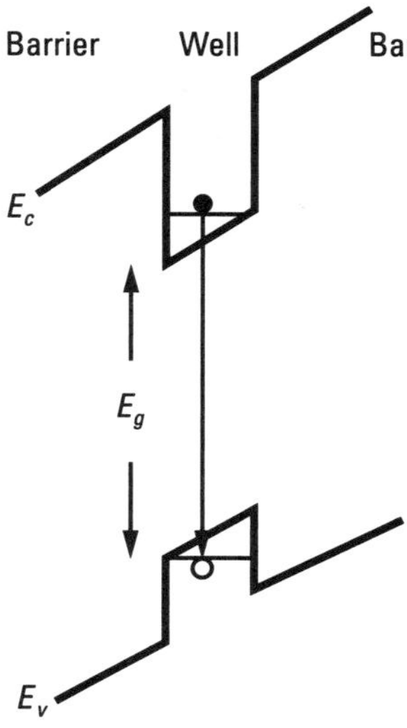


**Figure 2.17** Schematic diagram of the electron and hole energy level in QW with nonzero field.

#### 2.5.1.4 Finite Quantum Well with Applied Field

Finally, we consider this realistic configuration that we find in real microLEDs. Singh [61] derived a simple equation for the first confined energy level and is expressed by

$$\varepsilon_1 \approx \frac{qV_0}{2} - \frac{\pi^2\hbar^2}{4m_w d^2}\left(\left\{1+32\left[\left(\frac{qV_0}{\pi}\right)^2+\left(\frac{q\xi d}{\pi}\right)^2\right]\frac{d^4 m_w^2}{\pi^4\hbar^4}\right\}^{1/2}-1\right) \quad (2.12)$$

where $\xi$ is the electric field in the QW.

It should be noted that other models and methods may be used to calculate the ground state in a QW under the influence of an external field [60, 62–66].

### 2.5.2 Transition Energy

The transition energy is given by (2.1). For the $In_xGa_{1-x}N$ material, $E_g(x)$ is the energy gap of the active layer (QW) as a function of the indium mole fraction $x$ $(0 \leq x \leq 1)$, and

$$E_g(x) \approx 0.7x - 1.4x(1-x) + 3.45(1-x) \quad (2.13)$$

The energies $\varepsilon_{1n}$ and $\varepsilon_{1p}$ are given by

$$\varepsilon_{1n} \approx \frac{qV_{0,c}}{2} - \frac{\pi^2\hbar^2}{4m_{w,n}d^2}\left(\left\{1+32\left[\left(\frac{qV_{0,c}}{\pi}\right)^2+\left(\frac{q\xi d}{\pi}\right)^2\right]\frac{d^4m_{w,n}^2}{\pi^4\hbar^4}\right\}^{1/2}-1\right) \tag{2.14}$$

$$\varepsilon_{1p} \approx \frac{qV_{0,v}}{2} - \frac{\pi^2\hbar^2}{4m_{w,p}d^2}\left(\left\{1+32\left[\left(\frac{qV_{0,v}}{\pi}\right)^2+\left(\frac{q\xi d}{\pi}\right)^2\right]\frac{d^4m_{w,p}^2}{\pi^4\hbar^4}\right\}^{1/2}-1\right) \tag{2.15}$$

These equations assume quasi-bound states in the QW, and this is only valid when the field satisfies the following assumption:

$$q_0^2 = \frac{2m_w d^2}{\hbar^2}(V_0 - \varepsilon_0)\,. \tag{2.16}$$

$$\frac{q\xi d}{q_0} \ll \frac{q_0^2\hbar^2}{2m_w d^2} \tag{2.17}$$

where $q_0$ is a characteristic dimensionless wave vector, and $\varepsilon_0$ is the zero-field first quantum state.

The voltage across the QW has two components: (1) the voltage drop due to current flow is given by (2.18a), and (2) the built-in voltage due polarization field is given by (2.18b) [67–69]:

$$V_{w1} \approx \frac{kT}{q}\left(\frac{J}{J_0}\right)^{0.5} \tag{2.18a}$$

$$V_{w2} = \frac{(P_w - P_b)}{\epsilon_b / d_b + \epsilon_w / d} \tag{2.18b}$$

$$V_q = \frac{kT}{q}\left(\frac{J}{J_0}\right)^{0.5} \pm \frac{(P_w - P_b)}{\epsilon_b / d_b + \epsilon_w / d} \tag{2.18c}$$

where $J$ is the current density, $J_0$ is a characteristic current density, $k$ is the Boltzmann constant, $T$ is the temperature, $q$ is the electronic charge, $P(x)$ is the polarization charge density at the $In_xGa_{1-x}N/GaN$ interface, and $\epsilon_w(x)$ is the permittivity of the active layer, $\epsilon_b(x)$ is the permittivity of the barrier layer, plus sign corresponds to Ga-polar device and negative sign corresponds to N-polar device, $V_{0,c}(x)$ is the QW height in the conduction band, and $V_{0,v}(x)$ is the valence band height in the valence band, and they are given by

$$V_{0,c}(x) \approx 0.6\left[3.45 - E_g(x)\right] \tag{2.19}$$

$$V_{0,v}(x) \approx 0.4\left[3.45 - E_g(x)\right] \tag{2.20}$$

The characteristic current density is given by (as shown in Chapter 3)

$$J_0 = \frac{\epsilon_w^2 (kT/q)^2 B}{q^2 d^3} \tag{2.21}$$

with $B$ is the bimolecular radiative recombination coefficient.

The polarization charge density for the $In_xGa_{1-x}N/GaN$ system is given by (units $C/m^2$) [70]:

$$P_w = P_w^{PZ} + P_w^{SP} \tag{2.22}$$

$$P_b = P_b^{PZ} + P_b^{SP} \tag{2.23}$$

$$P_w^{SP}(x) = -0.042x - 0.034(1-x) + (1.06 - 0.0378)x(1-x) \tag{2.24}$$

$$P_b^{SP} = -0.034 \tag{2.25}$$

$$P_w^{PZ}(x) = 0.148x - 0.0424x(1-x) \tag{2.26}$$

$$P_b^{PZ} \approx 0 \tag{2.27}$$

The dielectric constant is of the $In_xGa_{1-x}N$ is given by [71]

$$\epsilon_w(x) \approx 4.33x + 10.28 \tag{2.28}$$

$$\epsilon_b \approx 10.28 \tag{2.29}$$

The binding energy is discussed after the derivation of the electron and hole wavefunctions.

### 2.5.3 Radiative Recombination Coefficient

The quantum efficiency of light emission depends on radiative and nonradiative recombination processes in the structures. An improvement in the efficiency of a structure can be achieved by either reducing nonradiative recombination of charge carriers or enhancing the radiative recombination rates. The radiative recombination processes are dominated by the physical properties of the semiconductor and the dimensionality of the structure. Assuming momentum conservation, the rate $R_r$ of radiative band-to-band recombination for free electrons and holes in a direct-gap semiconductor can be described by

$$R_r = B \bullet n \bullet p \tag{2.30}$$

where $B$ is radiative recombination coefficient, $n$ is the electron concentration per unit volume, and $p$ is the hole concentration per unit volume.

Considering a two-dimensional (2D) system like a QW, the charge carriers get quantized and are restricted to certain energy levels in the conduction and valence bands. In general, each possible transition from the $m$th induction band state to the $n$th valence band state will contribute to the total radiative rate $R_r$ (see Figure 2.18).

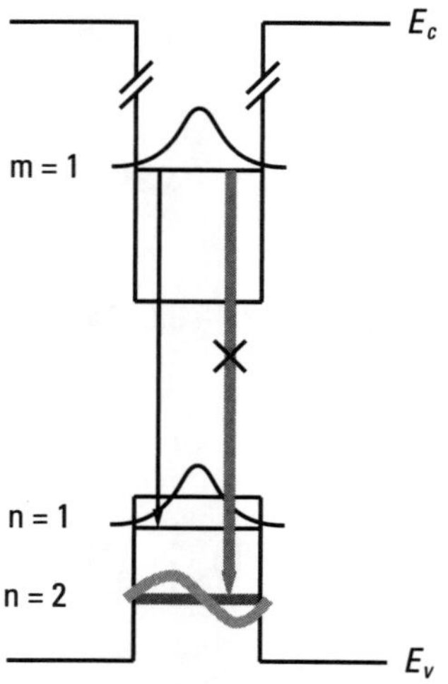


**Figure 2.18** Scheme showing allowed and forbidden transitions between the different quantized states in the conduction and valence bands. Exemplary energy separations are given for a thin (~2 nm) QW.

For the elementary analysis in this book, only first confined states in the conduction and valence bands will be considered for simplicity, and the 2D radiative recombination coefficient is given by the product of the 3D radiative recombination coefficient and the square of the wavefunction overlap [72–77].

#### 2.5.3.1 Electron and Hole Wavefunctions

The strategy to calculate the wavefunction is to transform the finite QW under the electric field problem into an equivalent infinite QW (with an increased effective QW width), then solve for the wavefunction inside the equivalent infinite QW. It can be demonstrated that the finite QW shown in Figure 2.19 can be converted into an equivalent infinite QW with modified width with the following expansion dimensions [78]:

$$\delta_L = \left[\frac{2m}{\hbar^2}\left(V_0 - q\frac{V_w}{2} - \varepsilon_{1n}\right)\right]^{-1/2} \tag{2.31}$$

$$\delta_R = \left[\frac{2m}{\hbar^2}\left(V_0 + q\frac{V_w}{2} - \varepsilon_{1n}\right)\right]^{-1/2} \tag{2.32}$$

Using the coordinate system introduced in Figure 2.20 we can find the wavefunctions associated with the motion of the carriers in the *x*-direction by solving Schrodinger's equation with an electron potential energy $V(x)$ given by

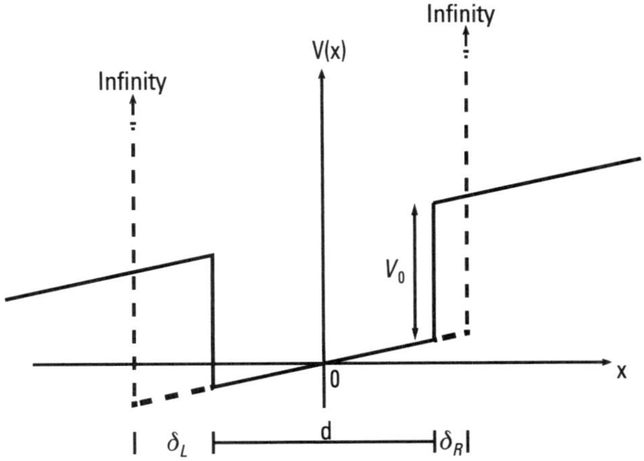


**Figure 2.19** A finite-height QW (solid line) with an applied electric field $\xi$ and its equivalent case of an infinite-height potential well (dashed line).

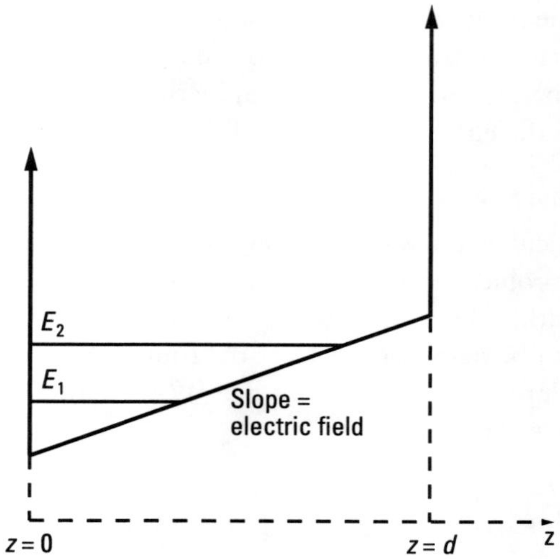


**Figure 2.20** An infinite-height QW with applied external electric field $\xi$.

$$\begin{aligned} V(x) &= q\xi x \quad 0 \le x \le L \\ V(x) &= \infty \quad\quad x > L \\ V(x) &= \infty \quad\quad x < 0 \end{aligned} \tag{2.33}$$

where $\xi$ is the electric field in the well and $q$ is the electronic charge. The electric field is assumed to be constant with $x$. The potential energy is arbitrarily set equal to zero at the interface:

$$V_w = q\xi d \tag{2.34}$$

The Schrodinger equation

$$-\frac{\hbar^2}{2m}\frac{d^2\psi}{dx^2} + (q\xi x)\psi = E\psi \tag{2.35}$$

where $m$ is the effective mass

$$\frac{d^2\psi}{dx^2} = \frac{2mq\xi}{\hbar^2}\left(x - \frac{E}{q\xi}\right)\psi \tag{2.36}$$

Let us define a new variable $z$ given by

$$z = \beta\left(x - \frac{E}{q\xi}\right) \tag{2.37}$$

where $\beta$ is a normalization factor to ensure that the equation ends up matching the Airy equation

$$\frac{dz}{dx} = \beta \tag{2.38}$$

Substitute $dx = dz/\beta$

$$\frac{d^2\psi(z)}{dz^2} = \left(\frac{2mq\xi}{\hbar^2} z\beta^{-3}\right)\psi \tag{2.39}$$

For this equation to be the Airy equation we must have

$$\left(\frac{2mq\xi}{\hbar^2}\beta^{-3}\right) = 1 \tag{2.40}$$

$$z = \left(\frac{2mq\xi}{\hbar^2}\right)^{\frac{1}{3}}\left(x - \frac{\varepsilon_1}{q\xi}\right) \tag{2.41}$$

The wavefunction is thus given by

$$\psi(z) = c \bullet Ai(z) \tag{2.42}$$

We compute the normalization constant $c$ from the condition

$$\int_0^\infty |\psi(x)|^2 \, dx = 1 \tag{2.43}$$

which leads to

$$|c|^2 = \left[\int_0^\infty \left\{ Ai\left[\left(\frac{2mq\xi}{\hbar^2}\right)^{\frac{1}{3}}\left(x - \frac{\varepsilon_1}{q\xi}\right)\right]\right\}^2\right]^{-1} \tag{2.44}$$

An analytical solution is possible in the form

$$c = \left( \frac{\left( \frac{2mq\xi}{\hbar^2} \right)^{1/3}}{\mathrm{Ai}'^2 \left[ -\left( \frac{2mq\xi}{\hbar^2} \right)^{1/3} \bullet \frac{\varepsilon_1}{q\xi} \right]} \right)^{1/2} \tag{2.45}$$

where Ai′ is the first derivative of the Airy function.

Now the wavefunction may be expressed by

$$\psi(x) = \left( \frac{\left( \frac{2mq\xi}{\hbar^2} \right)^{1/3}}{\mathrm{Ai}'^2 \left[ -\left( \frac{2mq\xi}{\hbar^2} \right)^{1/3} \bullet \frac{\varepsilon_1}{q\xi} \right]} \right)^{1/2} \bullet Ai\left[ \left( \frac{2mq\xi}{\hbar^2} \right)^{\frac{1}{3}} \left( x - \frac{\varepsilon_1}{q\xi} \right) \right] \tag{2.46}$$

The Airy function is defined as

$$Ai(x) = \frac{1}{\pi} \int_0^\infty \cos\left( \frac{u^3}{3} + xu \right) du \tag{2.47}$$

$$Ai(x) = \frac{1}{3^{2/3}\Gamma(2/3)} \left( 1 + \frac{x^3}{6} + \frac{x^6}{180} + \ldots \right) - \frac{1}{3^{1/3}\Gamma(1/3)} \left( x + \frac{x^4}{12} + \frac{x^7}{504} + \ldots \right) \tag{2.48}$$

$$\Gamma(x) = \int_0^\infty t^{x-1} \exp(-t)\, dt \tag{2.49}$$

By moving the left boundary to correct for the finite barrier height, we can now write the electron wavefunction as

$$\psi_n(x) = \left( \frac{\left( \frac{2m_{w,n}q\xi}{\hbar^2} \right)^{1/3}}{\mathrm{Ai}'^2 \left[ -\left( \frac{2m_{w,n}q\xi}{\hbar^2} \right)^{1/3} \frac{\varepsilon_{1n}}{q\xi} \right]} \right)^{1/2} Ai\left[ \left( \frac{2m_{w,n}q\xi}{\hbar^2} \right)^{\frac{1}{3}} \left( x + \delta_L - \frac{\varepsilon_{1n}}{q\xi} \right) \right] \tag{2.50}$$

Similarly, the hole wavefunction can be found from

$$\psi_p(x) = \left( \frac{\left( \frac{2m_{w,p} q\xi}{\hbar^2} \right)^{1/3}}{\mathrm{Ai}'^2 \left[ -\left( \frac{2m_{w,p} q\xi}{\hbar^2} \right)^{1/3} \frac{\varepsilon_{1p}}{q\xi} \right]} \right)^{1/2} Ai \left[ \left( \frac{2m_{w,p} q\xi}{\hbar^2} \right)^{\frac{1}{3}} \left( -x + d + \delta_R + \frac{\varepsilon_{1p}}{q\xi} \right) \right] \tag{2.51}$$

The wavefunction overlap is given by

$$\zeta = \int_0^d \psi_p(x) \bullet \psi_n(x) \bullet dx \tag{2.52}$$

The separation between the peak of the electron and hole wavefunctions is given by finding the difference of the zeros of the following functions

$$Ai' \left[ \left( \frac{2m_{w,n} q\xi}{\hbar^2} \right)^{\frac{1}{3}} \left( x_n + \delta_L - \frac{\varepsilon_{1n}}{q\xi} \right) \right] = 0 \tag{2.53}$$

$$Ai' \left[ \left( \frac{2m_{w,p} q\xi}{\hbar^2} \right)^{\frac{1}{3}} \left( -x_p + d + \delta_R + \frac{\varepsilon_{1p}}{q\xi} \right) \right] = 0 \tag{2.54}$$

The effective masses for electrons and holes in $In_xGa_{1-x}N$ are given in terms of the indium mole fraction by the following expressions [79–81]:

$$\frac{m_{w,n}}{m_0} \approx 0.07x + 0.2(1-x) \tag{2.55}$$

$$\frac{m_{w,p}}{m_0} \approx 0.4x + 2(1-x) \tag{2.56}$$

#### 2.5.3.2 Bulk Bimolecular Radiative Recombination Coefficient

The 3D bimolecular radiative recombination coefficient is given by [82]

$$B_{3D} = \frac{1}{\tau_r N_c} \left( \frac{m_{w,r}}{m_{w,p}} \right)^{3/2} \tag{2.57}$$

$$\tau_r = \frac{\pi \epsilon_0 \hbar^4 c^3}{q^5 x_{vc}^2 \sqrt{\epsilon_w} \left(E_t / q\right)^3} \tag{2.58}$$

$$x_{cv}^2 = \frac{\hbar^2 \varepsilon_P}{3m_0 E_{g,w}^2} \tag{2.59}$$

$$N_c = \frac{1}{4}\left(\frac{2m_{wn} k_B T}{\pi \hbar^2}\right)^{3/2} \tag{2.60}$$

$$\frac{1}{m_{w,r}} = \frac{1}{m_{w,n}} + \frac{1}{m_{w,p}} \tag{2.61}$$

where $\varepsilon_P$ is the Kane energy and is approximately 10 eV.

#### 2.5.3.3 Binding Exciton Energy

Excitons are charge-neutral quasi-particles created when light is absorbed by a semiconductor. A schematic showing the construction and formation of an exciton is shown in Figure 2.21. The exciton binding energy, the energy required to dissociate an excited electron–hole pair into free charge carriers, is one of the key factors to the optoelectronic performance of light-emitting diodes. These excitonic effects originate from electron-hole Coulombic interactions, which strongly enhance the oscillator strength between the electron and hole. The free exciton binding energy provides the necessary link between the energy threshold for valence to conduction band optical absorption and the bandgap determining electronic properties and is used in calculating the transition energy given by (2.1). In general, for common III-V semiconductors such as GaAs-based systems, the bulk exciton binding energy (~4.2 meV) is low compared to the thermal energy (~26 meV), which leads to the ionization of excitons. On the other hand, the binding energy of excitons in bulk GaN is ~20 meV. The free exciton binding energy is

$$E_0 = R_\infty \frac{\mu}{m_0} \frac{1}{\epsilon^2} \tag{2.62}$$

where $R_\infty = 13.6$ eV.

Excitons significantly increase the absorption slightly below the band edge. The interaction of photons and excitons creates a mixed state, the

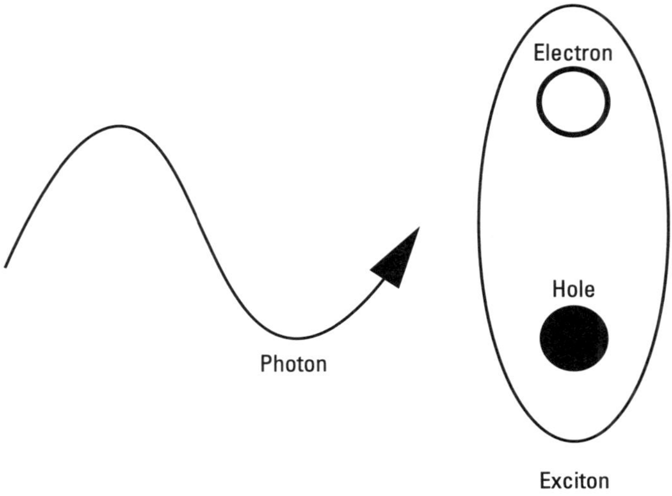


**Figure 2.21** Schematic illustration of the concept of an exciton. Optical band-to-band absorption can produce an electron and a hole in close proximity that attract each other via Coulomb interaction and can form a hydrogen-like bond state, the exciton. Both electron and hole do not have enough kinetic energy at low temperatures to separate. They form a bound state. This bound state is called an exciton.

exciton–polariton, with photon-like and exciton-like dispersion branches. With exciton contribution, a semiconductor with a direct bandgap between spherical parabolic bands has an increased absorption given by [83]

$$\alpha = \gamma_e \frac{e^{\gamma_e}}{\sinh \gamma_e} \tag{2.63}$$

$$\gamma_e = \pi \left( \frac{E_b}{E - E_g} \right)^{1/2} \tag{2.64}$$

In the case of GaN-based QWs, the exciton binding energies are expected to be quite large because quantum confinement causes an increase in the binding energy of excitons. However, the exciton binding energies were reported to be greatly reduced by the internal field due to the spontaneous and the piezoelectric polarizations.

The binding energy of excitons in QWs is usually obtained from the solution of the two-body Schrodinger equation (SE).

The binding energy in a finite QW can be approximated as [84]

$$E_b = \frac{E_0}{\left[1 - \frac{1}{2}\exp\left(-(d + \delta_L + \delta_R)/2a_0\right)\right]^2} \tag{2.65}$$

$$a_0 = \frac{\epsilon}{\epsilon_0}\frac{m_0}{\mu}a_H \tag{2.66}$$

$$a_H = \frac{4\pi\epsilon_0\hbar^2}{q^2 m_0} \tag{2.67}$$

where $E_0$ is the effective Rydberg constant, $a_0$ is the effective Bohr radius, $\delta_L$, and $\delta_R$ are given by (2.31) and (2.32).

An alternative formulation was given in [85]:

$$E_b = \frac{\hbar^2}{2\mu\lambda^2} - \frac{q^2}{2\pi\epsilon\lambda}\int_{-\infty}^{\infty}\int_{-\infty}^{\infty}\left|\psi_n(x_n)\right|^2\left|\psi_p(x_p)\right|^2 G\left(\left|x_n - x_p\right|\right)dx_n dx_p \tag{2.68}$$

$$G\left(\left|x_n - x_p\right|\right) = \frac{2\left|x_n - x_p\right|}{2}\left[\frac{\pi}{2}\left\{H_1\left(\frac{2\left|x_n - x_p\right|}{\lambda}\right) - N_1\left(\frac{2\left|x_n - x_p\right|}{\lambda}\right)\right\} - 1\right] \tag{2.69}$$

where $H_1(x)$ is the first-order Struve function and $N_1(x)$ is the first order Neumann function. A survey of free exciton binding energy for III-V and II-VI semiconductors is shown in Figure 2.22. Energy $E_b$ can be determined by adjusting $\lambda$ variationally to minimize $E_b$:

$$H_1(u) = \frac{u}{\sqrt{\pi}\Gamma(3/2)}\int_0^{\pi/2}\sin(u \bullet \sin\tau)\cos^2\tau\, d\tau \tag{2.70}$$

$$N_1(u) = \frac{1}{\pi}\int_0^{\pi}\sin(u \bullet \sin\theta - \theta)\, d\theta - \frac{2}{\pi}\int_0^{\infty} e^{-u\sinh t}\sinh t\, dt \tag{2.71}$$

### 2.5.4 Nonradiative Recombination Coefficients

Like the radiative recombination coefficient, a nonradiative recombination coefficient in 2D QW is the product of the bulk nonradiative recombination coefficient and the square of the wavefunction overlap [74, 86–92]. Empirically though, it was found that the Shockley-Read-Hall (SRH) nonradiative recombination coefficient is proportional to $\Gamma^{1.6}$ and the Auger nonradiative recombination coefficient is proportional to $\Gamma^{2.3}$ [88].

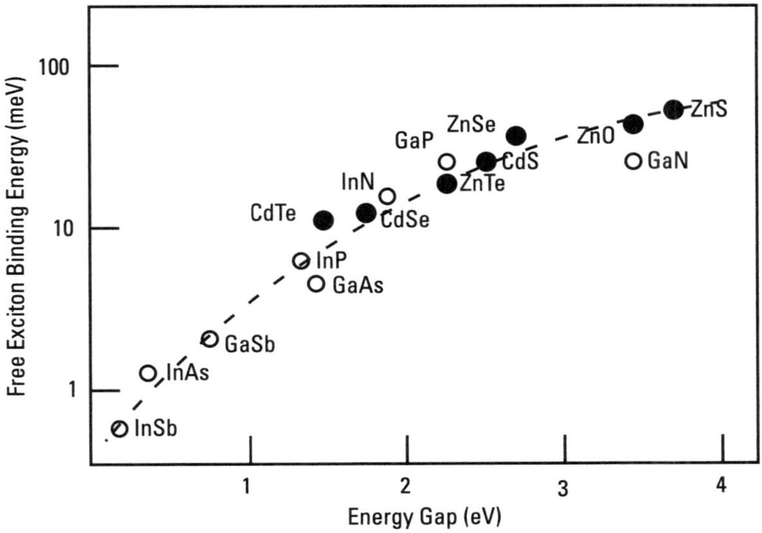


**Figure 2.22** Survey of free exciton binding energy for III-V and II-VI semiconductors.

Defect-assisted recombination is an important limitation on efficiency of optoelectronic devices. The classic SRH recombination picture considers a defect with a single energy level in the bandgap [93]. A complete recombination cycle requires capture of an electron by the neutral defect, followed by capture of a hole at the negatively charged defect. The overall recombination rate is thus governed by the slower of the two processes. In wide bandgap semiconductors such as InGaN, excited states drastically change the dynamics of SRH recombination [94, 95]. The inclusion of excited states enhances nonradiative recombination rates by many orders of magnitude.

SRH recombination is thought to be dependent on the microLED size due to a high density of surface states. The SRH recombination coefficient $A$ was found to sharply increase, by a factor of almost two decades, with decreasing LED dimensions from approximately 100 to 5-$\mu$m. The Auger nonradiative recombination coefficient $C$ was found to be nearly independent of LED size [96–99].

The recombination coefficients dependency on microLED size determines the dependence of the IQE on the microLED size. The role of defects at the sidewalls of a microLED is schematically illustrated in Figure 2.23.

To estimate the dependence of the SRH recombination coefficient on microLED size for a planar microLED, it is necessary to find the carrier density distribution along the microLED length. The carrier density along the length of the microLEDs inside the QW (with thickness $d$) is governed by the following rate equation:

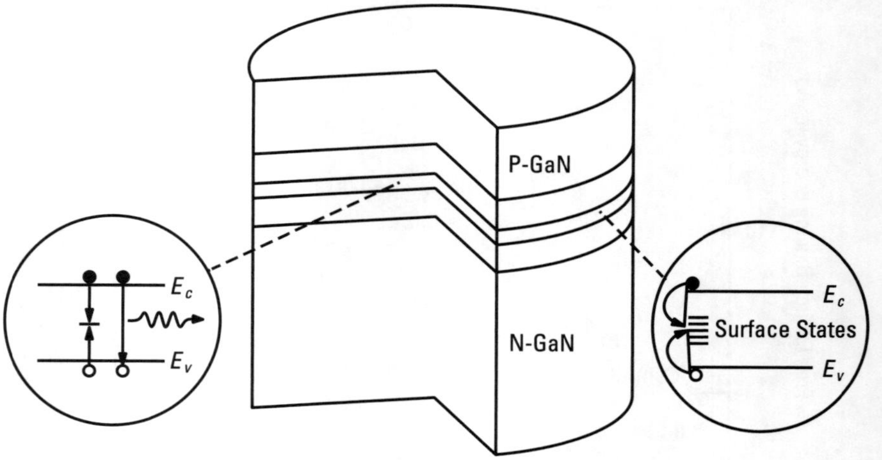


**Figure 2.23** Illustration of carrier recombination process of InGaN/GaN QW microLEDs in the middle of a microLED (left) and at the edge of the microLED (right) where defects result from etching the sidewalls to define a circular mesa in this example.

$$\frac{\partial n}{\partial t} = D\frac{\partial^2 n}{\partial x^2} - \frac{n}{\tau} = 0 \tag{2.72}$$

where $\tau$ is the recombination time constant and $D$ is the carrier diffusion coefficient. Equation (2.70) is subject to the following boundary conditions:

$$n\big|_{x=0} = n_b \tag{2.73}$$

$$q \bullet D \bullet \left.\frac{\partial n}{\partial x}\right|_{x=L/2} = q \bullet s \bullet n\big|_{x=L/2} \tag{2.74}$$

The solution of (2.70) is

$$n = n_b \bullet \exp\left(\frac{x}{\sqrt{D\tau}}\right) \tag{2.75}$$

where $n_b$ is the carrier density at the center point of the microLED length. The current through the microLED is composed of a bulk component and a surface leakage current according. If the total device current is due to SRH recombination, the total device current is given by

$$I_{SRH} = q \bullet d \bullet n_b \left[ A_b L^2 + \frac{4 \bullet s}{L} \exp\left( \frac{-L}{2\sqrt{D\tau}} \right) \right] \tag{2.76}$$

Dividing by the device area $L^2$, the current density is given by

$$J_{SRH} = q \bullet d \bullet n_b \left[ A_b + \frac{4 \bullet s}{L} \exp\left( \frac{-L}{2\sqrt{D\tau}} \right) \right] \tag{2.77}$$

If we define an effective SRH recombination coefficient, $A$, according to $J_{SRH} = q \cdot d \cdot A \cdot n_b$, then $A$ can be expressed by

$$A = A_b + \left( \frac{4 \bullet s}{L} \right) \exp\left( \frac{-L}{2\sqrt{D \bullet \tau}} \right) \tag{2.78}$$

where $A_b$ is the bulk SRC recombination coefficient.

Equation (2.76) reduces to the following classical expression when $L \ll 2\sqrt{D \bullet \tau}$ [100]:

$$A \approx A_b + \frac{4 \bullet s}{L} \tag{2.79}$$

For a nanowire microLED, it was shown that the effective SRH recombination coefficient for nanowires with radius $r$ can be expressed by [101]

$$A = A_b + \frac{\omega^2 \bullet D}{r^2} \tag{2.80}$$

$$\omega \bullet J_1(\omega) - \left( \frac{r \bullet s}{D} \right) \bullet \omega \bullet J_0(\omega) = 0 \tag{2.81}$$

where $D$ is the diffusion coefficient and $s$ is the surface recombination velocity, and $J_0$ and $J_1$ are the Bessel functions. For small $\omega$, (2.78) reduces to

$$A \approx A_b + \frac{2 \bullet s}{r} \tag{2.82}$$

A survey of measured surface recombination velocity for various semiconductor materials is depicted in Figure 2.24.

The surface states causing nonradiative recombination in microLEDs can be categorized into two types based on their formation: intrinsic and extrinsic.

Intrinsic surface states arise due to the termination of the ideal crystal structure at the surface as shown in Figure 2.25. This occurs when growing nanowires out of a sapphire of silicon substrate and on the sidewalls of nanowires. In this case the periodic potential field will be interrupted at the surface and cause additional energy levels in the forbidden band known as surface energy levels, whose corresponding electronic states are called surface states.

Extrinsic surface states result due to dry etch damage and ions adsorbed from the surrounding environment such as oxygen, carbon, and hydrogen, each with its unique energy level. A schematic of this case is shown in Figure 2.25.

A number of technological solutions to mitigate sidewall damage in scaled microLEDs have been proposed [102–112]. According to (2.76), mitigation technologies have two strategies: (1) prevent the electrons and holes from the bulk (near middle of the microLED mesa) to reach the sidewall traps, and (2) reduce the density of sidewall trap density by using a passivation technology such as chemical treatment or a deposition of a dielectric film.

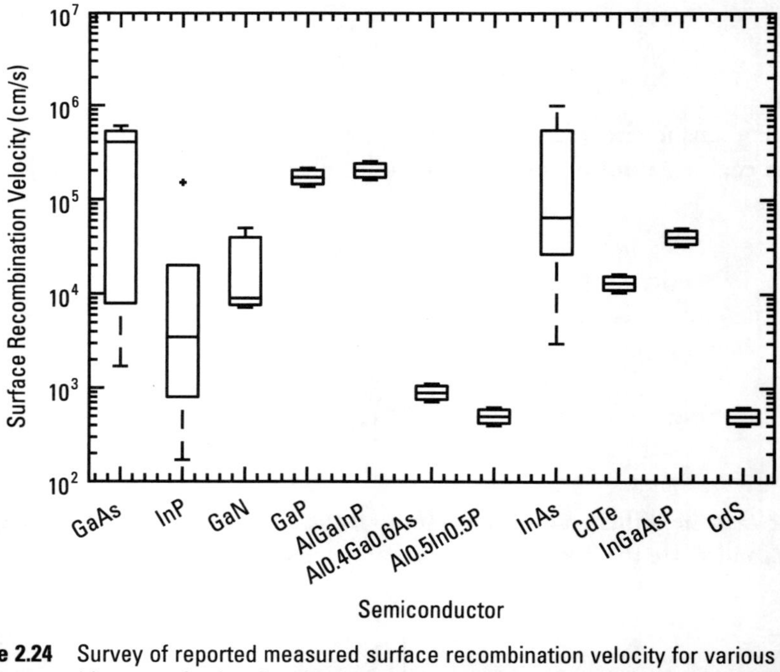


**Figure 2.24** Survey of reported measured surface recombination velocity for various semiconductors without passivation. Passivation could result in reduction of the surface recombination velocity. Large variance is seen for some materials.

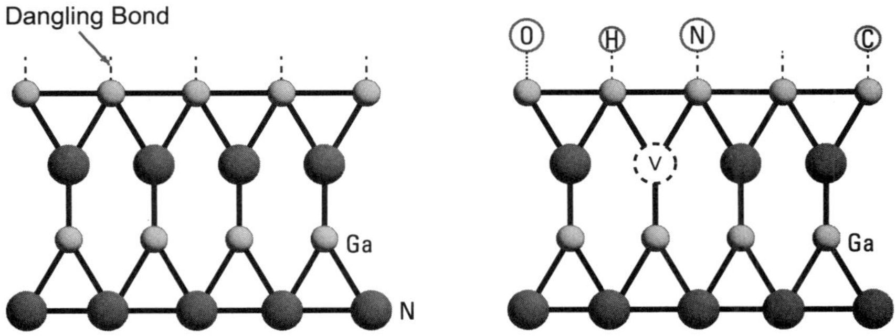


**Figure 2.25** Schematic ball and stick model of the GaN surface after epitaxial growth of, for example, nanowire GaN core. Dangling bonds at the surface are shown. Chemical bonding theory explains that the chemical bonds of GaN crystal break at the surface, and the unbounded electron pairs from dangling bonds, the corresponding electronic states being surface states.

## 2.6 MicroLED Efficiency Enhancement Measures

### 2.6.1 Carrier Localization

Carrier localization refers to the confinement of charge carriers (electrons and holes) within specific regions of the microLED structure, particularly within the QWs where light emission occurs. The physics of carrier localization and its design principles were discussed in Sections 2.3 to 2.5. Optimizing carrier localization in InGaN/GaN microLEDs is crucial for achieving high-efficiency light emission, precise control over emitted wavelengths, and improved overall microLED performance. This involves careful design of quantum well structures, precise material composition, and growth techniques during microLED fabrication. This localization has several effects. When carriers are confined within the quantum wells due to carrier localization, the probability of radiative recombination increases. This means that a higher percentage of electron-hole pairs recombine and emit photons, contributing to more efficient light emission. By confining carriers within the quantum wells and promoting radiative recombination, carrier localization contributes to higher microLED efficiency and brightness. It ensures that a larger portion of the injected carriers contribute to light emission rather than being lost to nonradiative processes. Carrier localization influences the energy band structure within the quantum wells, affecting the emitted wavelength of light. By precisely controlling the composition and thickness of the InGaN layers, carrier localization can be tuned to emit specific wavelengths, enabling the production of microLEDs covering a wide range of colors in the visible spectrum. Carrier localization can help mitigate efficiency droop by maintaining better control over carrier recombination processes, allowing for a more stable and efficient performance at higher operating currents. Effective carrier localization minimizes nonradiative recombination pathways. Nonradiative recombination processes, where carriers recombine without emitting photons, decrease the microLED's efficiency. Carrier localization helps prevent carriers from escaping and undergoing nonradiative processes, thus improving efficiency.

### 2.6.2 Carrier Leakage

In some cases, carriers may leak out of the active region of the microLED without contributing to light emission. This reduces the number of carriers available for radiative recombination. EBL helps prevent electron overflow, a phenomenon where excess electrons reach the p-type layers, causing efficiency losses and thermal issues. The EBL mitigates this by acting as a barrier that restricts the movement of excess electrons [113]. The EBL helps confine electrons within the active region of the microLED. It prevents the leakage of electrons into other parts of the device, ensuring that most electrons remain within the quantum wells where light generation occurs. This confinement enhances the efficiency of the microLED by maximizing the probability of electron-hole recombination in the active region.

### 2.6.3 Doping Concentration in p-GaN Electrode

High active doping density in the p-GaN layer enhances the conductivity of this region, reducing the contact resistance between the microLED's electrical contacts and the semiconductor material. Lower contact resistance results in improved electrical performance and reduced power losses, contributing to higher efficiency. High p-type active doping density creates a region with an excess of holes that can readily inject into the active region (InGaN/GaN multiple quantum wells). This facilitates the recombination process with electrons, promoting efficient light emission [114]. High active p-type doping also improves the mobility of holes in the p-GaN layer, allowing for more efficient transport of carriers towards the active region [114]. This ensures a higher probability of recombination, contributing to better light emission efficiency. P-type doping helps confine the current flow within the microLED structure, preventing lateral spreading of current and carriers. This confinement aids in maintaining a focused and efficient injection of carriers into the active region, optimizing the recombination process. Finally, properly doped p-GaN layers ensure more uniform injection of carriers into the active region across the microLED surface. This uniformity reduces localized nonradiative recombination, thereby enhancing overall efficiency and improving light output uniformity.

### 2.6.4 Temperature Effects

High operating temperatures can exacerbate nonradiative recombination processes, negatively impacting the efficiency of the microLED [115–120]. LEDs usually experience a decrease in their output power as the temperature rises. Temperature changes can also cause a shift in the peak wavelength of emitted light. This shift may not significantly affect the overall power output but could impact the perceived color or spectral characteristics of the emitted light. Proper thermal management is crucial for maintaining microLED performance. Heat generated within the LED should be efficiently dissipated to prevent excessive temperature rise, which can adversely affect the microLED's output power, lifespan, and reliability.

## References

[1] Sakalauskas, E., Ö. Tuna, A. Kraus, et al., "Dielectric Function and Bowing Parameters of InGaN Alloys," *physica status solidi (b)*, Vol. 249, No. 3, 2012, pp. 485–488.

[2] Moses, P., and C. Van de Walle, "Band Bowing and Band Alignment in InGaN Alloys," *Applied Physics Letters*, Vol. 96, No. 2, 2010.

[3] Liu, X., Y. Wu, Y. Malhotra, et al., "Submicron Full-Color LED Pixels for Microdisplays and Micro-LED Main Displays," *Journal of the Society for Information Display*, Vol. 28, No. 5, 2020, pp. 410–417.

[4] Sekiguchi, H., K. Kishino, and A. Kikuchi, " Emission Color Control from Blue to Red with Nanocolumn Diameter of InGaN/GaN Nanocolumn Arrays Grown on Same Substrate," *Applied Physics Letters*, Vol. 96, No. 23, 2010.

[5] Mi, Z., Y. Ra, R. Wang, and R. Rashid, "Multi-Color Nanowire LEDs on a Single Chip," in *2017 IEEE Photonics Conference (IPC)*, 2017.

[6] Kishino, K., A. Yanagihara, K. Ikeda, and K. Yamano, "Monolithic Integration of Four-Colour InGaN-Based Nanocolumn LEDs," *Electronics Letters*, Vol. 51, No. 11, 2015, pp. 852–854.

[7] Takeuchi, T., S. Sota, M. Katsuragawa, et al., "Quantum-Confined Stark Effect Due to Piezoelectric Fields in GaInN Strained Quantum Wells," *Japanese Journal of Applied Physics*, Vol. 36, 1997, pp. L382–L385.

[8] Miller, D. A. B., D. S. Chemla, T. C. Damen, A. C. Gossard, T. H. W. W. Wiegmann, and C. A. Burrus, "Band-Edge Electroabsorption in Quantum Well Structures: The Quantum-Confined Stark Effect," *Physical Review Letters*, Vol. 53, No. 22, 1984, p. 2173–2176.

[9] Der Maur, M., A. Pecchia, G. Penazzi, W. Rodrigues, and A. Di Carlo, "Efficiency Drop in Green InGaN/GaN Light Emitting Diodes: The Role of Random Alloy Fluctuations," *Physical Review Letters*, Vol. 116, No. 2, 2016, p. 027401.

[10] Fiorentini, V., F. Bernardini, F. Della Sala, A. Di Carlo, and P. Lugli, "Effects of Macroscopic Polarization in III-V Nitride Multiple Quantum Wells," *Physical Review B*, Vol. 60, No. 12, 1999, p. 8849.

[11] Bechstedt, F., U. Grossner, and J. F. Fuller, "Dynamics and Polarization of Group-III Nitride Lattices: A First-Principles Study," *Physical Review B*, Vol. 62, 2000, p. 8003.

[12] Piprek, J. (ed.), *Nitride Semiconductor Devices: Principles and Simulation,* Wiley, 2007.

[13] Ambacher, O., J. Majewski, C. Miskys, et al., "Pyroelectric Properties of Al(In) GaN/GaN Hetero-and Quantum Well Structures," *Journal of Physics: Condensed Matter*, Vol. 14, No. 13, 2002, p. 3399.

[14] Bernardini, F., V. Fiorentini, and D. Vanderbilt, "Spontaneous Polarization and Piezoelectric Constants of III-V Nitrides," *Physical Review B*, Vol. 56, No. 16, 1997, pp. 10024–10027.

[15] Monavarian, M., A. Rashidi, and D. Feezell, "A Decade of Nonpolar and Semipolar III-Nitrides: A Review of Successes and Challenges," *physica status solidi (a)*, Vol. 216, No. 1, 2019, p. 1800628.

[16] Feezell, D., A. Rashidi, M. Monavarian, et al., "III-Nitride High-Speed Optoelectronics," 2019 *Device Research Conference (DRC)*, 2019, pp. 77–78.

[17] Bi, Z., Z. Chen, F. Danesh, and L. Samuelson, "From NanoLEDs to the Realization of RGB-Emitting MicroLEDs," in *Semiconductors and Semimetals, Volume 106: MicroLEDS* (H. Jiang and J. Lin, eds.), Elsevier, 2021, pp. 223–251.

[18] Nami, M., I. Stricklin, K. DaVico, et al., "Carrier Dynamics and Electro-Optical Characterization of High-Performance GaN/InGaN Core-Shell Nanowire Light-Emitting Diodes," *Scientific Reports*, Vol. 8, No. 1, 2018, p. 501.

[19] Nami, M., A. Rashidi, M. Monavarian, et al., "Electrically Injected GHz-Class GaN/InGaN Core–Shell Nanowire-Based $\mu$LEDs: Carrier Dynamics and Nanoscale Homogeneity," *ACS Photonics*, Vol. 6, No. 7, 2019, pp. 1618–1625.

[20] Tchoulfian, P., U. Steegmueller, B. Amstatt, M. Broell, and P. Gilet, "GaN-on-Silicon Nanowire Technology for MicroLED Devices," *Proc. SPIE, Light-Emitting Devices, Materials, and Applications XXVII,* Vol. 12441, 2023, pp. 49–52.

[21] Rishinaramangalam, A., M. Nami, M. Fairchild, et al., "Semipolar InGaN/GaN Nanostructure Light-Emitting Diodes on c-Plane Sapphire," *Applied Physics Express*, Vol. 9, No. 3, 2016, p. 032101.

[22] Chuang, S., and D. Ahn, "Optical Transitions in a Parabolic Quantum Well with an Applied Electric Field—Analytical Solutions," *Journal of Applied Physics*, Vol. 65, No. 7, 1989, pp. 2822–2826.

[23] Zhang, Z., W. Liu, Z. Ju, et al., "InGaN/GaN Multiple Quantum-Well Light-Emitting Diodes with a Grading InN Composition Suppressing the Auger Recombination," *Applied Physics Letters*, Vol. 105, No. 3, 2014.

[24] Karan, H., A. Biswas, and M. Saha, "Improved Performance of InGaN/GaN MQW LEDs with Trapezoidal Wells and Gradually Thinned Barrier Layers Towards Anode," *Optics Communications*, Vol. 400, 2017, pp. 89–95.

[25] Lee, J., J. Leburton, and C. Bayram, "Design Tradeoffs Between Traditional Hexagonal and Emerging Cubic InXGa(1–X)N/GaN-Based Green Light-Emitting Diodes," *JOSA B*, Vol. 40, No. 5, 2023, pp. 1017–1023.

[26] Lee, L., "Cubic Zincblende Gallium Nitride for Green-Wavelength Light-Emitting Diodes," *Materials Science and Technology*, Vol. 33, No. 14, 2017, pp. 1570–1583.

[27] Binks, D., P. Dawson, R. Oliver, and D. Wallis, "Cubic GaN and InGan/GaN Quantum Wells," *Applied Physics Reviews*, Vol. 9, No. 4, 2022.

[28] Gundimeda, A., M. Frentrup, S. Fairclough, M. Kappers, D. Wallis, and R. Oliver, "Investigation of Wurtzite Formation in MOVPE-Grown Zincblende GaN Epilayers on AlxGa1- xN Nucleation Layers," *Journal of Applied Physics*, Vol. 131, No. 11, 2022, pp. 115703-1.

[29] Lee, J., Y. Chiu, M. Johar, and C. Bayram, "Structural and Optical Properties of Cubic GaN on U-Grooved Si (100)," *Applied Physics Letters*, Vol. 121, No. 3, 2022.

[30] F. Meier, M. Littmann, J. Bürger, et al., "Selective Area Growth of Cubic Gallium Nitride in Nanoscopic Silicon Dioxide Masks," *physica status solidi (b)*, 2022, p. 2200508.

[31] Feng, S., P. Liao, B. Leung, J. Han, F. Yang, and H. Wang, "Efficient Carrier Relaxation and Fast Carrier Recombination of N-Polar InGaN/GaN Light Emitting Diodes," *Journal of Applied Physics*, Vol. 118, No. 4, 2015.

[32] Muthuraj, V., C. Reilly, T. Mates, S. Keller, S. Nakamura, and S. DenBaars, "Inverted N-Polar Blue and Blue-Green Light Emitting Diodes with High Power Grown by Metalorganic Chemical Vapor Deposition," *Applied Physics Letters*, Vol. 120, No. 10, 2022.

[33] Akyol, F., D. Nath, E. Gür, P. Park, and S. Rajan, "N-Polar III–Nitride Green (540 nm) Light Emitting Diode," *Japanese Journal of Applied Physics*, Vol. 50, No. 5R, 2011, p. 052101.

[34] Zhuang, Z., D. Iida, and K. Ohkawa, "Enhanced Performance of N-Polar AlGaN-Based Deep-Ultraviolet Light-Emitting Diodes," *Optics Express*, Vol. 28, No. 21, 2020, pp. 30423–30431.

[35] Deng, G., Y. Zhang, Y. Yu, et al.,"Simulation and Fabrication of N-Polar GaN-Based Blue-Green Light-Emitting Diodes with p-Type AlGaN Electron Blocking Layer," *Journal of Materials Science: Materials in Electronics*, Vol. 29, 2018, pp. 9321–9325.

[36] Keller, S., H. Li, M. Laurent, et al., "Recent Progress in Metal-Organic Chemical Vapor Deposition of N-Polar Group-III Nitrides," *Semiconductor Science and Technology*, Vol. 29, No. 11, 2014, p. 113001.

[37] Muthuraj, V., C. Reilly, T. Mates, S. Keller, S. Nakamura, and S. DenBaars, "Inverted N-Polar Blue and Blue-Green Light Emitting Diodes with High Power Grown by Metalorganic Chemical Vapor Deposition," *Applied Physics Letters*, Vol. 120, No. 10, 2022, p. 101104.

[38] Ptak, A., T. Myers, L. Romano, C. G. Van de Walle, and J. Northrup, "Magnesium Incorporation in GaN Grown by Molecular-Beam Epitaxy," *Applied Physics Letters*, Vol. 78, No. 3, 2001, pp. 285–287.

[39] Sumiya, M., K. Yoshimura, K. Ohtsuka, and S. Fuke, "Dependence of Impurity Incorporation on the Polar Direction of GaN Film Growth," *Applied Physics Letters*, Vol. 76, No. 15, 2000, pp. 2098–2100.

[40] Pristovsek, M., I. Furuhashi, and P. Pampili, "Growth of N-Polar GaN in Metal–Organic Vapour Phase Epitaxy on Sapphire," *Crystals*, Vol. 13, No. 7, 2023, p. 1072.

[41] A. Ptak, L. Holbert, L. Ting, C. Swartz, M. Moldovan, N. Giles, T. Myers, P. Van Lierde, C. Tian, R. Hockett and S. Mitha, "Controlled Oxygen Doping of GaN Using Plasma Assisted Molecular-Beam Epitaxy," *Applied Physics Letters*, Vol. 79, No. 17, 2001, pp. 2740–2742.

[42] Fiorentini, V., F. Bernardini, F. D. Sala, A. D. Carlo, and P. Lugli, "Effects of Macroscopic Polarization in III-V Nitride Multiple Quantum Wells," *Physical Review B*, Vol. 60, No. 12, 1999, p. 8849.

[43] Young, N., R. Farrell, S. Oh, et al., " Polarization Field Screening in Thick (0001) InGaN/GaN Single Quantum Well Light-Emitting Diodes," *Applied Physics Letters*, Vol. 108, No. 6, 2016.

[44] Franssen, G., T. Suski, P. Perlin, et al., "Fully-Screened Polarization-Induced Electric Fields in Blue\Violet InGaN\GaN Light-Emitting Devices Grown on Bulk GaN," *Applied Physics Letters*, Vol. 87, No. 4, 2005, p. 041109.

[45] Chow, Y. C., C. Lynsky, F. Wu, et al., "Reduction of Efficiency Droop in c-Plane InGaN/GaN Light-Emitting Diodes Using a Thick Single Quantum Well with Doped Barriers," *Applied Physics Letters*, Vol. 119, No. 22, 2021, p. 221102.

[46] Chow, Y. C., C. Lynsky, S. Nakamura, S. P. DenBaars, C. Weisbuch, and J. S. Speck, "Impact of Doped Barriers on the Recombination Coefficients of c-Plane InGaN/GaN Single Quantum Well Light-Emitting Diodes," *Applied Physics Letters*, Vol. 121, No. 18, 2022, p. 181102.

[47] Y. Chow, C. Lynsky, S. Nakamura, S. DenBaars, C. Weisbuch and J. Speck, "Low-Efficiency-Droop c-plane InGaN/GaN Light-Emitting Diodes through the use of Thick Single Quantum Wells and Doped Barriers," *Journal of Applied Physics*, Vol. 133, No. 14, 2023, p. 143101.

[48] Park, B., J. Lee, C. Koch, M. Wölz, L. Geelhaar, and S. Oh, "High-Resolution Mapping of Strain Partitioning and Relaxation in InGaN/GaN Nanowire Heterostructures," *Advanced Science*, Vol. 9, No. 22, 2022, p. 2200323.

[49] Pandey, A., Y. Xiao, M. Reddeppa, et al., "A Red-Emitting Micrometer Scale LED with External Quantum Efficiency > 8%," *Applied Physics Letters*, Vol. 122, No. 15, 2023.

[50] Pandey, A., J. Min, M. Reddeppa, et al., "An Ultrahigh Efficiency Excitonic Micro-LED," *Nano Letters*, Vol. 23, No. 5, 2023, pp. 1680–1687.

[51] Guo, W., M. Zhang, A. Banerjee, and P. Bhattacharya, "Catalyst-Free InGaN/GaN Nanowire Light Emitting Diodes Grown on (001) Silicon by Molecular Beam Epitaxy," *Nano Letters*, Vol. 10, No. 9, 2010, pp. 3355–3359.

[52] Pandey, A., J. Min, Y. Malhotra, M. Reddeppa, Y. Xiao, Y. Wu, and Z. Mi, "Strain-Engineered N-Polar InGaN Nanowires: Towards High-Efficiency Red LEDs on the Micrometer Scale," *Photonics Research*, Vol. 10, No. 12, 2022, pp. 2809–2815.

[53] Glas, F., "Critical Dimensions for the Plastic Relaxation of Strained Axial Heterostructures in Free-Standing Nanowires," *Physical Review B*, Vol. 74, No. 12, 2006, p. 121302.

[54] Guo, L., X. Wang, H. Xiao, and B. Wang, "The Influence of Internal Electric Fields on the Transition Energy of InGaN/GaN Quantum Well," *Journal of Crystal Growth*, Vol. 298, 2007, pp. 522–526.

[55] Wei, S., Y. Jia, and C. Xia, "Excitonic Optical Absorption in Wurtzite InGaN/GaN Quantum Wells," *Superlattices and Microstructures*, Vol. 51, No. 1, 2012, pp. 9–15.

[56] Pieniak, K., M. Chlipala, H. Turski, et al., "Quantum-Confined Stark Effect and Mechanisms of Its Screening in InGaN/GaN Light-Emitting Diodes with a Tunnel Junction," *Optics Express*, Vol. 29, No. 2, 2021, pp. 1824–1837.

[57] Rodina, A., M. Dietrich, A. Göldner, et al., "Free Excitons in Wurtzite GaN," *Physical Review B*, Vol. 64, No. 11, 2001, p. 115204.

[58] Monemar, B., P. Paskov, J. Bergman, et al., "Recombination of Free and Bound Excitons in GaN," *physica status solidi (b)*, Vol. 245, No. 9, 2008, pp. 1723–1740.

[59] David, A., and C. Weisbuch, "Excitons in a Disordered Medium: A Numerical Study in InGaN Quantum Wells," *Physical Review Research*, Vol. 4, No. 4, 2022, p. 043004.

[60] Ahn, D., and S. Chuang, "Variational Calculations of Subbands in a Quantum Well with Uniform Electric Field: Gram–Schmidt Orthogonalization Approach," *Applied Physics Letters*, Vol. 49, No. 21, 1986, pp. 1450–1452.

[61] Singh, J., "Analytical Closed Form Expressions for the Effective Band Edges in Shallow Quantum Wells," *Applied Physics Letters*, Vol. 64, No. 20, 1994, pp. 2694–2696.

[62] Jonsson, B., and S. Eng, "Solving the Schrodinger Equation in Arbitrary Quantum-Well Potential Profiles Using the Transfer Matrix Method," *IEEE Journal of Quantum Electronics*, Vol. 26, No. 11, 1990, pp. 2025–2035.

[63] Ahn, D., and S. Chuang, "Exact Calculations of Quasibound States of an Isolated Quantum Well with Uniform Electric Field: Quantum-Well Stark Resonance," *Physical Review B*, Vol. 34, No. 12, 1986, p. 9034.

[64] Bastard, G., E. Mendez, L. Chang, and L. Esaki, "Variational Calculations on a Quantum Well in an Electric Field," *Physical Review B*, Vol. 28, No. 6, 1983, p. 3241.

[65] Bloss, W., "Electric Field Dependence of Quantum-Well Eigenstates," *Journal of Applied Physics*, Vol. 65, No. 12, 1989, pp. 4789–4794.

[66] Hutchings, D., "Transfer Matrix Approach to the Analysis of an Arbitrary Quantum Well Structure in an Electric Field," *Applied Physics Letters*, Vol. 11, No. 55, 1989, p. 1082.

[67] Z. Zhang, W. Liu, Z. Ju, et al., "Self-Screening of the Quantum Confined Stark Effect by the Polarization Induced Bulk Charges in the Quantum Barriers," *Applied Physics Letters*, Vol. 104, No. 24, 2014.

[68] Leroux, M., N. Grandjean, J. Massies, B. Gil, P. Lefebvre, and P. Bigenwald, "Barrier-Width Dependence of Group-III Nitrides Quantum-Well Transition Energies," *Physical Review B*, Vol. 60, No. 3, 1999, p. 1496.

[69] Grandjean, N., B. Damilano, S. Dalmasso, M. Leroux, M. Laügt, and J. Massies, "Built-in Electric-Field Effects in Wurtzite AlGaN/GaN Quantum Wells," *Journal of Applied Physics*, Vol. 86, No. 7, 1999, pp. 3714–3720.

[70] Y. Zhao, W. Han, J. Song, et al., "Spontaneous Emission Factor for Semiconductor Superluminescent Diodes," *Journal of Applied Physics,* Vol. 85, No. 8, 1999, pp. 3945–3948.

[71] Fan, W., M. Li, T. Chong, and J. Xia, "Valence Hole Subbands and Optical Gain Spectra of GaN/Ga1-xAlxN Strained Quantum Wells," *Journal of Applied Physics,* Vol. 80, No. 6, 1996, pp. 3471–3478.

[72] David, A., N. Young, C. Hurni, and M. Craven, "All-Optical Measurements of Carrier Dynamics in Bulk-GaN LEDs: Beyond the ABC Approximation," *Applied Physics Letters,* Vol. 110, No. 25, 2017.

[73] Jones, C., C. Teng, Q. Yan, P. Ku, and E. Kioupakis, "Impact of Carrier Localization on Recombination in InGaN Quantum Wells and the Efficiency of Nitride Light-Emitting Diodes: Insights from Theory and Numerical Simulations," *Applied Physics Letters,* Vol. 111, No. 11, 2017.

[74] David, A., N. Young, C. Lund, and M. Craven, "The Physics of Recombinations in III-Nitride Emitters," *ECS Journal of Solid-State Science and Technology,* Vol. 9, No. 1, 2019, p. 016021.

[75] Feezell, D., J. Speck, S. DenBaars, and S. Nakamura, "Semipolar InGaN/GaN Light-Emitting Diodes for High-Efficiency Solid-State Lighting," *Journal of Display Technology,* Vol. 9, No. 4, 2013, pp. 190–198.

[76] David, A., and M. Grundmann, "Influence of Polarization Fields on Carrier Lifetime and Recombination Rates in InGaN-Based Light-Emitting Diodes," *Applied Physics Letters,* Vol. 97, No. 3, 2010.

[77] Kioupakis, E., Q. Yan, and C. Van de Walle, "Interplay of Polarization Fields and Auger Recombination in the Efficiency Droop of Nitride Light-Emitting Diodes," *Applied Physics Letters,* Vol. 101, No. 23, 2012.

[78] Chuu, D., and Y. Shih, "Exciton Binding Energy in a GaAs/AlxGa1xAs Quantum Well with Uniform Electric Field," *Physical Review B,* Vol. 44, No. 15, 1991, p. 8054.

[79] Kojima, K., M. Funato, Y. Kawakami, and S. Noda, "Valence Band Effective Mass of Non-c-Plane Nitride Heterostructures," *Journal of Applied Physics,* Vol. 107, No. 12, 2010.

[80] Chuang, S., and C. Chang, "k·p Method for Strained Wurtzite Semiconductors," *Physical Review B,* Vol. 54, No. 4, 1996, p. 2491.

[81] Leung, M., A. Djurii, and E. Li, "Refractive Index of InGaN/GaN Quantum Well," *Journal of Applied Physics,* Vol. 84, No. 11, 1998, pp. 6312–6317.

[82] Nisoli, M., *Semiconductor Photonics: Principles and Applications,* Chapter 5, Società Editrice Esculapio, 2016.

[83] Bassani, F., and G. Pastori-Parravicini, *Electronic States and Optical Transitions in Solids,* Oxford: Pergamon Press, 1975.

[84] Mathieu, H., P. Lefebvre, and P. Christol, "Simple Analytical Method for Calculating Exciton Binding Energies in Semiconductor Quantum Wells," *Physical Review B,* Vol. 46, No. 7, 1992, p. 4092.

[85] Ishikawa, T., S. Nishimura, and K. Tada, "Quantum-Confined Stark Effect in a Parabolic-Potential Quantum Well," *Japanese Journal of Applied Physics*, Vol. 29, No. 8R, 1990, p. 1466.

[86] David, A., N. Young, C. Lund, and M. Craven, "Compensation Between Radiative and Auger Recombinations in III-Nitrides: the Scaling Law of Separated-Wavefunction Recombinations," *Applied Physics Letters*, Vol. 115, No. 19, 2019.

[87] David, A., C. A. Hurni, N. G. Young, and M. D. Craven, "Field-Assisted Shockley-Read-Hall Recombinations in III-Nitride Quantum Wells," *Applied Physics Letters*, Vol. 111, No. 23, 2017, p. 233501.

[88] David, A., N. Young, C. Hurni, and M. Craven, "Quantum Efficiency of III-Nitride Emitters: Evidence for Defect-Assisted Nonradiative Recombination and its Effect on the Green Gap," *Physical Review Applied*, Vol. 11, No. 3, 2019, p. 031001.

[89] Kioupakis, E., D. Steiauf, P. Rinke, K. Delaney, and C. Van de Walle, "First-Principles Calculations of Indirect Auger Recombination in Nitride Semiconductors," *Physical Review B*, Vol. 92, No. 3, 2015, p. 035207.

[90] Kioupakis, E., Q. Yan, D. Steiauf, and C. Van de Walle, "Temperature and Carrier-Density Dependence of Auger and Radiative Recombination in Nitride Optoelectronic Devices," *New Journal of Physics*, Vol. 15, No. 12, 2013, p. 125006.

[91] Karpov, S., "Effect of Carrier Localization on Recombination Processes and Efficiency of InGaN-Based LEDs Operating in the "Green Gap," *Applied Sciences*, Vol. 8, No. 5, 2018, p. 818.

[92] Weisbuch, C., S. Nakamura, Y. Wu, and J. Speck, "Disorder Effects in Nitride Semiconductors: Impact on Fundamental and Device Properties," *Nanophotonics*, Vol. 10, No. 1, 2020, pp. 3–21.

[93] Shockley, W., and W. Read Jr., "Statistics of the Recombinations of Holes and Electrons," *Physical Review*, Vol. 87, No. 5, 1952, p. 835.

[94] Alkauskas, A., C. Dreyer, J. Lyons, and C. Van de Walle, "Role of Excited States in Shockley-Read-Hall Recombination in Wide-Band-Gap Semiconductors," *Physical Review B*, Vol. 93, No. 20, 2016, p. 201304.

[95] Dreyer, C., A. Alkauskas, J. Lyons, J. Speck, and C. Van de Walle, "Gallium Vacancy Complexes as a Cause of Shockley-Read-Hall Recombination in III-Nitride Light Emitters," *Applied Physics Letters*, Vol. 108, No. 14, 2016.

[96] Olivier, F., A. Daami, C. Licitra, and F. Templier, "Shockley-Read-Hall and Auger Non-Radiative Recombination in GaN Based LEDs: A Size Effect Study," *Applied Physics Letters*, Vol. 111, No. 2, 2017.

[97] Daami, A., F. Olivier, L. Dupré, F. Henry, and F. Templier, "Electro-Optical Size-Dependence Investigation in GaN Micro-LED Devices," in 2018 *SID Symposium Digest of Technical Papers*, 2018.

[98] Li, Y., F. Lin, K. Chi, S. Weng, G. Lee, H. Kuo, and C. Lin, "Analysis of Size-Dependent Quantum Efficiency in AlGaInP Micro–Light-Emitting Diodes with Consideration for Current Leakage," *IEEE Photonics Journal*, Vol. 14, No. 1, 2021, pp. 1–7.

[99] Smith, J., R. Ley, M. Wong, et al., "Comparison of Size-Dependent Characteristics of Blue and Green InGaN MicroLEDs down to 1 $\mu$m in Diameter," *Applied Physics Letters*, Vol. 116, No. 7, 2020.

[100] Bulashevich, K. A., S. S. Konoplev, S. Y. Karpov, et al., "Effect of Die Shape and Size on Performance of III-Nitride Micro-LEDs: A Modeling Study," *Photonics*, Vol. 5, No. 4, 2018, p. 41.

[101] Joyce, H. J., J. Wong-Leung, C. D. Yong, et al., "Ultralow Surface Recombination Velocity in InP Nanowires Probed by Terahertz Spectroscopy," *Nano Letters*, 2012, p. 5325.

[102] Ley, R., J. Smith, M. Wong, et al., "Revealing the Importance of Light Extraction Efficiency in InGaN/GaN MicroLEDs via Chemical Treatment and Dielectric Passivation," *Applied Physics Letters*, Vol. 116, No. 25, 2020.

[103] Wong, M., J. Kearns, C. Lee, et al., "Improved Performance of AlGaInP Red Micro-Light-Emitting Diodes with Sidewall Treatments," *Optics Express*, Vol. 28, No. 4, 2020, pp. 5787–5793.

[104] P. Li, H. Li, H. Zhang, C. Lynsky, et al., "Size-Independent Peak External Quantum Efficiency (>2%) of InGaN Red Micro-Light-Emitting Diodes with an Emission Wavelength over 600 nm," *Applied Physics Letters*, Vol. 119, No. 8, 2021.

[105] Wong, M., J. Speck, S. Nakamura, and S. DenBaars, "High Efficiency of III-Nitride and AlGaInP Micro-Light-Emitting Diodes Using Atomic Layer Deposition," in *SPIE Light-Emitting Devices, Materials, and Applications XXV*, Vol. 11706, 2021.

[106] Cho, H., D. Kim, S. Lee, C. Yoo, and Y. Sim, "Efficiency Enhancement of Submicron-Size Light-Emitting Diodes by Triple Dielectric Layers," *Journal of the Society for Information Display*, Vol. 31, No. 5, 2023, p. 289.

[107] Baek, W., D. Geum, J. Park, and S. Kim, "Enhanced External Quantum Efficiency in the Low-Current Region Using Three Terminal GaN-Based Blue Micro-Light-Emitting Diodes," in *SID Symposium Digest of Technical Papers*, 2022.

[108] Bour, D., K. McGroddy, D. Haeger, J. Perkins, A. Chakraborty, and J. Drolet, LED Structures for Reduced Non-Radiative Sidewall Recombination, US Patent 9,484,492, 2016.

[109] Perkins, J., Diffusion Revealed Blocking Junction, US Patent 10,396,241, 2019.

[110] Hahn, B., T. Lauermann, and M. Broell, High-Efficiency Red Micro-LED with Localized Current Aperture, US Patent 11,362,237, 2022.

[111] Ahmed, K., Passivated Micro LED Structures Suitable for Energy Efficient Displays, US Patent 10,153,401, 2018.

[112] Margalith, T., M. Wong, L. Chan, and S. DenBaars, Micro-LEDs with Ultra-Low Leakage Current, US Patent 17/281,700, 2022.

[113] Lee, J., X. Li, X. Ni, et al., "On Carrier Spillover in c-and m-Plane InGaN Light Emitting Diodes," *Applied Physics Letters*, Vol. 95, No. 20, 2009.

[114] Nakamura, S., "Nobel Lecture: Background Story of the Invention of Efficient Blue InGaN Light Emitting Diodes," *Reviews of Modern Physics*, Vol. 87, No. 4, 2015, p. 1139.

[115] Schubert, E., N. Hunt, R. Malik, M. Micovic, and D. Miller, "Temperature and Modulation Characteristics of Resonant-Cavity Light-Emitting Diodes," *Journal of Lightwave Technology*, Vol. 14, No. 7, 1996, pp. 1721–1729.

[116] Zhao, L., D. Yan, Z. Zhang, et al., "Temperature-Dependent Efficiency Droop in GaN-Based Blue LEDs," *IEEE Electron Device Letters*, Vol. 39, No. 4, 2018, pp. 528–531.

[117] Wang, C., J. Chen, C. Chiu, et al., "Temperature-Dependent Electroluminescence Efficiency in Blue InGaN–GaN Light-Emitting Diodes with Different Well Widths," *IEEE Photonics Technology Letters*, Vol. 22, No. 4, 2010 pp. 236–238.

[118] Huh, C., W. Schaff, L. Eastman, and S. Park, "Temperature Dependence of Performance of InGaN/GaN MQW LEDs with Different Indium Compositions," *IEEE Electron Device Letters*, Vol. 25, No. 2, 2004, pp. 61–63.

[119] Titkov, I., S. Karpov, A. Yadav, et al., "Temperature-Dependent Internal Quantum Efficiency of Blue High-Brightness Light-Emitting Diodes," *IEEE Journal of Quantum Electronics*, Vol. 50, No. 11, 2014, pp. 911–920.

[120] Xi, Y., and E. Schubert, "Junction–Temperature Measurement in GaN Ultraviolet Light-Emitting Diodes using Diode Forward Voltage Method," *Applied Physics Letters*, Vol. 85, No. 12, 2004, pp. 2163–2165.

# 3

# MicroLED Forward Current-Voltage (I-V) Characteristics

## 3.1 Introduction

As microLED applications become more ubiquitous, physics-based models of their electrical behavior are required in order to bridge the gap between the fabrication process and circuit/system design. Physics-based analytical models for optoelectronic devices play two distinct roles. First, the kernel of the model serves as a compact mathematical representation of our understanding of the device operation. This compact form helps device engineers to interpret experiments and detailed numerical simulations. Second, the model can be extended to treat parasitic elements and with consideration of the practicalities that ensure that it runs robustly in a circuit simulator. A closed-form current-voltage (I-V) solution for microLEDs is not trivial but provides several advantages:

- Phenomenological parameters emerge that provide intuition on device operation;
- Simple parameter extraction methods;
- Better computational efficiency that is good for circuit simulations;
- Better computational efficiency for design for manufacturing (DFM) risk assessment based on measurements;
- Modular form that allows for including more physics as device structure is changed;

- Guides experimentation with different device designs;
- Allows for defining performance figure of merits;
- Can often explain the physics of phenomena and especially various paradoxical situations;
- Can help determine asymptotic trends that helps generate insights or result in new creative designs;
- Helps generate memorable heuristics;
- Can help in creating abstract understanding of problems and create breakthrough inventions;
- Easy to use to convince R&D management with new investments by simply communicating new benefits of new technologies;
- Helps detect and/or understand anomalies in measurements.

This chapter presents a model for the I-V characteristics of a quantum well microLED through the regional approximation method [1]. This scheme is based on the simple observation that where there are several terms in an equation competing with each other with each being a function of position (inside a device), it is generally possible to divide up the volume of the device into separate regions in each of which at least one or two terms dominate. Within each such region, the basic approximation is made of neglecting all terms within the competing group except the one or two terms, which dominate in that region. As a result, a simple approximate analytical expression for the current-voltage characteristics of a microLED is derived. The expression takes into account recombination in the InGaN/GaN quantum well. Model parameters include quantum well width or thickness, internal quantum efficiency, radiative recombination coefficient, and indium mole fraction in the quantum well. The model includes the effect of carrier localization. The derived expression is shown to fit experimental data for red, green, and blue microLED data. Five parameters are extracted by fitting experimental I-V data: liminal forward voltage, liminal forward current, two ideality factors, and series resistance. The model can also be used to probe measured variability of the liminal forward voltage with respect to variability is quantum well width and indium mole fraction in the quantum well across the wafer; a tool for quantifying the manufacturing risk based on measured variability in quantum well width and indium mole fraction.

## 3.2 Related Models

The models available in literature for GaN LEDs have limited focus on correlating model parameters to measurable physical device and material properties of the microLEDs. For example, the modified Shockley model [2–7] can fit the data and helps in circuit simulations but does not give insight into the dependence of the I-V parameters on the quantum well width and indium mole fraction, a tool that can help design for manufacturing efforts. David proposed a model that takes into account recombination in the quantum well, but no simple form was given for the I-V characteristics [8]. Han added a space-charge limited current component to model the S-shaped behavior of the I-V curve at high voltages but the equation used for the space-charge current is not accurate for quantum well devices with an ultranarrow well [2].

Our model is derived based on Poisson's equation, current continuity equation, and rate equation, with simplifying assumptions. The presented model does not have restrictive approximations on the device architecture (i.e., planar versus nanowire) or the growth plane (e.g., c-plane versus m-plane). We focus on the premise that a good compact model should be based on a physical model that accurately fits I-V data. Unlike existing LED models in the literature, the presented model is descriptive, predictive, and prescriptive. The model benefits from the groundwork down by David et al. [8] and includes a novel expression for the space-charge limited current due to recombination in the quantum well at current density higher than the liminal forward current.

We will derive the current through careful selection of approximations in order to achieve a pseudoanalytical solution while not compromising the accuracy of said solution.

The cross section of the device is shown in Figure 3.1. The device contains "n+ GaN" and "p+ GaN" with an InGaN QW in between. The resulting band diagram is also shown, which also includes key variables for the following derivation. For simplicity, ideal ohmic contacts are assumed to be at the n+ GaN and the p+ GaN.

In order to obtain an expression for the current, we must consider the governing physics of the device that determines its behavior. Once all of these physics are taken into account, we can write equations that describe the physics and solve them to get the current. We must consider unimportant physics that we can ignore to simplify the problem.

Gauss' law gives

$$qN_D^+x_n - qN_A^-x_p - qn_q + qp_q = 0 \tag{3.1}$$

where $N_D^+$ is the ionized density of donors in the n-GaN layer, $x_n$ is the depletion layer width in the n-GaN layer, $N_A^-$ is the ionized density of acceptors in the p-GaN layer, $x_p$ is the depletion layer width in the p-GaN layer, $n_q$ ($p_q$) is the two-dimensional electron (hole) density in the quantum well, and $q$ is the electronic charge.

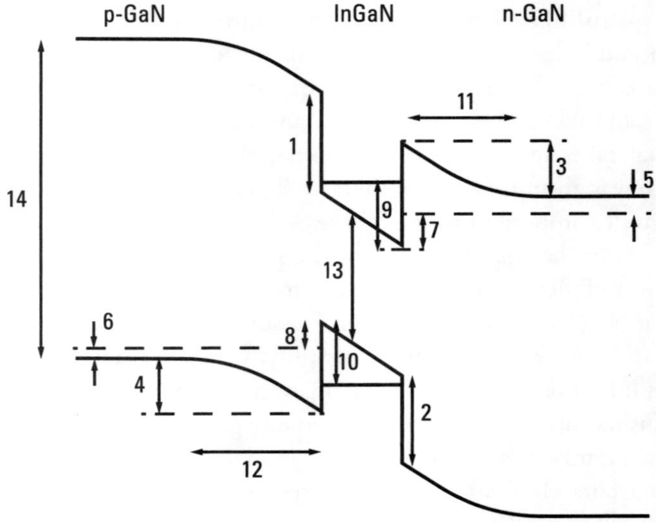


**Figure 3.1** Schematic illustrating general structure of a microLED. The parameters are: (1) $\Delta E_c$, (2) $\Delta E_v$, (3) $qN_D^+ x_n^2 / 2\epsilon$, (4) $qN_A^- x_p^2 / 2\epsilon$, (5) $\xi_n = E_{cN} - E_{fN}$, (6) $\xi_p = E_{fP} - E_{vP}$, (7) $\Delta E_{fn}$, (8) $\Delta E_{fp}$, (9) $E_{1,n}$, (10) $E_{1,p}$, (11) $x_n$, (12) $x_p$, (13) $E_{gq}$, (14) $E_g$. The polarization fields are not taken into account, which is good for nonpolar growth planes like m-plane. A correction term is provided at the end of the chapter for the polarization field.

In our device, the potential drop is distributed across both the n and p depletion regions, as well as across the quantum well. However, we will assume the width of the quantum well to be less than 6 nm, and thus the potential across the quantum well to be negligible, especially at low current density. This assumption is valid when the total depletion width is much greater than the quantum well width. At high current density we will later derive a simple expression for the voltage drop across the quantum well.

From the energy band diagram shown in Figure 3.1 and the Poisson's equation we can write the following three equations:

$$E_g = \xi_p + qN_A^- x_p^2 / 2\epsilon + \Delta E_{fp} + E_{gq} + \Delta E_c$$
$$E_g = \xi_n + qN_D^+ x_n^2 / 2\epsilon + \Delta E_{fn} + E_{gq} + \Delta E_v$$
$$qV_j = \Delta E_{fn} + E_{gq} + \Delta E_{fp}$$

where $V_j$ is the total junction voltage, $\xi_n = E_{cN} - E_{fN}$, and $\xi_p = E_{fP} - E_{vP}$ as shown in Figure 3.1.

Combining these equations, we get

$$qV_j = \left(E_g - \xi_n - \xi_p\right) - qN_D^+ x_n^2 / 2\epsilon - qN_A^- x_p^2 / 2\epsilon$$

where $\epsilon$ is the permittivity of the n-GaN or p-GaN layers.

The built-in voltage defined by

$$V_{bi} = E_g - \xi_n - \xi_p$$

Thus, the voltage equation is given by

$$\frac{qN_D^+ x_n^2}{2\epsilon} + \frac{qN_A^- x_p^2}{2\epsilon} = -\left(V_j - V_{bi}\right) \tag{3.2}$$

As with any LED, recombination within the quantum well is the dominant contributor to the current. The diffusion current in an LED is usually negligible. We write the following equations for the current at three points in the device. At the n-GaN/InGaN QW interface we can write the current using thermionic equation, modified by carriers coming out of the quantum well back into the n-GaN:

$$J = qn_n v_{th,n} \exp\left(-\frac{qN_D^+ x_n^2}{2\epsilon kT}\right)\left[1 - \exp\left(\frac{-\Delta E_{fn}}{kT}\right)\right] \tag{3.3}$$

where the thermal velocity is given by $(1/2)m_n v_{th,n}^2 = (3/2)kT/q$, and $m_n$ is the electron effective mass in GaN.

At the p-GaN/InGaN QW interface we can write the current using thermionic equation modified by carriers coming out of the quantum well back into the p-GaN:

$$J = qp_p v_{th,p} \exp\left(-\frac{qN_A^- x_p^2}{2\epsilon kT}\right)\left[1 - \exp\left(\frac{-\Delta E_{fp}}{kT}\right)\right] \tag{3.4}$$

where $(1/2)m_p v_{th,p}^2 = (3/2)kT/q$, and $m_p$ is the hole effective mass in GaN.

Inside the QW the current is dominated by the recombination

$$\eta \bullet J = q \bullet \left(\frac{n_q}{d} \bullet \frac{p_q}{d} - n_{i,q}^2\right) \bullet d \bullet B \tag{3.5}$$

where $\Delta E_{fn}$ and $\Delta E_{fp}$ are the change in the electron and hole quasi-Fermi levels going from their depletion regions into the QW (as defined in Figure 3.1), $B$ is the radiative recombination coefficient, $\eta$ is the internal quantum efficiency, $d$

is the width of the quantum well. $n_q$ and $p_q$ are the 2D carrier densities inside the quantum well, and can be written as [9]

$$n_q \approx \frac{\pi m_{nq} kT}{\hbar^2} \ln\left[1+\exp\left(-\frac{\Delta E_{1,n} - E_{fn}}{m \bullet kT}\right)\right] \tag{3.6}$$

$$p_q \approx \frac{\pi m_{pq} kT}{\hbar^2} \ln\left[1+\exp\left(-\frac{E_{1,p} - E_{fp}}{m \bullet kT}\right)\right] \tag{3.7}$$

where $E_{fn} = \Delta E_c - qN_D^+ x_n^2 / 2\epsilon - \xi_n$ and $E_{fp} = \Delta E_v - qN_A^- x_p^2 / 2\epsilon - \xi_p$ are the quasi-Fermi level for electrons and holes, respectively, and $E_{1,n}$ and $E_{1,p}$ are the distances from the ground state within the QW to the to (bottom) of the conduction (valence) band, added to the distance between the electron (hole) quasi-Fermi level and the conduction (valence) band in the bulk. Here, we approximate that the ground state is the only occupied state within the QW. This will not significantly change the value of the current: since we are assuming a narrow QW, the energy difference between the first two states in the QW will be large enough such that the ground state will have orders of magnitude larger carrier concentration. The masses $m_{pq}$ and $m_{nq}$ are for InGaN QW [10]. The ideality factor $m$ is added to account for the p-GaN/QW and n-GaN/QW junction quality [6].

The internal quantum efficiency $\eta$ is expressed as a function of radiative and nonradiative recombination using the definition [11–14]

$$\eta = \frac{B \bullet n_q \bullet p_q}{\dfrac{n_q \bullet p_q}{n_q \bullet \tau_n + p_q \bullet \tau_p} + B \bullet n_q \bullet p_q + \left(C_n \bullet n_q + C_p \bullet p_q\right) \bullet n_q \bullet p_q} \tag{3.8}$$

where $A \cdot n_q = n_q \cdot p_q/(n_q \cdot \tau_n + p_q \cdot \tau_p)$, $A$ is the Shockley-Read-Hall nonradiative recombination coefficient, $\tau_n$ is the SRH electron nonradiative recombination lifetime, $\tau_p$ is the SRH hole nonradiative recombination lifetime, $B$ is the radiative recombination coefficient, $C_n$ is the electron-electron-hole Auger nonradiative recombination coefficient, and $C_p$ is the hole-hole-electron Auger nonradiative recombination coefficient.

We need now to calculate $n_n p_p$, $N_A^-$, and $N_D^+$, as a function of temperature. These quantities are given by the following equations for carrier statistics [15]

$$p_p = N_V \bullet \mathcal{F}_{1/2}\left(-\xi_p / kT\right) \tag{3.9}$$

$$n_n = N_C \bullet \mathcal{F}_{1/2}\left(-\xi_n / kT\right) \tag{3.10}$$

$$N_C = 2 \bullet \left(\frac{m_e k_B T}{2\pi \bullet \hbar^2}\right)^{3/2} \tag{3.11}$$

$$N_V = 2 \bullet \left(\frac{m_h k_B T}{2\pi \bullet \hbar^2}\right)^{3/2} \tag{3.12}$$

$$\mathcal{F}_{1/2}(\xi) = \frac{2}{\sqrt{\pi}} \int_0^\infty \frac{x^{1/2}\ dx}{\exp(x-\xi)+1} \tag{3.13}$$

$$N_A^- = \frac{N_A}{1 + 4\exp\left[\left(E_a - \xi_p\right)/kT\right]} \tag{3.14}$$

$$N_D^+ = \frac{N_D}{1 + 2\exp\left[\left(E_d - \xi_n\right)/kT\right]} \tag{3.15}$$

$$n_i^2 = N_C N_V \exp\left(-\frac{E_g}{kT}\right) \tag{3.16}$$

$$E_g(T) = E_{g0} - \frac{\alpha \bullet T^2}{T + \beta} \tag{3.17}$$

$$n_{iq}^2 = N_{Cq} N_{Vq} \exp\left(-\frac{E_{gq}}{kT}\right) \tag{3.18}$$

$$E_{gq}(T) = E_{gq0} - \frac{\alpha \bullet T^2}{T + \beta} \tag{3.19}$$

Find $\xi_p$ (defined in Figure 3.1) by solving

$$p_p - \frac{n_i^2}{p_p} - N_A^- = 0 \quad (3.20)$$

Find $\xi_n$ (defined in Figure 3.1) by solving

$$-n_n + \frac{n_i^2}{n_n} + N_D^+ = 0 \quad (3.21)$$

The voltage drop across the QW is approximately correlated to the geometric capacitance $\epsilon_q/d$ by

$$\frac{\epsilon_q}{d} \approx \frac{q \bullet n_{q3D} \bullet d}{V_q} \quad (3.22)$$

with $n_{q3D}$ being the 3D carrier concentration in the QW, and $\epsilon_q$ is the permittivity of the QW material, and we have the approximation

$$\eta \bullet J \approx q \bullet n_{q3D}^2 \bullet B \bullet d \quad (3.23)$$

After straightforward algebra we find

$$V_q = \sqrt{\frac{q \bullet \eta \bullet J \bullet d^4}{\epsilon_q^2 \bullet B \bullet d}} \quad (3.24)$$

The terminal voltage can be written as

$$V = V_j + V_q \quad (3.25)$$

Typically, there is a finite contact resistance at the terminals of the microLEDs (i.e., between the cathode metal and the n-GaN, and between the anode metal and the p-GaN). This can be taken into effect by modifying (3.26) as

$$V = V_j + V_q + J \bullet \rho_C \quad (3.26)$$

where $\rho_C$ is the sum of the contact resistances at the cathode metal/n-GaN and anode metal/p-GaN interfaces and has the units of $\Omega$-cm$^2$.

Due to a mix of polynomial, logarithmic, and exponential terms, an exact closed form solution to the system of equations (3.1) to (3.26) is not possible. However, a numerical solution is possible. We used MATLAB® to solve the set of equations numerically after proper normalization.

In Figure 3.2 the calculated I-V curve for $T = 300K$ and zero nonradiative recombination is shown. The I-V curve is similar to drain current versus gate voltage of a MOSFET [16, 17] with a liminal forward voltage, $V_{FL}$, separating two conduction regimes: (1) a subliminal regime for voltages below the $V_{FL}$, and (2) a supraliminal regime for voltages above $V_{FL}$. The current at the liminal forward voltage is called liminal forward current or $J_{FL}$. In the subliminal conduction regime, the current increases exponentially with increasing voltage, and the slope of the curve there is characterized by an ideality factor or subliminal voltage swing. The ideality factor approaches one for ideal p-GaN/QW and n-GaN/QW junctions, and when nonradiative recombination is minimal. The subliminal swing ($S_{SL}$) approaches ~60 mV/decade for ideal junctions and minimal nonradiative recombination. In the supraliminal conduction regime, the current has a power-law dependence on the drive voltage that is given by the

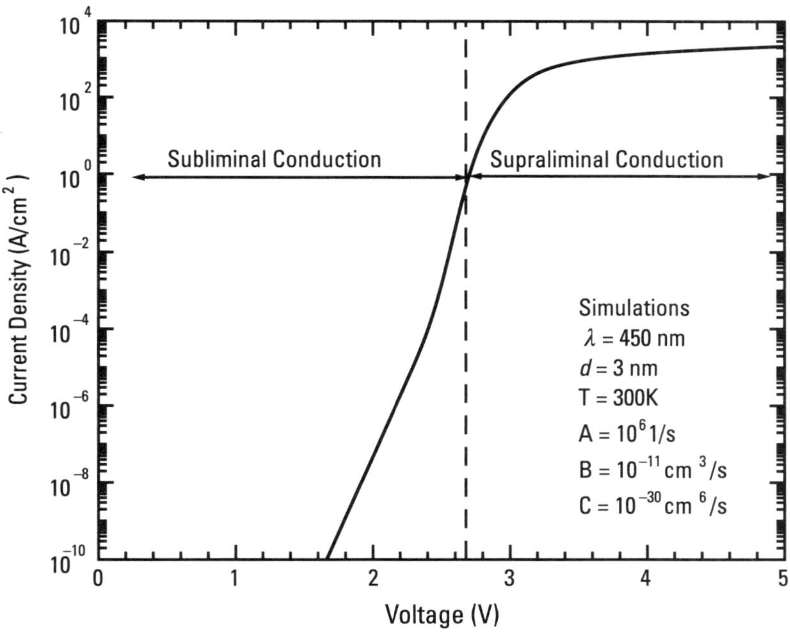


**Figure 3.2** Simulated I-V characteristics of a microLED. A liminal point (liminal voltage and liminal current) separates two conduction regimes: subliminal and supraliminal below and above the liminal point, respectively. The current increases exponentially with voltage in the subliminal conduction regime. The current increases according to a power law in the supraliminal conduction regime.

difference between the applied voltage and $V_{FL}$. Again, this behavior resembles a MOSFET drain current versus gate voltage curve despite the difference in the underlying physics.

The calculated I-V curves for microLEDs with zero and nonzero nonradiative recombination parameters $A$ and $C$ are shown with all other parameters fixed (e.g., $T = 300K$, quantum well thickness = 3 nm, and design wavelength = 470 nm). Nonradiative recombination results in excess current in the subliminal conduction regime as shown in Figure 3.3.

The liminal forward voltage ($V_{FL}$) can be determined by monitoring the peak of the function $F(V)$ given by [17]

$$F(V) = \frac{\partial}{\partial x}\left(\frac{\partial J / \partial V}{J}\right) \tag{3.27}$$

An example of the function $F(V)$ calculated for typical set of parameters is shown in Figure 3.4.

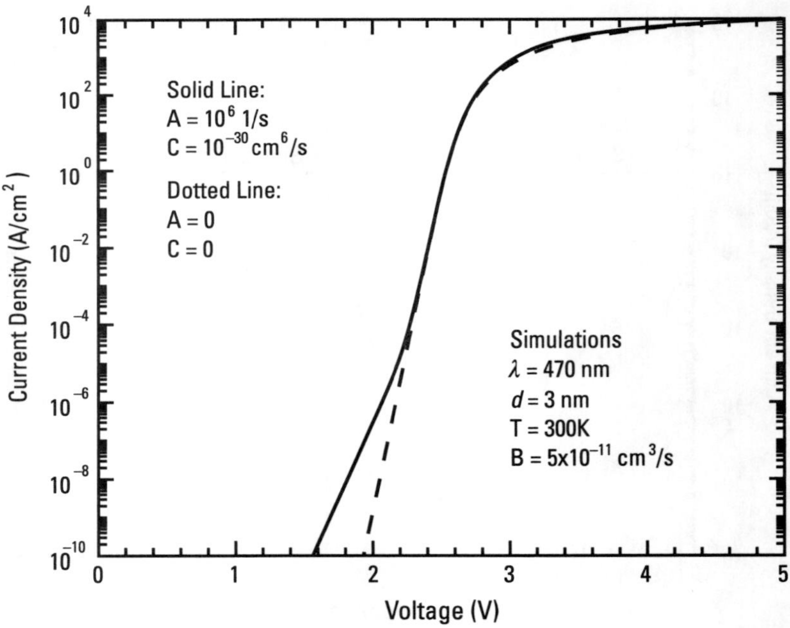


**Figure 3.3** Example simulation of the I-V curve of a microLED with ideal junction and zero nonradiative recombination, and more realistic microLED parameters (i.e., nonzero nonradiative recombination coefficients $A$ and $C$). The ideality factor or subliminal swing are 1.0 and 60 mV/decade for an ideal microLED. The ideality factor is greater than 1 and subliminal swing is greater than 60 mV/decade for the practical microLED.

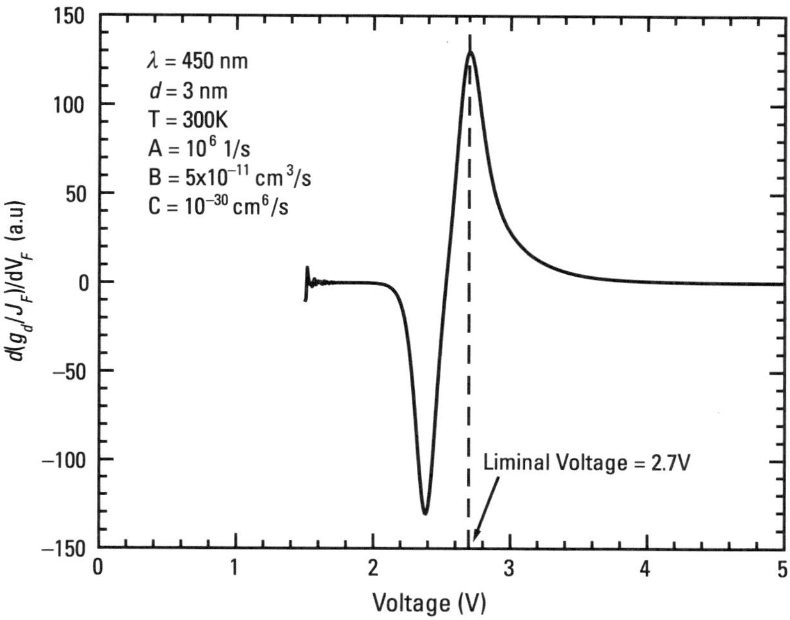


**Figure 3.4** Example plot of the function $F(V)$ as a function of voltage. The liminal forward voltage is the voltage at the peak of $F(V)$.

The liminal forward voltage can also be determined by fixing the current density at ~10 A/cm$^2$ and monitoring the corresponding voltage. The simulated I-V curves for three temperatures of 30K, 120K, and 300K are shown in Figure 3.5. A constant current of 10 A/cm$^2$ is used to monitor the liminal forward voltage. Smaller temperature corresponds to larger liminal forward voltage.

The simulated $V_{FL}$ versus temperature is shown in Figure 3.6, and the result is in excellent agreement with experimental data reported by [18–21].

## 3.3 Closed-Form Analytic I-V Model

The current is limited by the injection of carriers at the p-GaN/QW and n-GaN/QW junctions according to the Shockley formulae (i.e., $n_{q3D} \approx n_{iq}$ $\exp(qV_j/2kT)$ and $p_{q3D} \approx n_{iq} \exp(qV_j/2kT)$) [6]. The voltage drop across the device is the superposition of the voltages across junction and the voltage drop across the quantum well. If the voltage across the P-N junction is $V_j$ and the current at that junction is $J$, the internal quantum efficiency is $\eta$, the quantum well thickness is $d$, the intrinsic carrier concentration in the QW is $n_{iq}$, and the radiative recombination coefficient is $B$, then $V_j$ is given by the current continuity equation at that junction (i.e., injection current is equal to the recombination current):

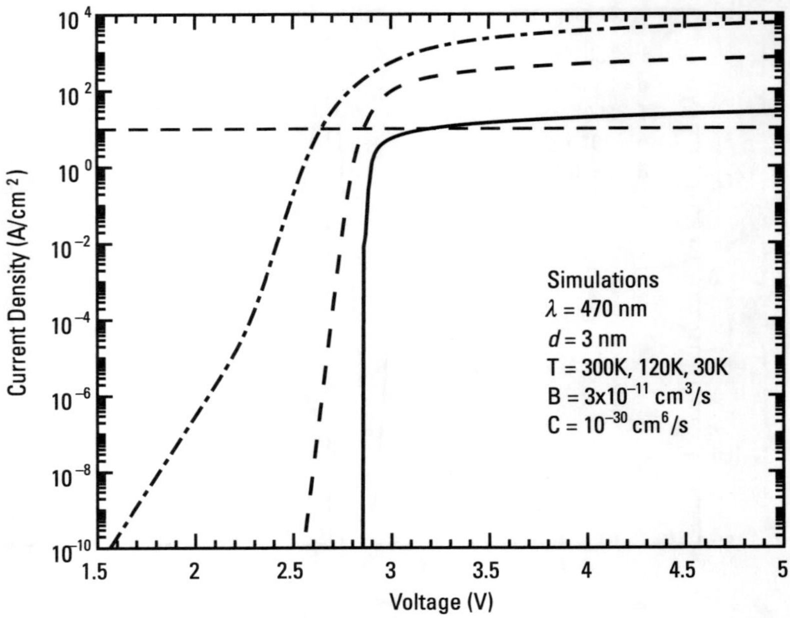


**Figure 3.5** Simulated I-V curves for three different temperatures of 300K (left), 120K (center), and 30K (right). A constant current density (e.g., 10 A/cm$^2$) may be used to track the forward voltage.

$$\eta \bullet J \approx q \bullet B \bullet d \bullet n_{iq} \bullet \exp\left(\frac{qV_j}{2kT}\right) \bullet n_{iq} \bullet \exp\left(\frac{qV_j}{2kT}\right) \tag{3.28}$$

In (3.28), it is assumed, for simplicity, that the junction voltage is divided equally between the p-GaN/QW and n-GaN/QW junctions.

The voltage drop across the quantum well is approximately correlated to the geometric capacitance by

$$\frac{\epsilon_q}{d} \approx \frac{q \bullet n_{q3D} \bullet d}{V_q} \tag{3.29}$$

with $n_{q3D}$ being the volume carrier concentration in the quantum well, and $\epsilon_q$ is the permittivity of the quantum well material, and we have the approximation:

$$\eta \bullet J \approx q \bullet n_{q3D}^2 \bullet B \bullet d \tag{3.30}$$

After straightforward algebra of (3.29) and (3.30), we find

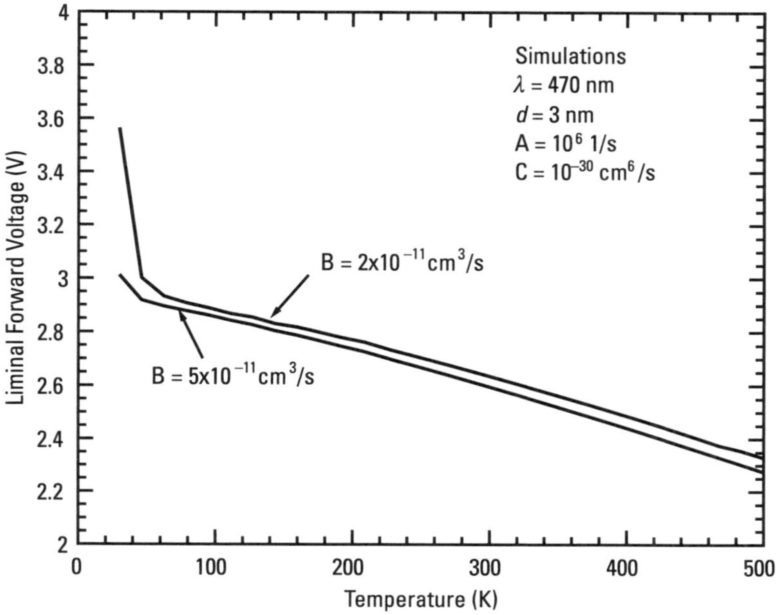


**Figure 3.6** Simulated liminal forward voltage (taken at current density of 10 A/cm²) versus junction temperature.

$$V_q = \sqrt{\frac{q \bullet \eta \bullet J \bullet d^4}{\epsilon_q^2 \bullet B \bullet d}} \tag{3.31}$$

The terminal voltage can be written as

$$V = V_j + V_q \tag{3.32}$$

Substituting (3.28) and (3.31) in (3.32) we find

$$V = E_{g,q} + \frac{kT}{q}\ln\left(\frac{J}{J_L}\right) + \frac{kT}{q}\left(\frac{J}{J_0}\right)^{\frac{1}{2}} \tag{3.33}$$

where

$$J_L = \frac{q \bullet N_{Cq} \bullet N_{Vq} \bullet B \bullet d}{\eta} \tag{3.34}$$

$$J_0(\eta) = \frac{\epsilon_q^2 \bullet B \bullet (kT/q)^2}{q \bullet \eta \bullet d^3} \quad (3.35)$$

$$n_{iq} = N_{Cq} N_{Vq} \exp\left(qE_{gq}/2kT\right) \quad (3.36)$$

Now the I-V relationship can be written as

$$V \cong V_F + \frac{kT}{q}\ln\left(\frac{J}{J_0}\right) + \frac{kT}{q}\left(\frac{J}{J_0}\right)^{\frac{1}{2}} \quad (3.37)$$

where

$$V_F \equiv E_{gq} + \frac{kT}{q}\ln\left(\frac{\epsilon_q^2 \bullet (kT/q)^2}{q^2 \bullet d^4 \bullet N_{Cq} \bullet N_{Vq}}\right) \quad (3.38)$$

Here, $V_F$ is the liminal forward voltage of the microLED, and it is a function of the energy gap of the quantum well material $E_{g,q}$, junction temperature $T$, and quantum well thickness $d$. The conduction and valence band density of states are given by

$$N_{Vq} = 2 \bullet \left(\frac{m_{pq} k_B T}{2\pi \bullet \hbar^2}\right)^{3/2} \quad (3.39a)$$

$$N_{Cq} = 2 \bullet \left(\frac{m_{nq} k_B T}{2\pi \bullet \hbar^2}\right)^{3/2} \quad (3.39b)$$

In order to take into account the internal resistance due to the depletion layers barrier heights at the n-GaN/QW and p-GaN/QW junctions, we introduce a series resistance term in (3.37): $J \cdot \rho_{TE}$ due to thermionic barriers [22]. Also, in order to take the contact series resistances into account we add the following term to (3.37): $J \cdot \rho_C$:

$$V \cong V_F + \frac{kT}{q}\ln\left(\frac{J}{J_0}\right) + \frac{kT}{q}\left(\frac{J}{J_0}\right)^{\frac{1}{2}} + J \bullet \rho_C + J \bullet \rho_{TE} \quad (3.40)$$

Equation (3.40) can be regarded as providing the correct form for the I-V characteristics but calculated in a simplified way. The model parameters can be allowed to depart from their ideal values so as to compensate for the approximations and omissions in the model. For example, the dependence of $J_0$ on internal quantum efficiency can result in deviation from a square root dependence in the third term, which will impact the supraliminal power $n_2$, as shown in (3.42). Specifically, the internal quantum efficiency is a function of the current density according to the ABC model, and is given by [13]

$$\eta = 1 - \left(\frac{1-\eta_{max}}{2}\right) \bullet \left(1 + \frac{\eta}{\eta_{max}} \bullet \frac{J}{J_{max}}\right) \bullet \left(\frac{\eta / \eta_{max}}{J / J_{max}}\right)^{1/2} \quad (3.41)$$

with $\eta_{max} = B / \left(B + 2\sqrt{A \bullet C}\right)$ and $J_{max} = q \bullet d \bullet A \bullet \left(B + 2\sqrt{A \bullet C}\right) / C$.

Based on the above discussion, (3.40) can be rewritten as

$$V \cong V_{FL} + n_1 \frac{kT}{q} \ln\left(\frac{J}{J_{FL}}\right) + \frac{kT}{q}\left(\frac{J}{J_{FL}}\right)^{n_2} + J \bullet \rho_s \quad (3.42)$$

In (3.42), $J_{FL}$ and $V_{FL}$ are independent of the current density, and $\rho_s$ is a total series resistance (composed of the thermionic internal junction resistance and the terminal contact resistance).

Figure 3.7 shows an example comparison between the numerical model results and the analytical model given by (3.42) for ideal microLEDs with zero values of the nonradiative recombination coefficients. Excellent agreement is observed for both subliminal and supraliminal conduction regimes using ideal values of $V_{FL}$, $J_{FL}$, $n_1$, and $n_2$. Figure 3.8 shows an example comparison between the numerical model when the nonradiative recombination coefficients $A$ and $C$ were nonzero. The analytical model was based on ideal model parameters used in Figure 3.7. A deviation is observed between an ideal analytical model and more realistic numerical calculations. The difference can be recovered if we allow the model parameters ($V_{FL}$, $J_{FL}$, $n_1$, and $n_2$) to slightly deviate from their ideal values, as given in (3.42).

In Figure 3.9, nonlinear least-squares fitting (using MATLAB) was used to fit the numerical I-V data to the analytical expression given by (3.42). Best fit resulted in the following model parameters: $V_{FL} = 2.975\,V$, $J_{FL} = 86.6A/\text{cm}^2$, $n_1 = 1.97$, $n_2 = 1.6$, and $r_s = 5 \times 10^{-4}\Omega\text{-cm}^2$. The ideal parameters used in Figures 3.7 and 3.8 to produce the analytical curve were $V_{FL} = 2.5407\,V$, $J_{FL} = 0.2117A/\text{cm}^2$, $n_1 = 1.0$, $n_2 = 0.5$, and $r_s = 5 \times 10^{-4}\Omega\text{-cm}^2$. In other words, nonradiative recombination results in larger apparent liminal forward voltage $V_{FL}$, liminal forward current $J_{FL}$, subliminal ideality factor $n_1$, and supraliminal power $n_2$, according to model equation (3.42).

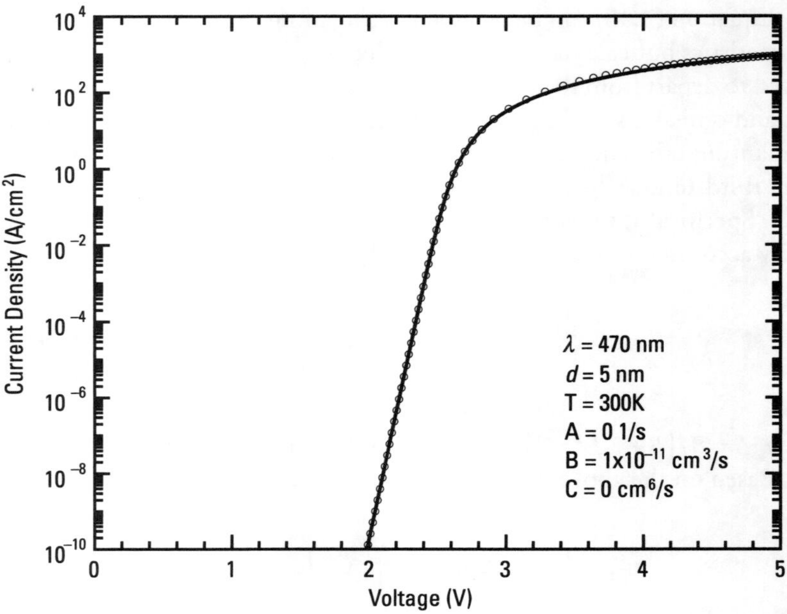


**Figure 3.7** Comparison between numerical and analytics I-V models. Excellent agreement is observed for the subliminal and supraliminal regimes. Lines are the analytical model and symbols are the numerical model. The liminal forward voltage was 2.54V, the liminal forward current was 0.2 A/cm$^2$, the subliminal ideality factor was 1.0, and the supraliminal power was 0.5. It is noted here that nonradiative recombination coefficients $A$ and $C$ were set to zero.

The thermionic series resistance is extracted by fitting various numerical data calculated at different temperatures is shown as a function of the junction temperature in Figure 3.10. It is assumed here that $A = C = 0$ to illustrate the origin of the thermionic resistance. Indeed, $\rho_{TE}$ decreases exponentially with increasing the junction temperature in accordance with the thermionic theory [22].

## 3.4 Comparison with Experimental Data

Now that we have compared numerical data and closed-form analytical expression for the I-V characteristics, it is important that we compare the model (3.42) with experimental data. We use data published in the literature to show the ability of the analytical model to capture a wide set of I-V curves from various sources. Experimental I-V data can be fitted to (3.42) by adjusting five parameters: (1) liminal forward voltage ($1 \precsim V \precsim 3.5V$), (2) a liminal forward current ($10^{-3} \precsim J_{FL} \precsim 10A/cm^2$), (3) a subliminal ideality factor ($n_1 \geq 1$), (4) a supraliminal exponent ($0 \leq n_2 \leq 1$), and (5) a series resistance ($10^{-6} \precsim \rho_s \precsim 10^{-2}$ Ù-cm$^2$).

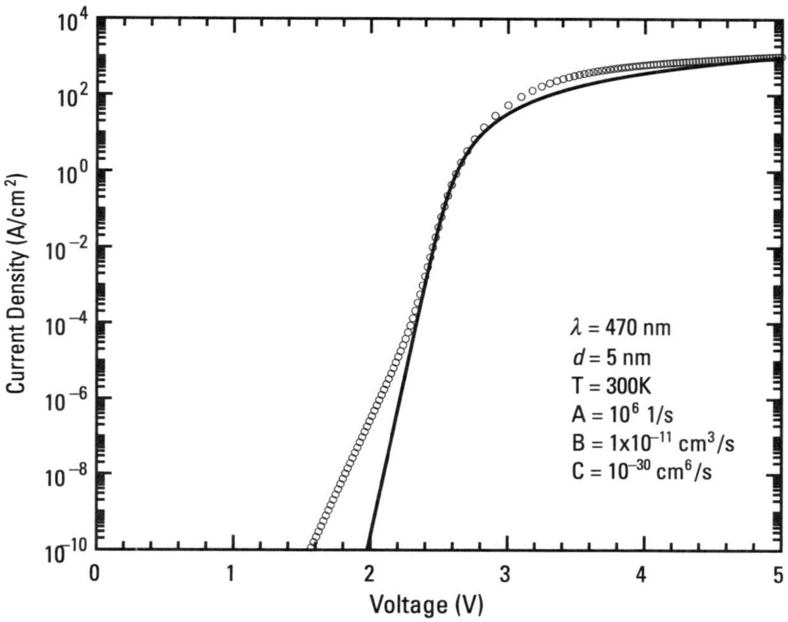


**Figure 3.8** Comparison between numerical and analytics I-V models. Lines are analytical model and symbols are numerical model. The liminal forward voltage was 2.54V, the liminal forward current was 0.2 A/cm$^2$, the subliminal ideality factor was 1.0, and the supraliminal power was 0.5. The nonradiative recombination coefficients *A* and *C* had typical experimental values, causing differences between numerical model and analytical model when ideal model parameters (given in Figure 3.7) were used to calculate the analytical model.

The parameters values are based on numerous analyses of experimental data on InGaN/GaN microLEDs reported in the literature as will be shown below. The curves shown in Figures 3.11 to 3.18 cover the visible light spectrum (red, green, and blue). The fitted parameters are shown for each graph. The model is able to capture various curves with model parameters within physical ranges expected based on the theory.

## 3.5 Incorporation of a Polarization Field

The above models were derived assuming that there is no polarization field between an InGaN quantum well and GaN. This is valid for m-plane-grown microLEDs. However, for c-plane-grown microLEDs, there is a finite polarization field at the InGaN/GaN interface as shown in Figure 3.19. The effect of the polarization field is taken into account by modifying (3.2) using a term for the polarization field [14, 31]

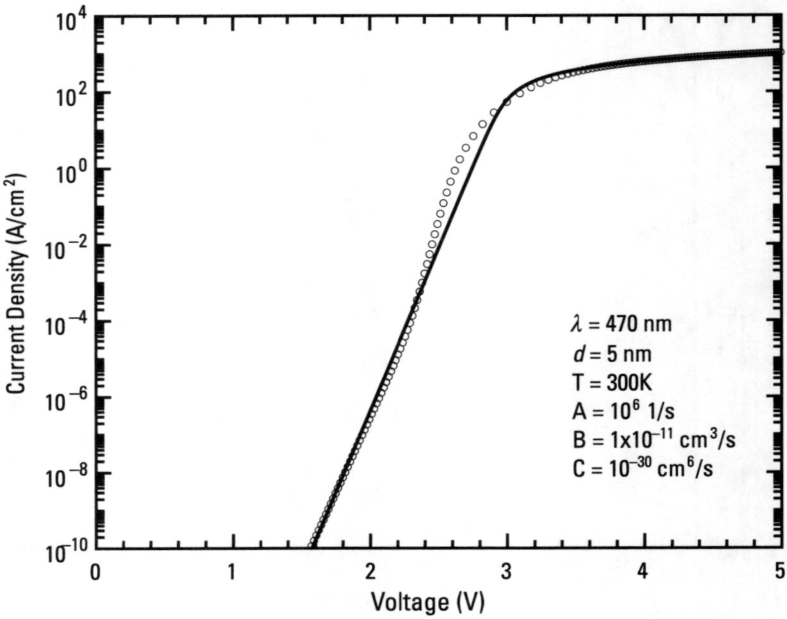


**Figure 3.9** Comparison between numerical and analytics I-V models. Lines are analytical model and symbols are numerical model. Nonlinear least-squares fitting was used to obtain an effective set of model parameters that produce the best fit with numerical data generated with nonzero nonradiative recombination. The nonradiative recombination coefficients *A* and *C* had typical experimental values, resulting in higher apparent liminal forward voltage, higher apparent liminal forward current, higher apparent subliminal ideality factor, and higher supraliminal power.

$$\frac{qN_D^+ x_n^2}{2\epsilon} + \frac{qN_A^- x_p^2}{2\epsilon} = -\left(V_j - \frac{\Delta P}{\epsilon} \bullet d - V_{bi}\right) \tag{3.43}$$

where $\Delta P/\epsilon$ represents the electric field in the quantum well, $\epsilon$ represents the dielectric constant of the quantum well material, and $\Delta P$ represents the net polarization charge density. Here, $\Delta P$ is a function of the indium mole fraction in InGaN quantum wells [32, 33].

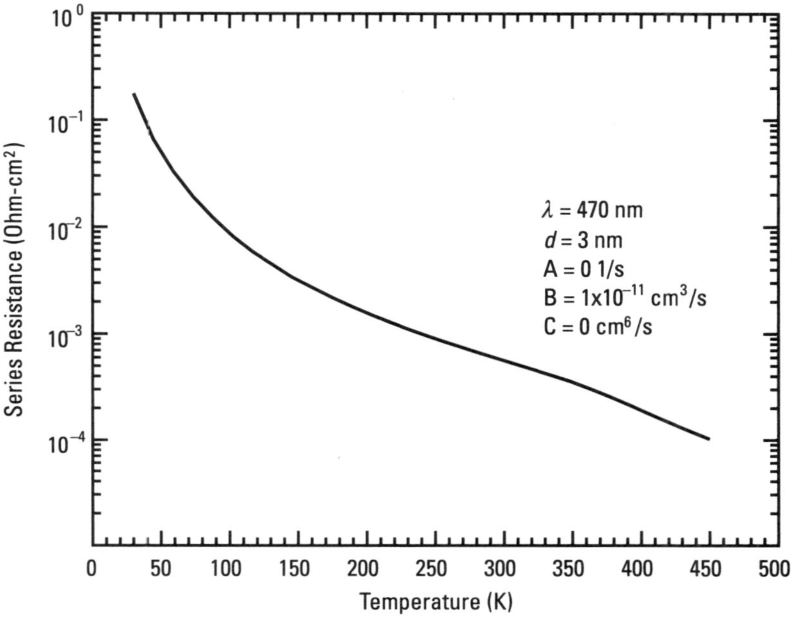


**Figure 3.10** Thermionic series resistance extracted by fitting numerical I-V data to the analytical formula (3.42) for various junction temperatures. Exponential dependence of $\rho_{TE}$ explains that the physical origin of this series resistance is the thermionic emission resistance at the p-GaN/QW and n-GaN/QW junctions.

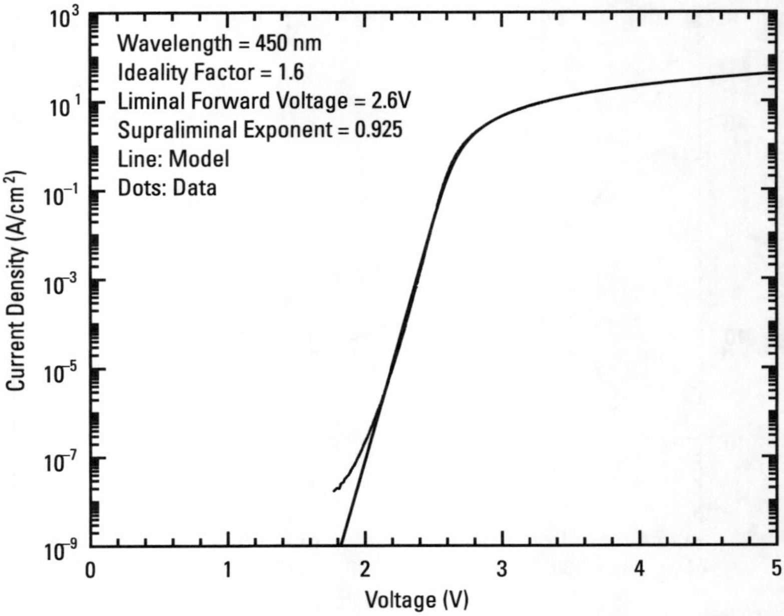


**Figure 3.11** Experimental data [23] and analytical model fit for InGaN/GaN LEDs emitting a wavelength of 450 nm.

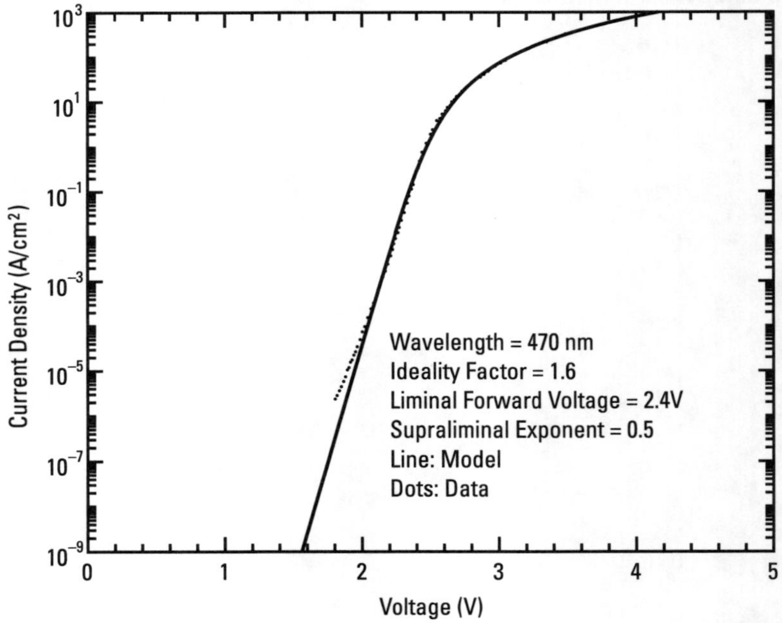


**Figure 3.12** Experimental data [24] and analytical model fit for InGaN/GaN LEDs emitting a wavelength of 470 nm.

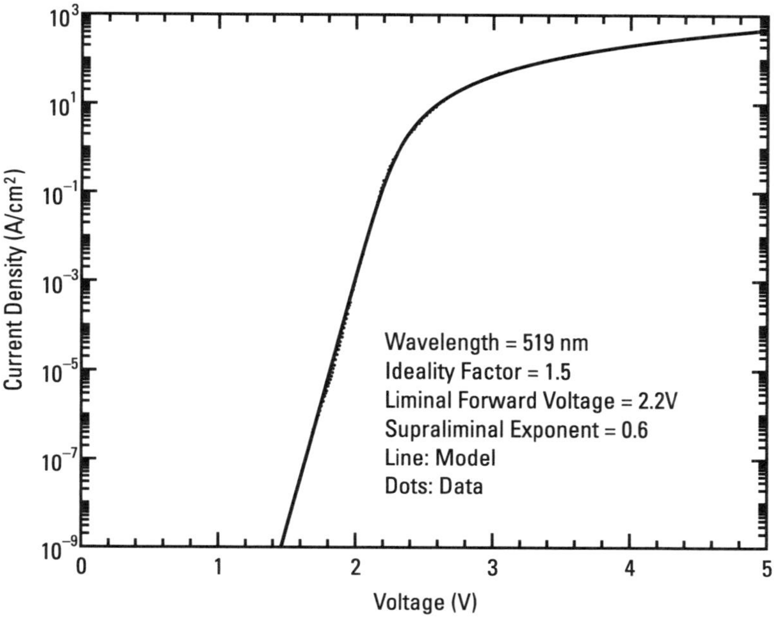


**Figure 3.13** Experimental data [25] and analytical model fit for InGaN/GaN LEDs emitting a wavelength of 519 nm.

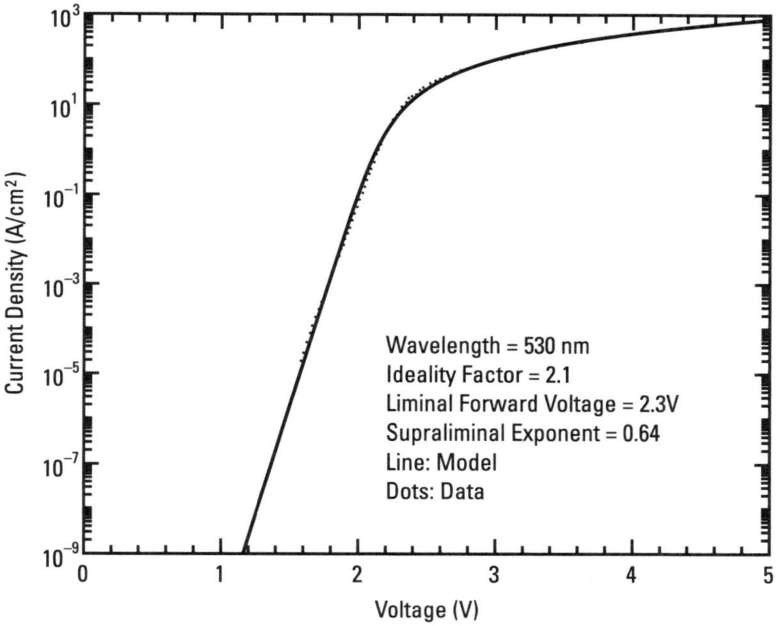


**Figure 3.14** Experimental data [26] and analytical model fit for InGaN/GaN LEDs emitting a wavelength of 530 nm.

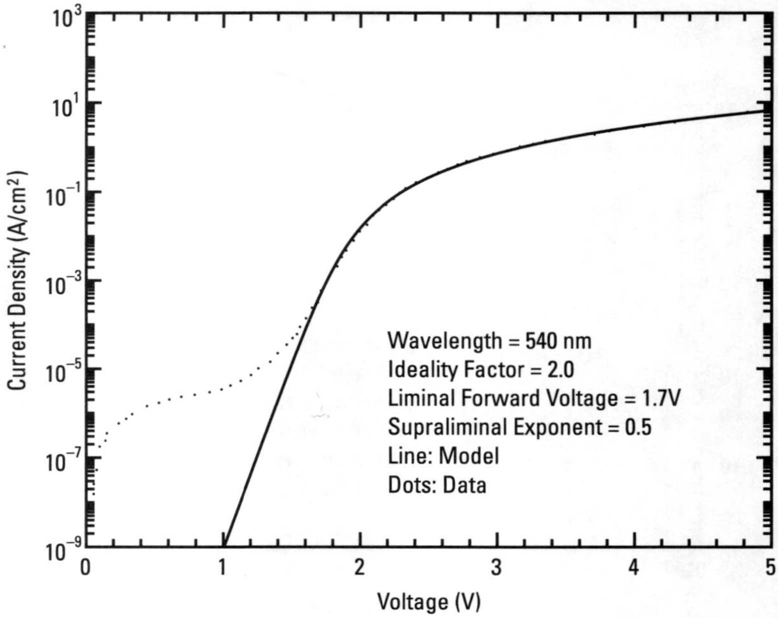


**Figure 3.15** Experimental data [27] and analytical model fit for InGaN/GaN LEDs emitting a wavelength of 540 nm.

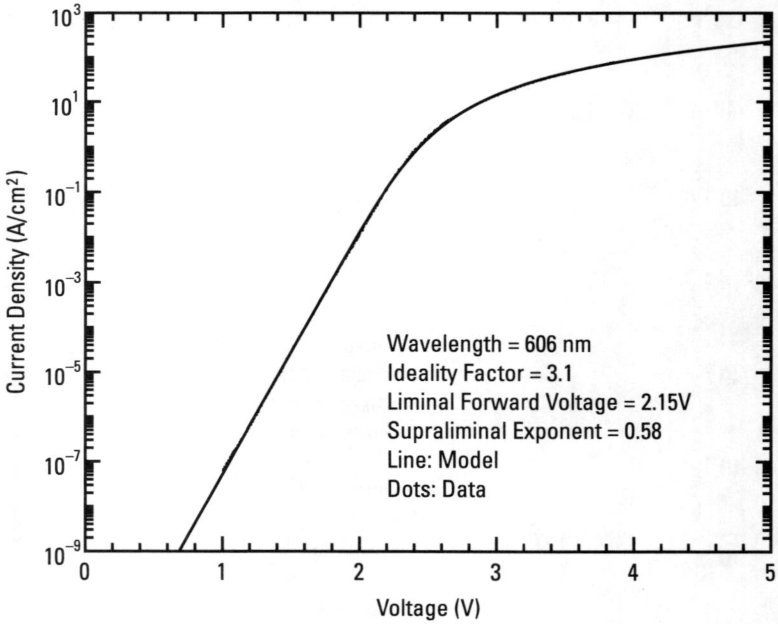


**Figure 3.16** Experimental data [28] and analytical model fit for InGaN/GaN LEDs emitting a wavelength of 606 nm.

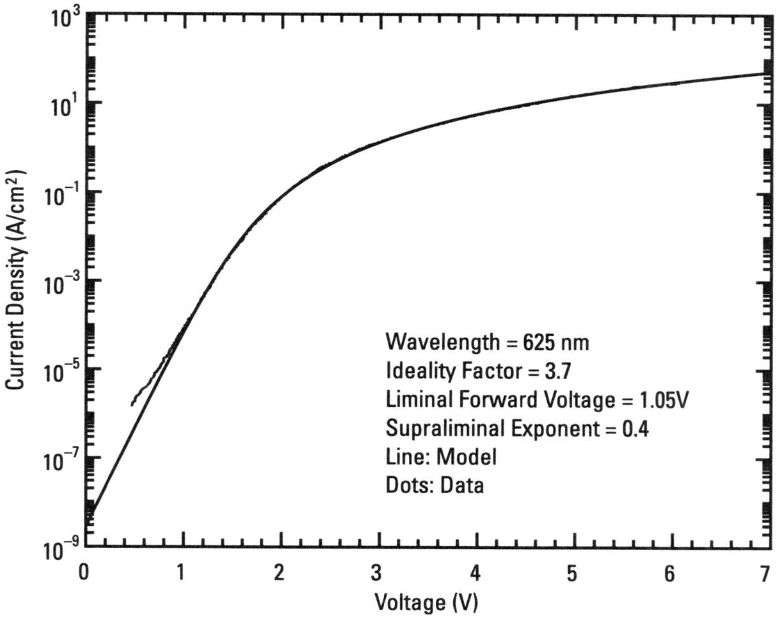


**Figure 3.17** Experimental data [29] and analytical model fit for InGaN/GaN LEDs emitting a wavelength of 625 nm.

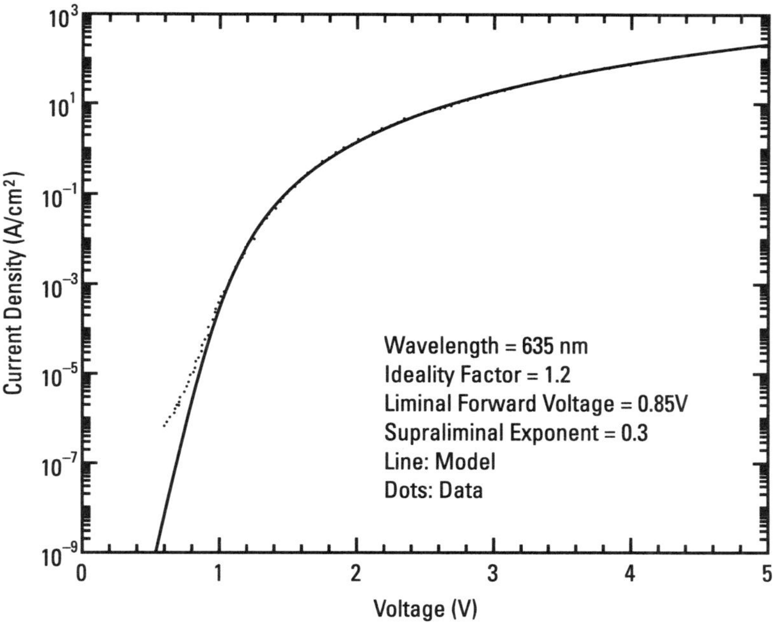


**Figure 3.18** Experimental data [30] and analytical model fit for InGaN/GaN LEDs emitting a wavelength of 635 nm.

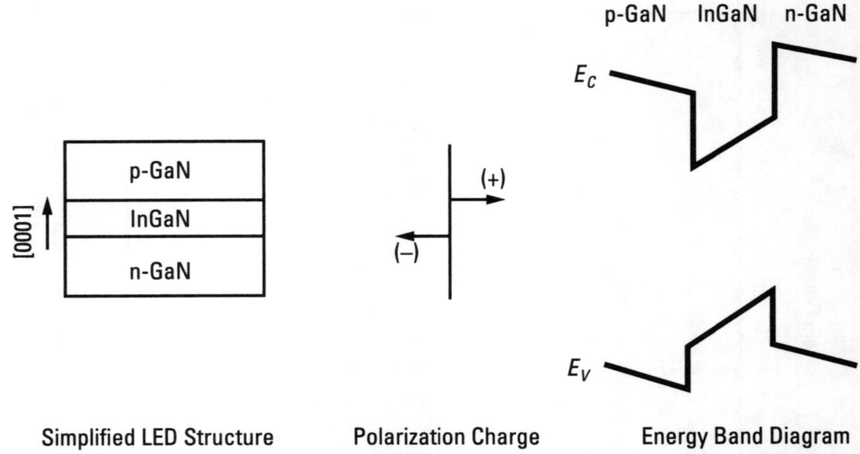


**Figure 3.19** Energy band diagram showing the polarization field due to InGaN/GaN along polar [0001] plane.

# References


[1] Lampert, M., and R. Schilling, "Current Injection in Solids: The Regional Approximation Method," in *Semiconductors and Semimetals* Vol. 6, Elsevier, 1970, pp. 1–96.

[2] Han, D.- P., D.-S. Shin, J.-I. Shim, et al., "Modified Shockley Equation for GaInN-Based Light-Emitting Diodes: Origin of the Power-Efficiency Degradation under High Current Injection," *IEEE Journal of Quantum Electronics*, Vol. 55, No. 4, 2019, pp. 1–11.

[3] Li, C. C., J. L. Zhan, Z. Z. Chen, et al., "Operating Behavior of Micro-LEDs on a GaN Substrate at Ultrahigh Injection Current Densities," *Optics Express*, Vol. 27, No. 16, 2019, pp. A1146–A1155.

[4] Musolino, M., A. Tahraoui, D. van Treeck, L. Geelhaar, and H. Riechert, "A Modified Shockley Equation Taking into Account the Multi-Element Nature of Light Emitting Diodes Based on Nanowire Ensembles," *Nanotechnology*, Vol. 27, No. 27, 2016, p. 275203.

[5] Prudaev, I., O. Tolbanov, and S. Khludkov, "Low-Temperature Transport of Charge Carriers in InGaN/GaN Multiple Quantum Well Light-Emitting Diodes," *physica status solidi (a)*, Vol. 212, No. 5, 2015, pp. 930–934.

[6] Sah, C., T. R. N. Noyce, and W. Shockley, "Carrier Generation and Recombination in PN Junctions and PN Junction Characteristics," *Proceedings of the IRE*, Vol. 45, No. 9, 1957, pp. 1228–1243.

[7] Zhu, D., J. Xu, A. N. Noemaun, et al., "The Origin of the High Diode-Ideality Factors in GaInN/GaN Multiple Quantum Well Light-Emitting Diodes," *Applied Physics Letters*, Vol. 94, No. 8, 2009, p. 081113.

[8] David, A., C. A. Hurni, N. G. Young, and M. D. Craven, "Electrical Properties of III-Nitride LEDs: Recombination-Based Injection Model and Theoretical Limits to Electrical Efficiency and Electroluminescent Cooling," *Applied Physics Letters*, Vol. 109, No. 8, 2016, p. 083501.

[9] Weisbuch, C., and B. Vinter, *Quantum Semiconductor Structures: Fundamentals and Applications,* Boston: Academic Press, 1991, p. 44.

[10] Leung, M., A. Djurisic, and E. Li, "Refractive Index of InGaN/GaN Quantum Well," *Journal of Applied Physics,* Vol. 84, No. 11, 1998, pp. 6312–6317.

[11] Karpov, S., "ABC-Model for Interpretation of Internal Quantum Efficiency and Its Droop in III-Nitride LEDs: A Review," *Optical and Quantum Electronics,* 2015, p. 1293.

[12] David, A., N. Young, C. Lund, and M. Craven, "The Physics of Recombinations in III-Nitride Emitters," *ECS Journal of Solid-State Science and Technology,* Vol. 9, No. 1, 2019, p. 016021.

[13] Ryu, H., H. Kim, and J. Shim, "Rate Equation Analysis of Efficiency Droop in InGaN Light-Emitting Diodes," *Applied Physics Letters,* Vol. 95, No. 8, 2009, p. 081114.

[14] Yuan, Z., Y. Li, X. Lu, et al., "Investigation of Modulation Bandwidth of InGaN Green Micro-LEDs by Varying Quantum Barrier Thickness," *IEEE Transactions on Electron Devices,* Vol. 69, No. 8, 2022, pp. 4298–4305.

[15] Nisoli, M., *Semiconductor Photonics: Principles and Applications,* Società Editrice Esculapio, 2016.

[16] G. T. Wright, "Threshold Modelling of MOSFETs for CAD of CMOS-VLSI," *Electronics Letters,* 1985, p. 223.

[17] Flandre, D., V. Kilchytska, and T. Rudenko, "gm/Id Method for Threshold Voltage Extraction Applicable in Advanced MOSFETs with Nonlinear Behavior Above Threshold," *IEEE Electron Device Letters,* Vol. 31, No. 9, 2010, pp. 930–932.

[18] Xi, Y., and E. Schubert, "Junction–Temperature Measurement in GaN Ultraviolet Light-Emitting Diodes Using Diode Forward Voltage Method," *Applied Physics Letters,* Vol. 85, No. 12, 2004, pp. 2163–2165.

[19] Wang, Y., B. Lu, C. Liu, H. Kuo, B. Hyun, and Z. Liu, "Temperature-Dependent Forward Voltage of AlGaInP-Based Red Micro-LEDs," *SID Symposium Digest of Technical Papers,* Vol. 51, No. 1, 2020, pp. 129–131.

[20] Meyaard, D., J. Cho, E. Fred Schubert, S. Han, M. Kim, and C. Sone, "Analysis of the Temperature Dependence of the Forward Voltage Characteristics of GaInN Light-Emitting Diodes," *Applied Physics Letters,* Vol. 103, No. 12, 2013, p. 121103.

[21] Xi, Y., T. Gessmann, J. Xi, et al., "Junction Temperature in Ultraviolet Light-Emitting Diodes," *Japanese Journal of Applied Physics,* Vol. 44, No. 10R, 2005, p. 7260.

[22] Sze, S. M., Physics of Semiconductor Devices, New York: Wiley, 1982, pp. 250–254, 304–306.

[23] Han, D., Y. Kim, J. Shim, and D. Shin, "Forward-Capacitance Measurement on Wide-Bandgap Light-Emitting Diodes," *IEEE Photonics Technology Letters,* Vol. 28, No. 21, 2016, pp. 2407–2410.

[24] Ley, R., J. Smith, M. Wong, et al., "Revealing the Importance of Light Extraction Efficiency in InGaN/GaN MicroLEDs via Chemical Treatment and Dielectric Passivation," *Applied Physics Letters,* Vol. 116, No. 25, 2020, p. 251104.

[25] Liu, Y., K. Zhang, J. Chan, S. Yeung, Z. Liu, and H. Kwok, "The Size and Temperature Effect of Ideality Factor in GaN/InGaN Multiple Quantum Wells Micro Light Emitting Diodes (Micro-LEDs)," *SID Symposium Digest of Technical Papers*, Vol. 52, No. 1, 2021, pp. 387–390.

[26] Zhanghu, M., Y. Feng, and Z. Liu, "Size-Dependence Characterization of GaN-Based Green Micro-LED," *SID Symposium Digest of Technical Papers*, Vol. 52, No. 1, 2021, pp. 247–250.

[27] Wu, Y., B. Liu, F. Xu, et al., "High-Efficiency Green Micro-LEDs with GaN Tunnel Junctions Grown Hybrid by PA-MBE and MOCVD," *Photonics Research*, Vol. 9, No. 9, 2021, pp. 1683–1688.

[28] Zhuang, Z., D. Iida, M. Velazquez-Rizo, and K. Ohkawa, "606-nm InGaN Amber Micro-Light-Emitting Diodes with an On-Wafer External Quantum Efficiency of 0.56%," *IEEE Electron Device Letters*, Vol. 42, No. 7, 2021, pp. 1029–1032.

[29] Dussaigne, A., P. Le Maitre, H. Haas, et al., "Full InGaN Red (625 nm) Micro-LED (10 $\mu$m) Demonstration on a Relaxed Pseudo-Substrate," *Applied Physics Express*, Vol. 14, No. 9, 2021, p. 092011.

[30] Zhuang, Z., D. Iida, M. Velazquez-Rizo, and K. Ohkawa, "630-nm Red InGaN Micro-Light-Emitting Diodes ($<20\mu m \times 20\mu m$) Exceeding 1mW/mm2 for Full-Color Micro-Displays," *Photonics Research*, Vol. 9, No. 9, 2021, pp. 1796–1802.

[31] Shen, H., G. G. M. Wraback, H. Zhong, et al., "Polarization Field Crossover in Semi-Polar InGaN/GaN Single Quantum Well," *physica status solidi (c)*, Vol. 7, No. 10, 2010, pp. 2378–2381.

[32] Guo, L. X., Wang, H. Xiao, and B. Wang, " The Influence of Internal Electric Fields on the Transition Energy of InGaN/GaN Quantum Well," *Journal of Crystal Growth*, Vol. 298, 2007, pp. 522–526.

[33] Shapiro, N., H. Feick, W. Hong, M. Cich, R. Armitage, and E. Weber, "Luminescence Energy and Carrier Lifetime in InGaN/GaN Quantum Wells as a Function of Applied Biaxial Strain," *Journal of Applied Physics*, Vol. 94, No. 7, 2003, pp. 4520–4529.

# 4

# High-Speed Modulation of MicroLEDs

## 4.1 Introduction

Discovery of novel light sources that do not require exotic cooling would result in breakthrough optical interconnects that achieve both high figure of merit (speed/energy) with low total interconnect cost. For more than a decade now, visible light microLEDs that are being developed for display applications have been considered as a suitable candidate for realizing short reach optical interconnects between integrated circuit chips [1–5]. An example schematic of such a system is shown in Figure 4.1.

Visible-light communication (VLC) is based on the principle of modulating the light intensity of microLEDs at high speed. In a VLC system, the information-carrying signal is imposed as an ac signal on the microLED drive current. The modulation bandwidth of the microLED is dependent on the carrier (recombination) lifetime, which is the average time spent by an excess minority carrier to recombine radiatively or nonradiatively.

In order for decision makers to make more investments to convert this concept to actual products, a set of design heuristics for microLEDs have to be established. The heuristics should be based on as much physics and empirical data as possible to be credible. Heuristic modeling relies on a combination of rules with well-known linear or nonlinear equations relating physical quantities that have first-principles theory with simplifying approximations. The advantage of heuristic modeling is that it can give us important insight into the device that would not be possible to see just observing the equations.

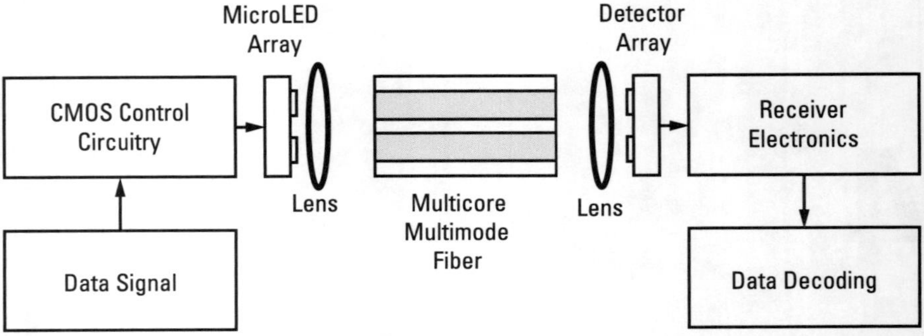


**Figure 4.1** Schematic IP block diagram of a parallel communication system utilizing microLEDs as light sources.

## 4.2 Small-Signal Modulation

The small-signal modulation bandwidth is directly related to the differential carrier lifetime, not carrier lifetime that is typically measured using time-resolved photoluminescence (TRPL) [6]. The differential carrier lifetime represents the response to a small signal and depends on the local slope of the recombination versus carrier density curve and takes into account carrier recombination dynamics including internal fields and electron and hole wavefunction overlap and their dependence on injected current.

Accurate small-signal model parameters extraction techniques for microLEDs are extremely important for optimizing the device performance and understanding the device physical mechanisms. A good circuit model is not only useful for predicting the modulation bandwidth of microLEDs but also convenient for parameter extraction.

In the microLED, since electrons and holes are injected in pairs and recombine in pairs, it is enough to consider the rate equation for only one type of charge carrier. Let $N$ be the number of electrons. The rate of increase of the number of electrons in the active region is given by

$$\frac{dN}{dt} = \frac{I}{q} - \frac{N}{\tau} \tag{4.1}$$

where $q$ is the electronic charge, $I$ is the injected current, and $\tau$ is the differential carrier lifetime. The first term on the right-hand side of (4.1) is the rate of electrons injected into the active region and the last term is the rate of electron-hole recombination, including radiative and nonradiative recombination.

Consider an injected current composed of a DC bias and a sinusoidal modulation

$$I = I_b + I_m e^{-i\omega t} \tag{4.2}$$

Substituting this current into (4.1) and solving for the steady state carrier number gives

$$N(t) = N_b + N_m e^{-i\omega t} \tag{4.3}$$

$$N_b = I_b \tau / q \tag{4.4}$$

$$N_m = \frac{(I_m / q)\tau}{1 + i\omega\tau} \tag{4.5}$$

Note that $N_b$ is the carrier number due to the bias current, and $N_m$ is the amplitude of the modulated carrier number.

It is clear from (4.5) that the modulated amplitude decreases as the modulation frequency increases. Physically, this may be interpreted as that, at high modulation frequencies, the pumping current changes so rapidly that there is insufficient time for some of the charge carriers to recombine.

Rewriting (4.5) as

$$H(\omega) = \frac{qN_m / \tau}{I_m} = \frac{1}{1 + i\omega\tau} \tag{4.6}$$

This is the transfer characteristic of the microLED: output current divided by the input modulation current.

If we assume that the quantum efficiency is 100% so that recombination is entirely radiative, then this current may be regarded as the AC photon generating current,

$$I_p = qN_m / \tau \tag{4.7}$$

We note that the frequency response is identical to that of a single-pole parallel RC circuit. Such a circuit is shown in Figure 4.2.

Next, we must find appropriate representation for $R$ and $C$ of the equivalent circuit. So far all we know is that the $RC$ time constant is equal to $\tau$. From junction current theory, we note that the differential resistance for small signals at low frequencies is given by $R_D = \partial V / \partial I$. This is applicable to the microLED under the condition of low-frequency, small-amplitude modulation. Therefore,

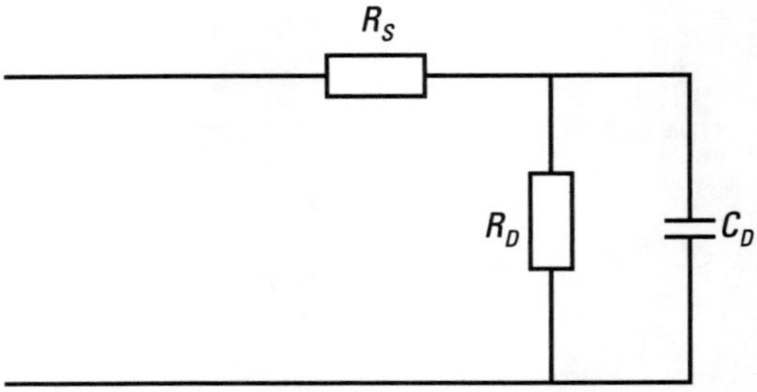


**Figure 4.2** Single pole model of a microLED including the series resistance. $R_D$ is the forward differential resistance and $C_D$ is the forward differential capacitance.

we have $R = R_D$ and, consequently, the parallel capacitance is given by $C_D = \tau/R_D$ [7, 8].

In addition to the ideal light emitting junction, a practical microLED will also have a contact series resistance $R_S$. The single port equivalent circuit of a light-emitting diode is thus as shown in Figure 4.1. This equivalent circuit has been commonly used to describe LEDs [6, 9–11] and VCSELs [12].

The contact series resistance $R_S$ and the differential resistance $R_D$ can be separately extracted from the DC current voltage device characteristic or, as shown below, from the low-frequency input impedance measurements of the microLED.

The device time constant $\tau = R_D C_D$ will determine the operating bandwidth.

### 4.2.1 Modulation Bandwidth Definition

The modulated optical power is linearly related to the modulated current $I_p$, whose transfer function is described by (4.6). The electro-optic bandwidth (E-O bandwidth) is defined as the frequency at which the output power is reduced by half. According to (4.6), this means $\left|H\left(\omega_c = 2\pi f_c\right)\right| = 1/2$. The E-O bandwidth is thus given by

$$f_c = \frac{\sqrt{3}}{2\pi\tau} \tag{4.8}$$

The E-O bandwidth is different from the electrical –3-dB bandwidth defined by $\left|H\left(\omega_c = 2\pi f_{3dB}\right)\right| = 1/\sqrt{2}$, and is described by [13]

$$f_{3dB} = \frac{1}{2\pi\tau} \tag{4.9}$$

### 4.2.2 Measurement Setup for E-O Modulation Bandwidth

Figure 4.3 shows the setup for measuring the modulation bandwidth of a microLED. Here, a network analyzer is used for providing an alternating-current (AC) voltage signal of 100 mV in modulation depth to combine with a direct-current (DC) voltage signal from a power supply. The mixed voltage signal drives the microLED to emit light, which is collected by a fiber and detected by a photoreceiver. Then, the modulation bandwidth is monitored by the network analyzer. The modulated signal pattern may also be monitored by an oscilloscope for making sure that it is not distorted.

### 4.2.3 Model for Small-Signal Equivalent Circuit Parameters

The differential resistance may be obtained using the definition

$$r_D = \frac{R_D}{A_c} = \frac{\partial V}{\partial J} \tag{4.10}$$

where $V$ and $J$ are the applied dc voltage and measured microLED current density, and $A_c$ is the area of the microLED. The specific resistance $r_D$ has the units of $\Omega$-cm$^2$. A model for the $J-V$ characteristics was given in Chapter 3 and is summarized here for convenience:

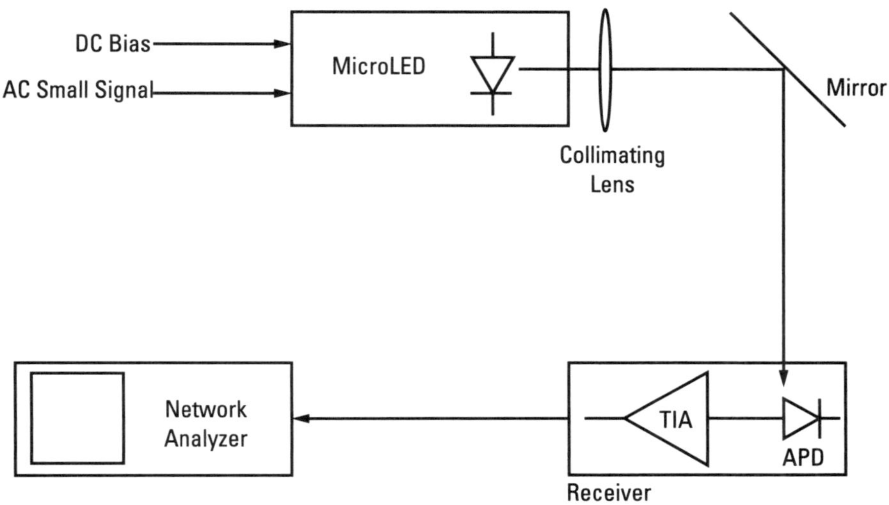


**Figure 4.3** Schematic of the measurement setup of the E-O modulation bandwidth of a microLED.

$$V \approx V_F + n\frac{kT}{q}\ln\left(\frac{J}{J_0}\right) + \frac{kT}{q}\left(\frac{J}{J_0}\right)^{\alpha} + J \bullet \rho_{TE} \tag{4.11}$$

where $V_F$ is the forward voltage; independent of $J$, $n$ is an ideality factor ($n \geq 1$), $k$ is the Boltzmann constant, $T$ is the junction temperature, $\alpha$ is supraliminal exponent ($0 < \alpha \preceq 1$), $\rho_{TE}$ is the thermionic series resistance at the heterojunction of the microLED, and $J_0$ is a characteristic current density and is given by

$$J_0 \approx \frac{\epsilon_q^2 \bullet (kT / q)^2 \bullet B}{q \bullet d^3} \tag{4.12}$$

where $d$ is the width of the quantum well, $\epsilon_q$ is the permittivity of the quantum well material, and $B$ is the radiative recombination coefficient. A typical value for $J_0$ is $0.1 - 10\text{A/cm}^2$ for GaN microLEDs.

The forward voltage is given by

$$V_F \approx E_{gq} + \frac{kT}{q}\ln\left(\frac{\epsilon_q^2 \bullet (kT / q)^2}{q^2 \bullet d^4 \bullet N_{Cq} \bullet N_{Vq}}\right) \tag{4.13}$$

where $E_{gq}$ is the energy gap of the quantum well material, $d$ is the quantum well thickness, $N_{Cq}$ is the conduction band density of states, and $N_{Vq}$ is the valence band density of states.

The differential carrier lifetime is obtained by differentiating the total recombination rate ($R_{total}$) with respect to carrier density. The total recombination rate can be approximated by the ABC model as

$$R_{total} = A \bullet n + B \bullet n \bullet (p_0 + n) + C \bullet n^2 \bullet (p_0 + n) \tag{4.14}$$

where $n$ is the injected carrier density, $A$ is the trap-assisted nonradiative recombination coefficient (also known as the SRH recombination coefficient), $B$ is the bimolecular radiative recombination coefficient, $C$ is the Auger nonradiative recombination coefficient, and $p_0$ is the active layer background doping.

The differential carrier lifetime is expressed by

$$\frac{1}{\tau} = \frac{\partial R_{total}}{\partial n} \tag{4.15}$$

The current density is related to the carrier density via the following equation:

$$J = q \bullet d \bullet \left[ A \bullet n + B \bullet n \bullet (p_0 + n) + C \bullet n^2 \bullet (p_0 + n) \right] \tag{4.16}$$

The internal quantum efficiency is given by

$$\eta = \frac{B \bullet n \bullet (p_0 + n)}{A \bullet n + B \bullet n \bullet (p_0 + n) + C \bullet n^2 \bullet (p_0 + n)} \tag{4.17}$$

It is therefore clear that there is a trade-off between efficiency and modulation bandwidth. The modulation bandwidth can be increased by increasing *A* and *C*, for example. But increasing these nonradiative recombination coefficients will also decrease the internal quantum efficiency.

The diffusion capacitance can now be obtained in terms of current density using

$$C_D = \frac{\tau}{R_D} \tag{4.18}$$

The parasitic series resistance is dominated by the specific contact resistance between the metal electrode at the cathode or anode and the semiconductor. If the specific contact resistance between the cathode and "n$^+$ GaN" is $\rho_{c,n}$ and the specific contact resistance between the anode and "p$^+$ GaN" is $\rho_{c,p}$, then the parasitic series resistance is given by

$$R_S = A_c \bullet (\rho_{c,n} + \rho_{c,p}) \tag{4.19}$$

This is independent of the current density *J*.

Now that we have expressions of the equivalent circuit parameters as a function of current density, we can calculate the E-O modulation bandwidth as a function of current density using circuit analysis. The addition of parasitic parallel capacitance is shown in Figure 4.4.

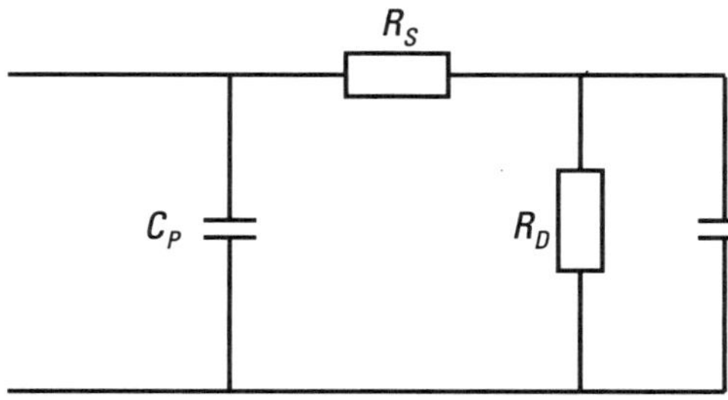


**Figure 4.4** Schematic of equivalent small-signal circuit of a microLED including parasitic parallel capacitance.

### 4.2.4 Scaling of E-O Modulation Bandwidth with MicroLED Size

It has been hypothesized that microLEDs with a diameter of less than 100 $\mu$m can achieve the higher modulation bandwidth as their *RC* time constant and differential carrier lifetime are reduced [14]. Using (4.1) through (4.19) it is now possible to calculate the modulation bandwidth from conventional circuit analysis of the circuit shown in Figure 4.4. It is found that there is a slight reduction of microLED E-O modulation bandwidth due to the series resistance increase with decreasing the microLED size. These calculations are consistent with recent data [15, 16]. The size effect appears when one plots the E-O modulation bandwidth versus energy per bit as shown in Figure 4.5 and Figure 4.6 for microLEDs with different sizes. For a given E-O modulation bandwidth, smaller microLEDs will result in much reduced energy per bit.

### 4.2.5 Scaling of E-O Modulation Bandwidth with Current Density

Without parasitic resistance and capacitance, the modulation bandwidth can be expressed by

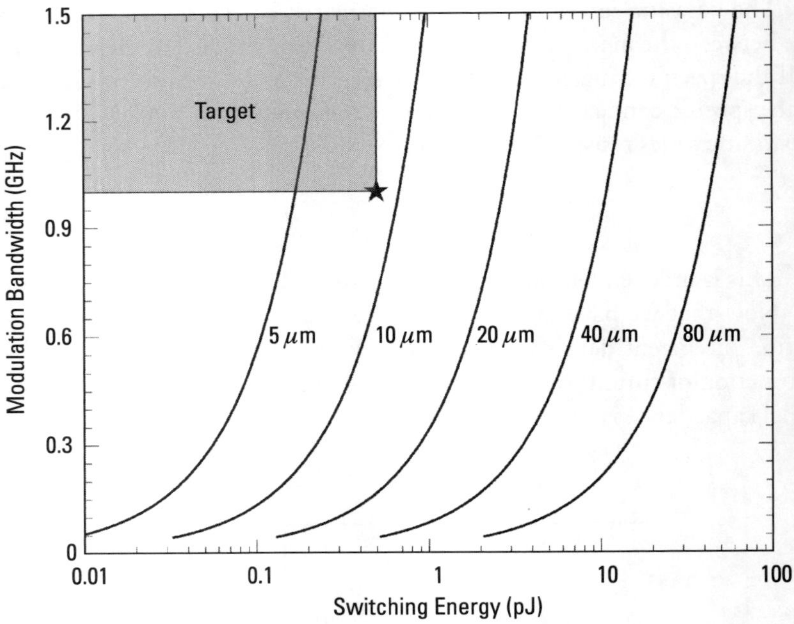


**Figure 4.5** Calculated E-O modulation bandwidth versus energy per bit for small- and large-size microLEDs. For a given microLED size, the current density is varied from 1 A/cm$^2$ to 1,000 A/cm$^2$ and the total microLED current is calculated. Then the energy per bit was calculated by dividing the electrical power (voltage x current) by twice the modulation speed for a non-return-to-zero modulation scheme. Active layer doping is zero, and a nonpolar device is assumed.

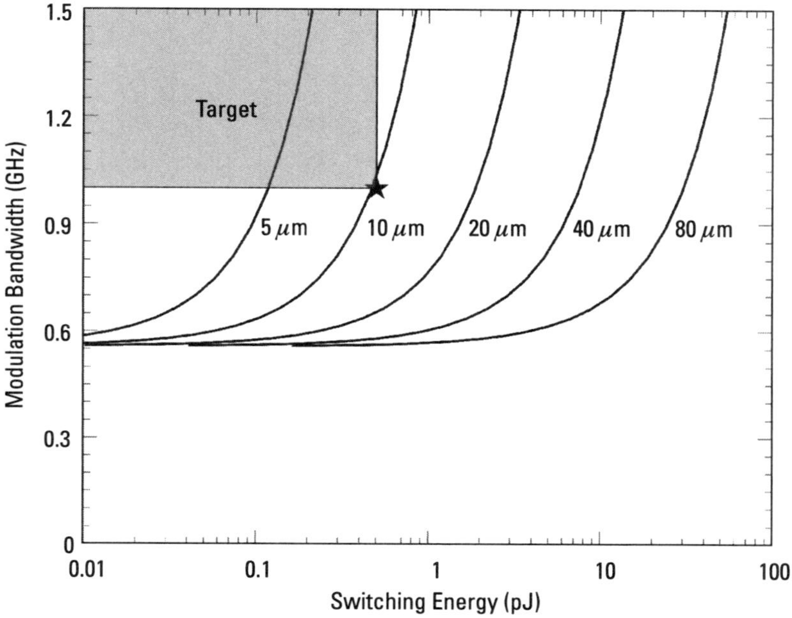


**Figure 4.6** Calculated E-O modulation bandwidth versus energy per bit for small- and large-size microLEDs. For a given microLED size, the current density is varied from 1 A/cm$^2$ to 1,000 A/cm$^2$ and the total microLED current is calculated. Then the energy per bit was calculated by dividing the electrical power (voltage x current) by twice the modulation speed for non-return-to-zero modulation scheme. Active layer doping is 10$^{19}$ cm$^{-3}$, and a nonpolar device is assumed.

$$f_c = \frac{\sqrt{3}}{2\pi}\left( A + 2B\sqrt{\frac{\eta \bullet J}{q \bullet d \bullet B}} + 3C\frac{\eta \bullet J}{q \bullet d \bullet B} \right) \tag{4.20}$$

Equation (4.22) states that the E-O modulation bandwidth approximately scales with the square root of the current density when the coefficients $A$ and $C$ are negligible.

An approximation in terms of internal quantum efficiency can be derived as [11]

$$f_c \approx \frac{\sqrt{3}}{2\pi}\left( \frac{3}{\sqrt{\eta}} - \sqrt{\eta} \right)\sqrt{\frac{B \bullet J}{q \bullet d}} \tag{4.21}$$

It should be pointed out that the internal quantum efficiency is a function of the current density.

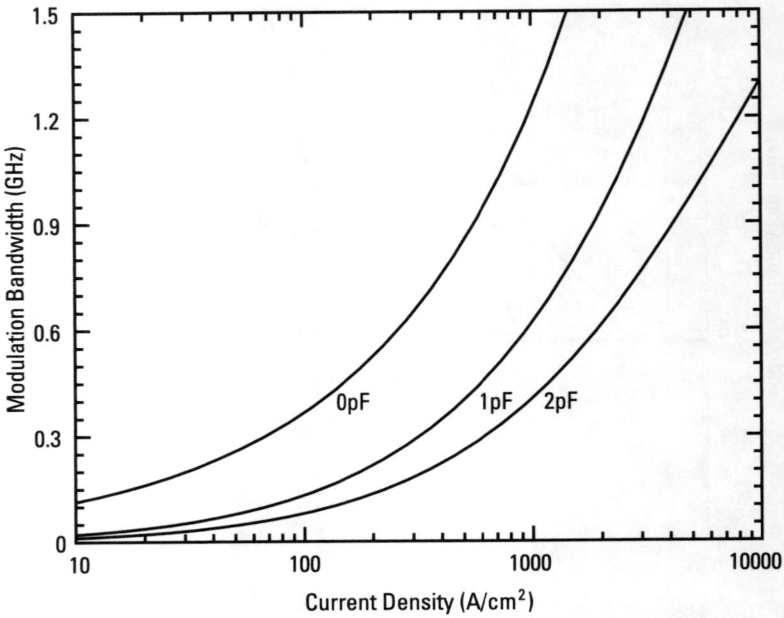


**Figure 4.7** Calculated E-O modulation bandwidth versus current density for a given set of values for the recombination coefficients *A*, *B*, and *C*. The microLED size was fixed at 5 $\mu$m. A nonpolar device is assumed. The parasitic capacitance was varied to demonstrate the importance of minimizing the parasitic parallel capacitance on obtaining an accurate measurement of the E-O modulation bandwidth.

## 4.3 Large-Signal Modulation

Large-signal modulation of microLEDs is characterized using a setup shown in Figure 4.8. Here, a pulse is applied to the microLED and light is detected with a high-speed APD connected to a TIA. An oscilloscope is used to measure the transient response.

### 4.3.1 Large-Signal Modulation Configurations

Two large signal modulation configurations will be discussed. A schematic comparison of the two large-signal bias configurations is shown in Figure 4.9. Configuration A is when a pulse is applied to the microLED starting from zero current (i.e., zero bias current). Configuration B is when a bias is applied to the microLED then a small amplitude pulse is superimposed on the bias.

### 4.3.2 Exact Numerical Model

The rate equation describing the large-signal behavior of a microLED is given by

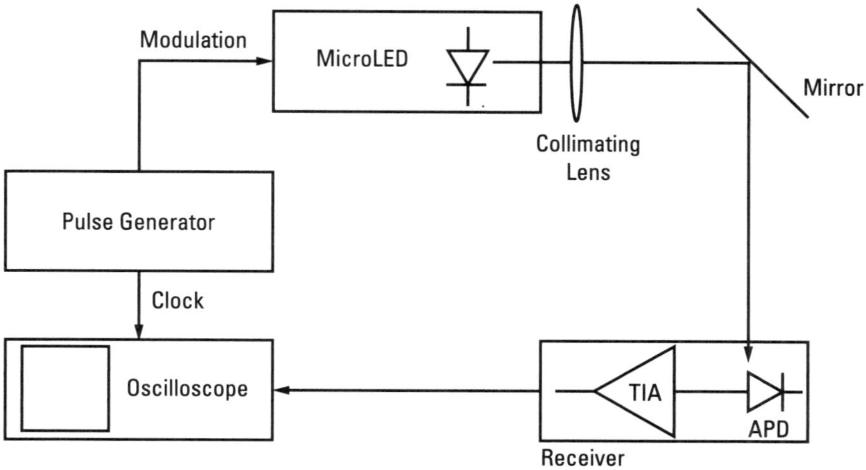


**Figure 4.8** Schematic of a setup used to characterize the large-signal response of a microLED. APD = avalanche photodiode; TIA = transimpedance amplifier.

$$\frac{dn}{dt} = \frac{J}{q \bullet d} - A \bullet n - B \bullet n \bullet (p_0 + n) - C \bullet n^2 \bullet (p_0 + n) \tag{4.22}$$

where $n$ is the volumetric electron density injected into the quantum well, $J$ is the injected current density, $q$ is the electronic charge, $d$ is the width of the quantum well, $A$ is the SRH nonradiative recombination coefficient, $B$ is the bimolecular radiative coefficient, $C$ is the Auger nonradiative recombination coefficient, and $p_0$ is the background doping in the quantum well. A numerical solution of this equation is possible. Here, MATLAB was used to solve this equation to give the carrier density $n$ as a function of time in response to one of the two modulation configurations shown in Figure 4.9. Once $n(t)$ is found, the optical power can be calculated using the definition

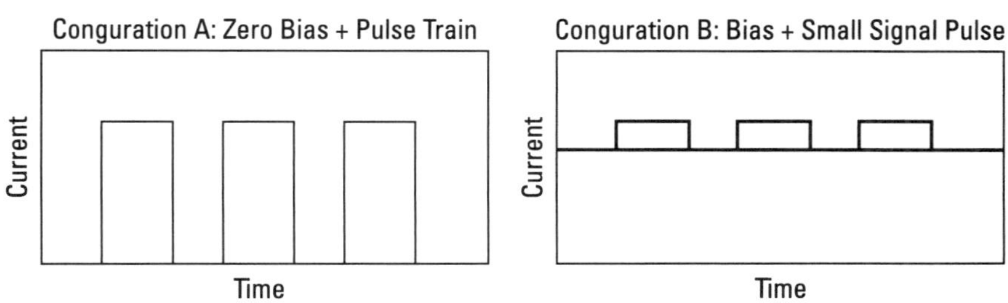


**Figure 4.9** Schematic of two driving configurations: applying a current pulse over zero bias current (configuration A), and applying a small signal current pulse over a nonzero bias current (configuration B). As explained in the text, configuration B results in 40% reduction of rise time relative to configuration A.

$$P_o(t) = q \bullet A_c \bullet d \bullet \frac{1240}{\lambda} \bullet \eta \bullet B \bullet n(t) \bullet [n(t) + p_0] \tag{4.23}$$

where $q$ is the electronic charge, $A_c$ is the microLED chip area, $d$ is the width of the quantum well, $\lambda$ is the emission wavelength in nanometers, and $B$ is the bimolecular recombination coefficient.

Example simulation of pulse response of a microLED with nonpolar growth plane and 5-$\mu$m size is shown in Figure 4.10. It is observed that the rise and fall times are greater than zero and they are slightly different from each other. The rise and fall times versus the magnitude of the current density are shown in Figure 4.11. Higher pulse current results in reduction of the rise and fall times.

### 4.3.3 Approximate Numerical Models

#### 4.3.3.1 Configuration A

If nonradiative recombination and doping of the quantum well are assumed negligible, the following rate equation describes the large-signal behavior of a microLED:

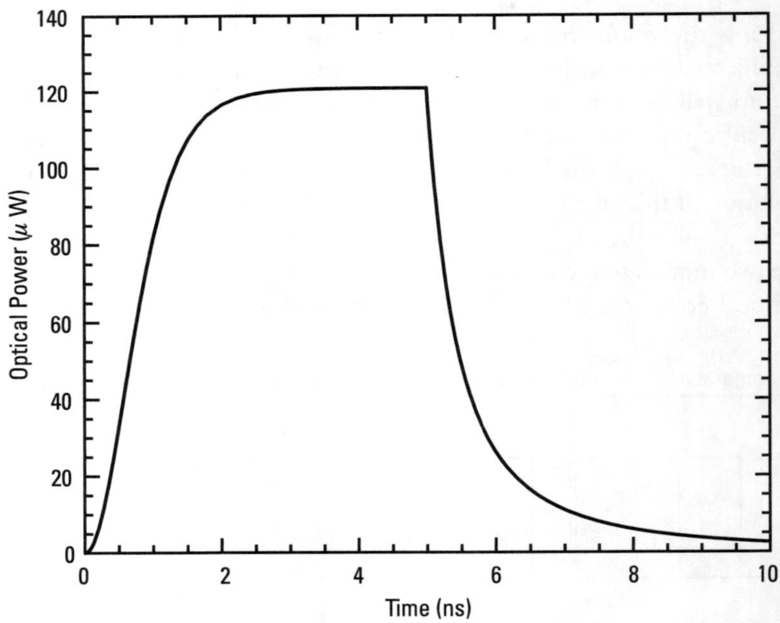


**Figure 4.10** Simulated large-signal response to a pulse of current with magnitude 1,000 A/cm$^2$ and pulse width of 5 ns. The rise and fall times are nonzero and they are not equal for this example.

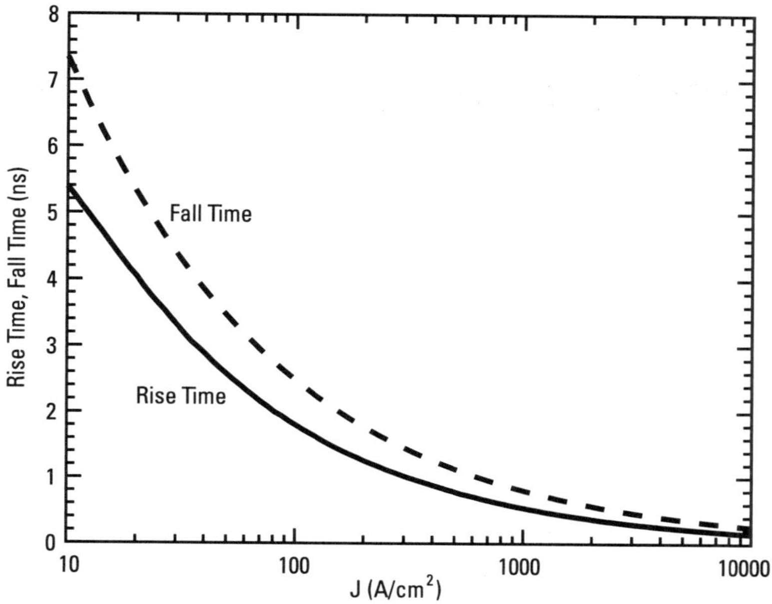


**Figure 4.11** Numerically calculated rise time and fall time versus pulse current density for a nonpolar device. The microLED size was fixed at 5 $\mu$m.

$$\frac{dn}{dt} = \frac{J}{q \bullet d} - B \bullet n^2 \tag{4.24}$$

where $n$ is the volumetric electron density in the quantum well, $J$ is the injected current density, $q$ is the electronic charge, $d$ is the width of the quantum well, and $B$ is the bimolecular radiative recombination coefficient. The first term on the right-hand side is the injection rate of carriers into the quantum well, and the second term is the recombination rate of carriers inside the quantum well. The solution for (4.22) when a step-function current with amplitude $J$ and starting from zero current is injected into the microLED is given by

$$n(t) = \frac{d}{2B} \tanh\left(\sqrt{\frac{J \bullet B}{q \bullet d}} \bullet t\right) \tag{4.25}$$

The optical output power is given by

$$P_o(t) = q \bullet A_c \bullet d \bullet \frac{1240}{\lambda} \bullet B \bullet \left[n(t)\right]^2 \tag{4.26}$$

Which can be written explicitly as a function of time as

$$P_o(t) = q \bullet A_c \bullet d \bullet \frac{1240}{\lambda} \bullet B \bullet \left(\frac{d}{2B}\right)^2 \tanh^2\left(\sqrt{\frac{J \bullet B}{q \bullet d}} \bullet t\right) \tag{4.27}$$

This can be used to estimate the rise as [17]

$$t_r \approx 1.5 \bullet \sqrt{\frac{q \bullet d}{J \bullet B}} \tag{4.28}$$

The E-O modulation bandwidth is related to the rise time via the relationship

$$f_c \approx \frac{\sqrt{3} \bullet \ln 9}{2\pi \bullet t_r} = \frac{0.7}{t_r} \tag{4.29}$$

#### 4.3.3.2 Configuration B

When a microLED is modulated by applying a bias current $J_b$ and a small pulse with amplitude $\Delta J$, the rate equation for the modulated carrier concentration $\Delta n$ (imposed on a bias carrier density of $n_b$) is

$$\frac{d(\Delta n)}{dt} \approx \frac{\Delta J}{q \bullet d} - (2 \bullet B \bullet n_b) \bullet \Delta n \tag{4.30}$$

where

$$n_b = \sqrt{\frac{J_b}{q \bullet d \bullet B}} \tag{4.31}$$

$$n_\infty = n_b + \Delta n_\infty = \sqrt{\frac{J_b + \Delta J}{q \bullet d \bullet B}} \tag{4.32}$$

The solution takes the form

$$\Delta n(t) = a \bullet \exp\left(-\frac{t}{\tau_{ss}}\right) + b \quad (4.33)$$

where $a$ and $b$ are constants, and

$$\tau_{ss} = \frac{1}{2 \bullet B \bullet n_b} = \frac{1}{2}\sqrt{\frac{q \bullet d}{J_b \bullet B}} \quad (4.34)$$

The initial condition is $\Delta n(0) = 0$. Substituting (4.31) and (4.30) into (4.28) we get

$$a = \sqrt{\frac{J_b + \Delta J}{q \bullet d \bullet B}} - \sqrt{\frac{\eta \bullet J_b}{q \bullet d \bullet B}} \quad (4.35)$$

The transient response is thus given by

$$\Delta n(t) = \left[\sqrt{\frac{J_b + \Delta J}{q \bullet d \bullet B}} - \sqrt{\frac{J_b}{q \bullet d \bullet B}}\right] \bullet \left[1 - \exp\left(-\frac{t}{\tau_{ss}}\right)\right] \quad (4.36)$$

The rise time is obtained from

$$t_r = \ln 9 \bullet \tau_{ss} \approx 1.1 \bullet \sqrt{\frac{q \bullet d}{J_b \bullet B}} \quad (4.37)$$

Comparing (4.37) to (4.28) we see that the rise time decreased by approximately 40% if small-signal modulation on top of a bias current is used instead of using a pulse that starts at zero initial current. This conclusion was verified by numerical calculations explained earlier.

## 4.4 Technological Implications

Throughout the above mathematical models, it has become clear that improving the modulation speed at a given current density (i.e., energy consumption) is dependent on the quantum well thickness and the bimolecular radiative recombination coefficient. As shown in Chapter 2, the same two parameters also impact the internal quantum efficiency of a microLED. $B$ depends on the wavefunction overlap, which is limited by the polarization field in polar devices. Several technological approaches were discussed to minimize or eliminate the polarization field. These include semipolar or nonpolar orientations, N-polar orientation, cubic GaN, graded gap active layer, and doped barriers.

### 4.4.1 Semipolar or Nonpolar Orientations

MicroLEDs on nonpolar and semipolar orientations are potential candidates for achieving higher bandwidth at lower current density due to their larger electron-hole wavefunction overlaps and shorter carrier lifetimes [18–22]. Non-c-plane orientations, including nonpolar and semipolar orientations, exhibit reduced or eliminated internal electric fields in quantum well devices. The reduction or elimination of this field in nonpolar and semipolar crystal orientations can result in improved device performance. This is shown with simulations in Figure 4.12. However, the lack of native bulk substrates has limited the application of these crystal orientations. Moreover, nonpolar InGaN growth has proven challenging [22].

### 4.4.2 N-Polar Orientation

MicroLEDs on nitrogen-polar orientation are potential candidates for achieving higher bandwidth at lower current density due to their polarization field being opposite to the applied external forward field, and thus the existence of

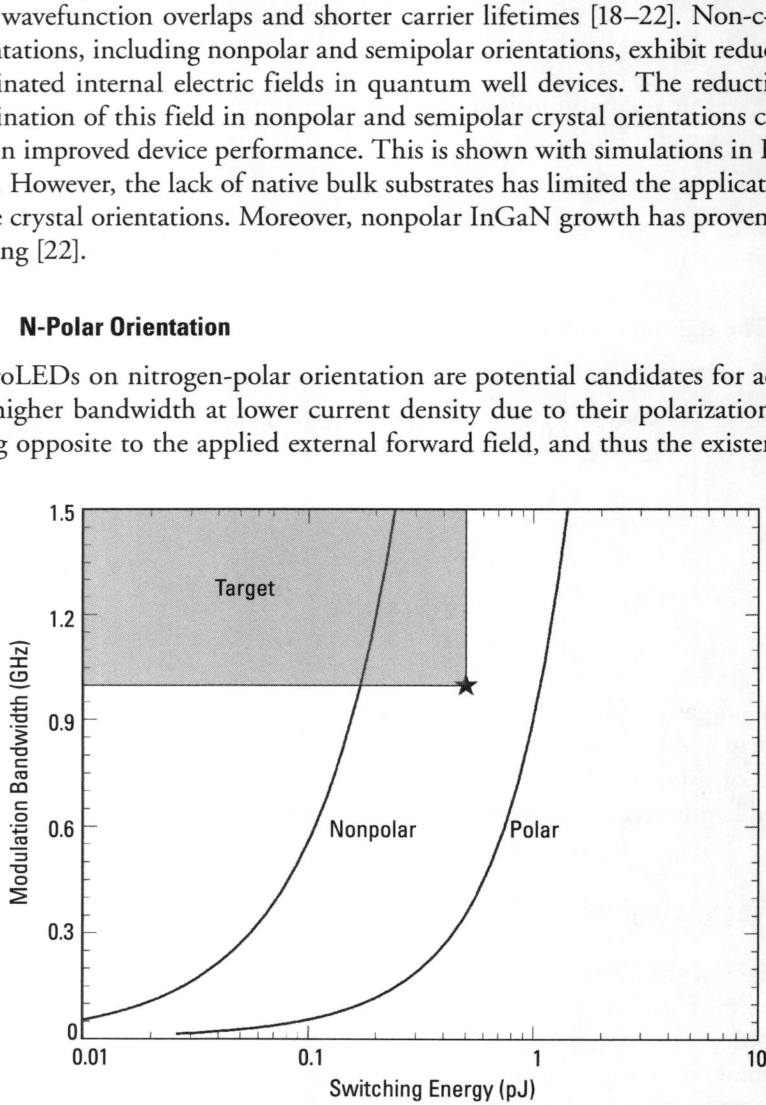


**Figure 4.12** Calculated E-O modulation bandwidth versus energy per bit polar and nonpolar devices. A desired target box is shown in gray. A nonpolar device easily meets the requirements for E-O modulation bandwidth and switching energy.

a bias point where electron-hole wavefunction overlap hits a peak [23–28]. At this point, the E-O modulation bandwidth can be maximized. Despite intensive research, the growth of micrometer-thick high-quality N-polar GaN based materials remains challenging [29–33]. For example, growth with smooth surface morphology is relatively harder for the N-polar surface. It is also known that under a fixed growth condition, the N-polar growth exhibits higher O incorporation and much lower Mg incorporation by almost an order of magnitude compared to metal-polar surface growth, which can make p-doping of N-polar GaN difficult.

### 4.4.3 Cubic GaN

MicroLEDs with cubic GaN are potential candidates for achieving higher bandwidth at lower current density due to their zero polarization field, larger electron-hole wavefunction overlaps, and shorter carrier lifetimes. The <001> direction (i.e., the direction of growth on the {001} crystal face) is not only free of spontaneous polarization, but also free of piezoelectric polarization. The bandgap of the cubic nitrides is slightly smaller than that of the wurtzite polytypes, and therefore the band-edge emission in bulk crystals of cubic InGaN has longer wavelength than in wurtzite crystals with the same indium concentration. The general absence of internal electric fields in c-GaN LEDs can eliminate the blueshift associated with the QCSE [34–36]. However, approaches to avoid the preferential [0001] wurtzite crystal growth are challenging as they often produce a reduced crystal quality frequently combined with comparably lower deposition rates [37–39].

### 4.4.4 Core-Shell Nanowires

MicroLEDs made with arrays of core-shell nanowires are potential candidates for achieving higher bandwidth at lower current density due to their zero polarization field, larger electron-hole wavefunction overlaps, and shorter carrier lifetimes [40]. One method to alleviate the problems with planar nonpolar device fabrication is to use GaN nanowires [41–45]. The diameter of the nanowires is typically small enough that the threading dislocation density is significantly reduced, increasing the IQE and lifetime. By controlling the crystallographic orientation of the GaN nanowires, nonpolar or semipolar planes can be used for device fabrication, thereby reducing the effect of the QCSE, which, in turn, can also lead to improvements in the IQE [46].

### 4.4.5 Graded Indium in InGaN

MicroLEDs made with a graded bandgap of the InGaN quantum well are potential candidates for achieving higher bandwidth at lower current density due to their zero polarization field, larger electron-hole wavefunction overlaps, and shorter carrier lifetimes [40]. Adjusting the shape of the bandgap of the quantum well layer has been proposed to minimize the influence of the polarization field by spreading the polarization-induced sheet charge into a quasi-volume space charge [47–49].

### 4.4.6 Doped Barriers

Theoretical and experimental efforts have shown that it is possible to reduce the internal electric fields in the c-plane InGaN/GaN QWs through the use of doped barriers [50–55]. Placing heavily doped p- and n-type GaN barriers close to the QW leads to an increase in the p–n junction electric field, which counteracts the opposite polarization-induced electric field in the QW, resulting in a smaller net internal electric field, thereby improving the electron–hole wavefunction overlap and IQE of the microLED. The technique has been employed in thick and thin c-plane single QW microLEDs, and improved efficiency droop has been observed.

### 4.4.7 Axial Nanowire (Disk-in-Wire) Architecture

A much reduced polarization field has been predicted by theory and realized by experiments using axial nanowire architecture [56–61]. Here, a nanowire with flat-top forming an n-GaN c-plane growth template is grown out of a silicon or sapphire wafer using selective area epitaxial growth. Then MBE is used to grow the barrier and quantum well structure, and finally the p-GaN contact layer. When the diameter of the nanowire is less than a critical value, strain is relaxed, which is the root cause for the piezoelectric field in conventional c-plane light-emitting diode structures.

### 4.4.8 Doped Active Layer

The simulated large-signal pulse response of a microLED with zero and nonzero background doping is shown in Figure 4.13. The simulations were done using a numerical solution of the rate equation given by (4.22). Higher background doping results in smaller rise and fall times in response to a current pulse.

### 4.4.9 Thin Quantum Well

Thinner quantum well results in significant improvement of the switching energy for a given E-O modulation bandwidth, as shown in Figure 4.15. Thinner quantum well also means more efficient recombination of carriers due to better wavefunction overlap and higher volumetric density of carriers in the quantum well.

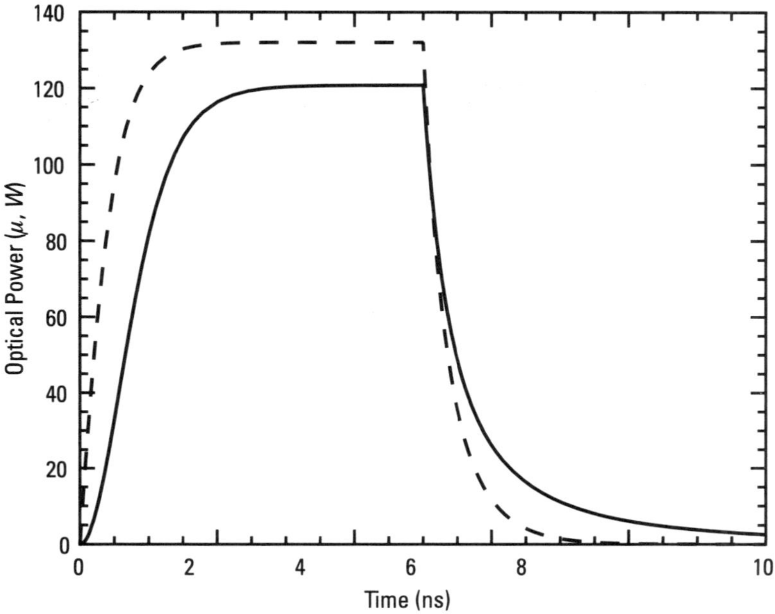


**Figure 4.13** Calculated pulse response of a microLED for zero (solid) and nonzero (dotted) active layer background doping. The current density was 100 A/cm$^2$.

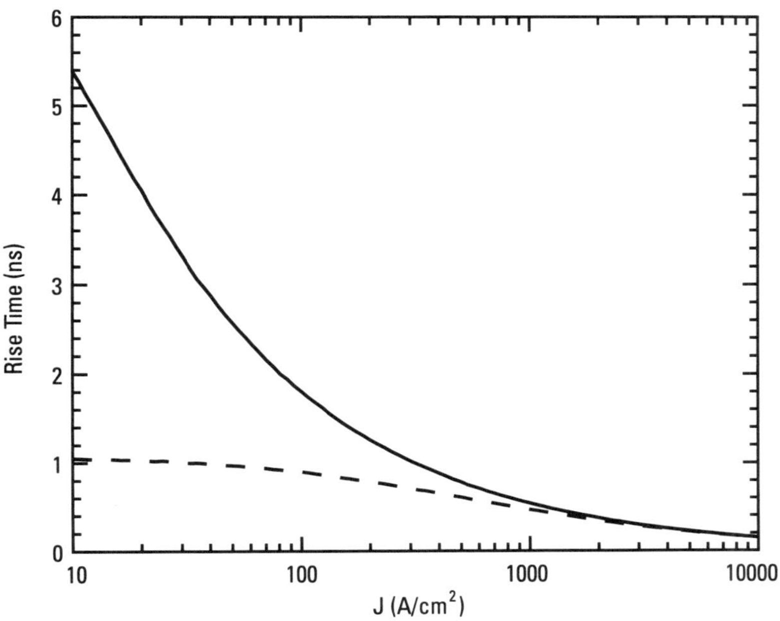


**Figure 4.14** Calculated rise time versus pulse magnitude current density for microLEDs with zero (solid line) and nonzero (dotted line) active layer background doping.

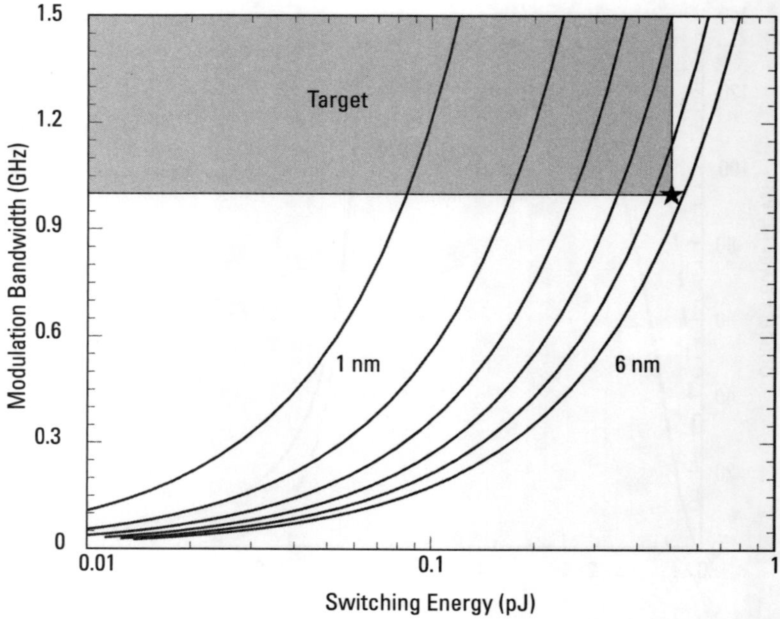


**Figure 4.15** Calculated E-O modulation bandwidth versus energy per bit for microLEDs with different quantum well width (1 to 6 nm). Thinner quantum well results in large reduction in switching energy for a given value of E-O modulation bandwidth.

# References


[1] Pezeshki, B., R. Kalman, A. Tselikov, and C. Danesh, "High Speed Light MicroLEDs for Visible Wavelength Communication," in *Light-Emitting Devices, Materials, and Applications XXV*, 2021.

[2] Pezeshki, B., F. Khoeini, A. Tselikov, R. Kalman, C. Danesh, and E. Afifi, "LED-Array Based Optical Interconnects for Chip-to-Chip Communications with Integrated CMOS Drivers, Detectors, and Circuitry," in *Optical Interconnects XXII*, 2022.

[3] Pezeshki, B., A. Tselikov, R. Kalman, and E. Afifi, "Sub 1pJ/bit Dense Optical Interconnects Using MicroLEDs on CMOS Transceiver ICs," in *Light-Emitting Devices, Materials, and Applications XXVII*, 2023.

[4] Pezeshki, B., A. Tselikov, R. Kalman, and C. Danesh, "Wide and Parallel LED-Based Optical Links Using Multi-Core Fiber for Chip-to-Chip Communication," in *Optical Fiber Communication Conference*, 2021.

[5] Pezeshki, B., F. Khoeini, A. Tselikov, R. Kalman, C. Danesh, and E. Afifi, "MicroLED Array-Based Optical Links Using Imaging Fiber for Chip-to-Chip Communications," in *Optical Fiber Communication Conference*, 2022.

[6] Rashidi, A., M. Nami, M. Monavarian, et al., "Differential Carrier Lifetime and Transport Effects in Electrically Injected III-Nitride Light-Emitting Diodes," *Journal of Applied Physics*, Vol. 122, No. 3, 2017.

[7] Kisacik, R., A. Yalcinkaya, A. Pusane, T. Baykas, and M. Uysal, "Characterization of LEDs for Visible-Light Communications," *Optical Engineering,* Vol. 60, No. 2, 2021, pp. 024102–024102.

[8] Cheung, W., P. Edwards, and G. French, "Determination of LED Equivalent Circuits Using Network Analyser Measurements," in *1998 Conference on Optoelectronic and Microelectronic Materials and Devices,* 1998.

[9] Rashidi, A., M. Monavarian, A. Aragon, et al., "High-Speed Nonpolar InGaN/GaN LEDs for Visible-Light Communication," *IEEE Photonics Technology Letters,* Vol. 29, No. 4, 2017, pp. 381–384.

[10] Song, P., Z. Wu, X. An, and J. Wang, "Energy Efficiency Analysis of Light-Emitting Diodes with High Modulation Bandwidth," *IEEE Electron Device Letters,* Vol. 42, No. 7, 2021, pp. 1025–1028.

[11] Ryu, H., and G. Ryu, "Small Signal Analysis of the Modulation Bandwidth of Light-Emitting Diodes for Visible Light Communication," *Optics & Laser Technology,* Vol. 152, 2022, p. 108170.

[12] Chen, Z., J. He, Z. Chen, J. Xu, and H. Li, "Impedance Characteristics of High Speed VCSELs," in *2021 International Conference on Optical Instruments and Technology: Advanced Laser Technology and Applications,* 2022.

[13] Yu, L., L. Wang, Z. Hao, Y. Luo, et al., "High-Speed Micro-LEDs for Visible Light Communication: Challenges and Progresses," *Semiconductor Science and Technology,* Vol. 37, No. 2, 2021, p. 023001.

[14] Yang, W., S. Zhang, J. McKendry, et al., "Size-Dependent Capacitance Study on InGaN-Based Micro-Light-Emitting Diodes," *Journal of Applied Physics,* Vol. 116, No. 4, 2014.

[15] Haemmer, M., B. Roycroft, M. Akhter, et al., "Size-Dependent Bandwidth of Semipolar Light-Emitting-Diodes," *IEEE Photonics Technology Letters,* Vol. 30, No. 5, 2018, pp. 439-442.

[16] Tian, P., J. McKendry, J. Herrnsdorf, et al., "Micro-LED Based Optical Wireless Communications Systems," in *Semiconductors and Semimetals* Vol. 106, Elsevier, 2021, pp. 281–321.

[17] Windisch, R., A. Knobloch, M. Kuijk, et al., "Large-Signal-Modulation of High-Efficiency Light-Emitting Diodes for Optical Communication," *IEEE Journal of Quantum Electronics,* Vol. 36, No. 12, 2000, pp. 1445–1453.

[18] Monavarian, M., A. Rashidi, A. Aragon, et al., "Impact of Crystal Orientation on the Modulation Bandwidth of InGaN/GaN Light-Emitting Diodes," *Applied Physics Letters,* Vol. 112, No. 4, 2018.

[19] Chen, S., Y. Huang, Y. Chang, et al., "High-Bandwidth Green Semipolar (20–21) InGaN/GaN Micro Light-Emitting Diodes for Visible Light Communication," *ACS Photonic,* Vol. 7, No. 8, 2020, pp. 2228–2235.

[20] Rashidi, A., M. Monavarian, A. Aragon, et al., "High-Speed Nonpolar InGaN/GaN LEDs for Visible-Light Communication," *IEEE Photonics Technology Letters,* Vol. 29, No. 4, 2017, pp. 381–384.

[21] Rashidi, A., M. Monavarian, A. Aragon, A. Rishinaramangalam, and D. Feezell, "Nonpolar m-Plane InGaN/GaN Micro-Scale Light-Emitting Diode with 1.5 GHz Modulation Bandwidth," *IEEE Electron Device Letters*, Vol. 39, No. 4, 2018, pp. 520–523.

[22] Monavarian, M., A. Rashidi, and D. Feezell, "A Decade of Nonpolar and Semipolar III-Nitrides: A Review of Successes and Challenges," *physica status solidi (a)*, Vol. 216, No. 1, 2019, p. 1800628.

[23] Feng, S., P. Liao, B. Leung, J. Han, F. Yang, and H. Wang, "Efficient Carrier Relaxation and Fast Carrier Recombination of N-Polar InGaN/GaN Light Emitting Diodes," *Journal of Applied Physics*, Vol. 118, No. 4, 2015.

[24] Muthuraj, V., C. Reilly, T. Mates, S. Keller, S. Nakamura, and S. DenBaars, "Inverted N-Polar Blue and Blue-Green Light Emitting Diodes with High Power Grown by Metalorganic Chemical Vapor Deposition," *Applied Physics Letters*, Vol. 120, No. 10, 2022.

[25] Akyol, F., D. Nath, E. Gür, P. Park, and S. Rajan, "N-Polar III–Nitride Green (540 nm) Light Emitting Diode," *Japanese Journal of Applied Physics*, Vol. 50, No. 5R, 2011, p. 052101.

[26] Zhuang, Z., D. Iida, and K. Ohkawa, "Enhanced Performance of N-Polar AlGaN-Based Deep-Ultraviolet Light-Emitting Diodes," *Optics Express*, Vol. 28, No. 21, 2020, pp. 30423–30431.

[27] Deng, G., Y. Zhang, Y. Yu, et al., "Simulation and Fabrication of N-Polar GaN-Based Blue-Green Light-Emitting Diodes with p-Type AlGaN Electron Blocking Layer," *Journal of Materials Science: Materials in Electronics*, Vol. 29, 2018, pp. 9321–9325.

[28] Keller, S., H. Li, M. Laurent, et al., "Recent Progress in Metal-Organic Chemical Vapor Deposition of N-Polar Group-III Nitrides," *Semiconductor Science and Technology*, Vol. 29, No. 11, 2014, p. 113001.

[29] Muthuraj, V., C. Reilly, T. Mates, S. Keller, S. Nakamura, and S. DenBaars, "Inverted N-Polar Blue and Blue-Green Light Emitting Diodes with High Power Grown by Metalorganic Chemical Vapor Deposition," *Applied Physics Letters*, Vol. 120, No. 10, 2022, p. 101104.

[30] Ptak, A., T. Myers, L. Romano, C.G. Van de Walle, and J. Northrup, "Magnesium Incorporation in GaN Grown by Molecular-Beam Epitaxy," *Applied Physics Letters*, Vol. 78, No. 3, 2001, pp. 285–287.

[31] Sumiya, M., K. Yoshimura, K. Ohtsuka, and S. Fuke, "Dependence of Impurity Incorporation on the Polar Direction of GaN Film Growth," *Applied Physics Letters*, Vol. 76, No. 15, 2000, pp. 2098–2100.

[32] Pristovsek, M., I. Furuhashi, and P. Pampili, "Growth of N-Polar GaN in Metal–Organic Vapour Phase Epitaxy on Sapphire," *Crystals*, Vol. 13, No. 7, 2023, p. 1072.

[33] Ptak, A., L. Holbert, L. Ting, et al., "Controlled Oxygen Doping of GaN Using Plasma Assisted Molecular-Beam Epitaxy," *Applied Physics Letters*, Vol. 79, No. 17, 2001, pp. 2740–2742.

[34] Lee, J., J. Leburton, and C. Bayram, "Design Tradeoffs Between Traditional Hexagonal and Emerging Cubic InXGa(1–X)N/GaN-Based Green Light-Emitting Diodes," *Journal of the Optical Society of America B*, Vol. 40, No. 5, 2023, pp. 1017–1023.

[35] Lee, L., "Cubic Zincblende Gallium Nitride for Green-Wavelength Light-Emitting Diodes," *Materials Science and Technology*, Vol. 33, No. 14, 2017, pp. 1570–1583.

[36] Binks, D., P. Dawson, R. Oliver, and D. Wallis, "Cubic GaN and InGan/GaN Quantum Wells," *Applied Physics Reviews*, Vol. 9, No. 4, 2022.

[37] Gundimeda, A., M. Frentrup, S. Fairclough, M. Kappers, D. Wallis, and R. Oliver, "Investigation of Wurtzite Formation in MOVPE-Grown Zincblende GaN Epilayers on AlxGa1- xN Nucleation Layers," *Journal of Applied Physics*, Vol. 131, No. 11, 2022, pp. 115703-1.

[38] Lee, J., Y. Chiu, M. Johar, and C. Bayram, "Structural and Optical Properties of Cubic GaN on U-Grooved Si (100)," *Applied Physics Letters*, Vol. 121, No. 3, 2022.

[39] Meier, F., M. Littmann, J. Bürger, et al., "Selective Area Growth of Cubic Gallium Nitride in Nanoscopic Silicon Dioxide Masks," *physica status solidi (b)*, 2022, p. 2200508.

[40] Nami, M., "Nanowire-Based Light-Emitting Diodes: A New Path Towards High-Speed Visible Light Communication," Doctoral Dissertation, The University of New Mexico, 2017.

[41] D. Feezell, A. Rashidi, M. Monavarian, et al., "III-Nitride High-Speed Optoelectronics," *2019 Device Research Conference (DRC)*, 2019, pp. 77–78.

[42] Bi, Z., Z. Chen, F. Danesh, and L. Samuelson, "From NanoLEDs to the Realization of RGB-Emitting MicroLEDs," in *Semiconductors and Semimetals*, Elsevier, 2021, pp. 223–251.

[43] Nami, M., I. Stricklin, K. DaVico, et al., "Carrier Dynamics and Electro-Optical Characterization of High-Performance GaN/InGaN Core-Shell Nanowire Light-Emitting Diodes," *Scientific Reports*, Vol. 8, No. 1, 2018, p. 501.

[44] Nami, M., A. Rashidi, M. Monavarian, et al., "Electrically Injected GHz-Class GaN/InGaN Core–Shell Nanowire-Based $\mu$LEDs: Carrier Dynamics and Nanoscale Homogeneity," *ACS Photonics*, Vol. 6, No. 7, 2019, pp. 1618–1625.

[45] Tchoulfian, P., U. Steegmueller, B. Amstatt, M. Broell, and P. Gilet, "GaN-on-Silicon Nanowire Technology for MicroLED Devices," *SPIE Light-Emitting Devices, Materials, and Applications XXVII*, Vol. 12441, 2023, pp. 49–52.

[46] A. Rishinaramangalam, M. Nami, M. Fairchild, et al., "Semipolar InGaN/GaN Nanostructure Light-Emitting Diodes on c-Plane Sapphire," *Applied Physics Express*, Vol. 9, No. 3, 2016, p. 032101.

[47] Chuang, S., and D. Ahn, "Optical Transitions in a Parabolic Quantum Well with an Applied Electric Field—Analytical Solutions," *Journal of Applied Physics*, Vol. 65, No. 7, 1989, pp. 2822–2826.

[48] Zhang, Z., W. Liu, Z. Ju, et al., "InGaN/GaN Multiple Quantum-Well Light-Emitting Diodes with a Grading InN Composition Suppressing the Auger Recombination," *Applied Physics Letters*, Vol. 105, No. 3, 2014.

[49] Karan, H., A. Biswas, and M. Saha, "Improved Performance of InGaN/GaN MQW LEDs with Trapezoidal Wells and Gradually Thinned Barrier Layers Towards Anode," *Optics Communications*, Vol. 400, 2017, pp. 89–95.

[50] V. Fiorentini, F. Bernardini, F. D. Sala, A. D. Carlo and P. Lugli, "Effects of Macroscopic Polarization in III-V Nitride Multiple Quantum Wells," *Physical Review B,* Vol. 60, No. 12, p. 8849, 1999.

[51] Young, N., R. Farrell, S. Oh, et al., "Polarization Field Screening in Thick (0001) InGaN/GaN Single Quantum Well Light-Emitting Diodes," *Applied Physics Letters,* Vol. 108, No. 6, 2016.

[52] Franssen, G., T. Suski, P. Perlin, et al., "Fully-Screened Polarization-Induced Electric Fields in Blue/Violet InGaN/GaN Light-Emitting Devices Grown on Bulk GaN," *Applied Physics Letters,* Vol. 87, No. 4, 2005, p. 041109.

[53] Chow, Y. C., C. Lynsky, F. Wu, et al., "Reduction of Efficiency Droop in c-Plane InGaN/GaN Light-Emitting Diodes Using a Thick Single Quantum Well with Doped Barriers," *Applied Physics Letters,* Vol. 119, No. 22, 2021, p. 221102.

[54] Chow, Y. C., C. Lynsky, S. Nakamura, S. P. DenBaars, C. Weisbuch, and J. S. Speck, "Impact of Doped Barriers on the Recombination Coefficients of c-plane InGaN/GaN Single Quantum Well Light-Emitting Diodes," *Applied Physics Letters,* Vol. 121, No. 18, 2022, p. 181102.

[55] Chow, Y., C. Lynsky, S. Nakamura, S. DenBaars, C. Weisbuch, and J. Speck, "Low-Efficiency-Droop c-Plane InGaN/GaN Light-Emitting Diodes through the Use of Thick Single Quantum Wells and Doped Barriers," *Journal of Applied Physics,* Vol. 133, No. 14, 2023, p. 143101.

[56] Park, B., J. Lee, C. Koch, M. Wölz, L. Geelhaar, and S. Oh, "High-Resolution Mapping of Strain Partitioning and Relaxation in InGaN/GaN Nanowire Heterostructures," *Advanced Science,* Vol. 9, No. 22, 2022, p. 2200323.

[57] Pandey, A., Y. Xiao, M. Reddeppa, et al., "A Red-Emitting Micrometer Scale LED with External Quantum Efficiency > 8%," *Applied Physics Letters,* Vol. 122, No. 15, 2023.

[58] Pandey, A., J. Min, M. Reddeppa, et al., "An Ultrahigh Efficiency Excitonic Micro-LED," *Nano Letters,* Vol. 23, No. 5, 2023, pp. 1680–1687.

[59] Guo, W., M. Zhang, A. Banerjee, and P. Bhattacharya, "Catalyst-Free InGaN/GaN Nanowire Light Emitting Diodes Grown on (001) Silicon by Molecular Beam Epitaxy," *Nano letters,* Vol. 10, No. 9, 2010, pp. 3355–3359.

[60] Pandey, A., J. Min, Y. Malhotra, et al., "Strain-Engineered N-Polar InGaN Nanowires: Towards High-Efficiency Red LEDs on the Micrometer Scale," *Photonics Research,* Vol. 10, No. 12, 2022, pp. 2809–2815.

[61] Glas, F., "Critical Dimensions for the Plastic Relaxation of Strained Axial Heterostructures in Free-Standing Nanowires," *Physical Review B,* Vol. 74, No. 12, 2006, p. 121302.

# 5

# MicroLED Display System

## 5.1 Introduction

A microLED ($\mu$LED) display is a type of display technology that uses a matrix of individually switched self-illuminating inorganic diodes that can be controlled and lit without a master backlight. Inorganic microLEDs have a number of potential advantages over OLEDs for display applications, which include the possibility of high brightness. Pioneering inorganic microLED microdisplays have been demonstrated by the research group at Kansas State University [1] and augmented by others.

A microLED display is similar in architecture to an OLED display. They are both emissive displays where the display is made of a two-dimensional array of pixels. Each pixel is composed of at least three microscopic-size light emitters (LEDs) that are controlled by electronic circuits for each pixel. For RGB displays, the three emitters produce red, green, and blue lights with different intensities so that the mixing of the three emissions produces a specific color according to the image to be displayed. The image data is provided to the 2D array of pixels from data drivers along the columns of the 2D array. A particular pixel is enabled using row scanning signals provided by scan drivers external to the 2D pixel array. A typical display architecture is shown in Figure 5.1.

The display device using microLEDs can be advantageously used in a variety of devices, such as smartwatches, mobile devices, virtual reality devices,

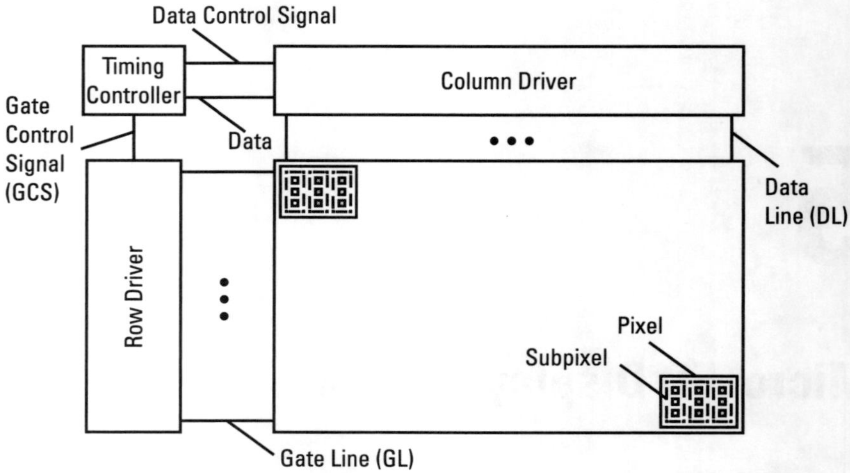


**Figure 5.1** Architecture of a microLED display showing a 2D array of pixels. Gate lines select a row, and a column line provides image data to the pixel. A pixel is composed of three subpixels. A subpixel is composed of one emitter (red, green, or blue) that is connected to a pixel driver circuit. A pixel driver circuit is enabled by row drivers and image data is provided from column drivers.

augmented reality devices, and flexible devices, since their size and weight can be reduced due to such microLEDs being used as pixels.

For example, a microLED display device may be implemented by growing microLEDs on a sapphire or silicon substrate, removing the microLED from the sapphire or silicon substrate, and transferring the removed microLED to a transistor substrate (also known as display backplane).

When a microLED is implemented using such a transfer method, there is a problem because the microLED is very small, so the transfer process may be relatively complicated, making it difficult to improve the precision and yield of the process.

Further, since for production of light, the transfer process is performed after microLEDs for red (R), green (G), and blue (B) lights are grown, the number of transfer steps and process times increases, causing increased defects due to misalignments, which are problematic.

In this chapter, we will discuss the advantage of microLED displays for reducing power consumption of the platform using it (e.g., smartphone or a laptop) using a physics-based model. We will also discuss challenges and potential solutions associated with the manufacturing yield using a physics-based yield model. Two key methods of transferring the microLEDs from growth wafer to a display backplane are discussed, highlighting the advantages and disadvantages.

## 5.2 Battery Gap in Mobile Devices

In laptop and smartphone displays, the display consumes around 50% to 70% of the total system power. This presents a major challenge for battery lifetime. A survey of smartphone products over the past 20 years shows a gap between what a battery can supply and the power demand of a device (see Figure 5.2). This data-driven battery gap requires power efficient displays with about 2× reduction in display power.

The display power efficiency depends on the use condition for each device. For example, laptop applications use largely white backgrounds, which means that the emitter power in the case of emissive displays dominate power consumption. On the other hand, smartphones rely less on white background and the lm/W metric is influenced more equally between the emitter power and display electronics power. High emitter power efficiency is therefore very important to overall display power consumption, especially for outdoor use when the required luminance is high. Currently, mobile displays made of OLEDs have power efficiency of ~13 lm/W under all-white condition, as shown in Figure 5.3. It is observed that lm/W efficiency has saturated over the past 7 years. Displays made of GaN microLEDs promise ~25 lm/W under an all-white condition. The promised higher efficiency relies on fundamental differences in

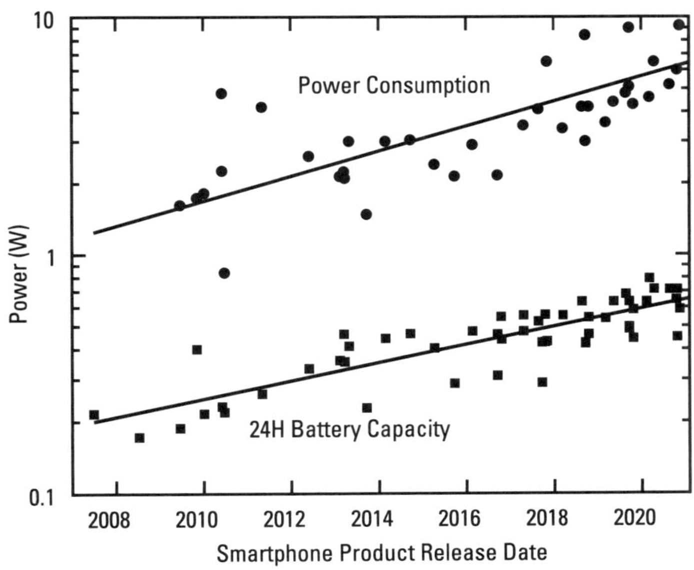


**Figure 5.2** Power consumed by display of several commercial smartphone devices and battery power capacity versus time of product introduction. A battery gap exists and presents a user experience challenge.

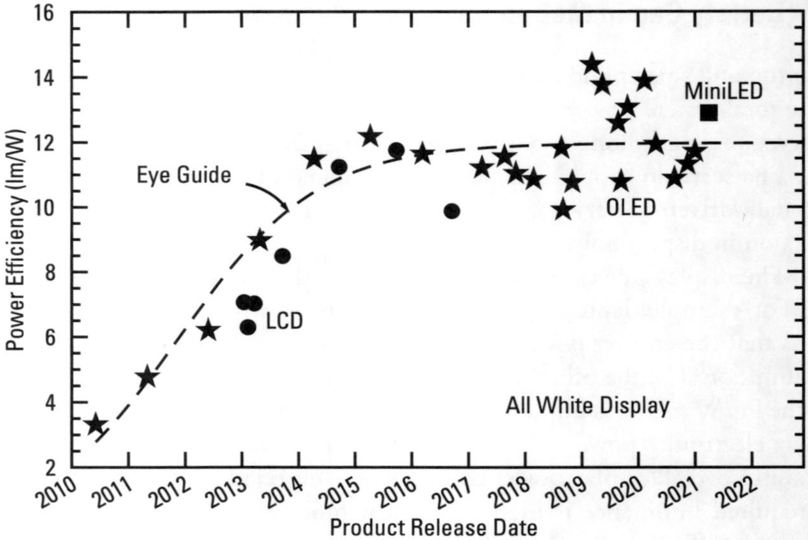


**Figure 5.3** Historical power efficiency of smartphones and laptops with LCDs, OLEDs, and miniLEDs. The dotted line is a guide to the eye. Raw data for power was obtained from www.displaymate.com and analyzed using the methodology published in [2]. The displays had all-white images.

materials used. As such, it is argued that OLEDs' power efficiency and luminance cannot be simply optimized to reach parity with microLEDs' promised lm/W.

Power efficiency envelope curves for OLEDs and microLEDs are shown in Figure 5.4. GaN microLEDs are superior to OLEDs for blue and green colors, but inferior to OLED for red color. The red GaN LED efficiency is much less than 6%, which was found to be the minimum required efficiency to achieve sizable improvement of lm/W metric [3]. Improvements in red GaN efficiency may be accomplished by low-temperature InGaN epitaxy [4].

## 5.3 MicroLED Display Power Calculations

In microLED displays a desired color and luminance value are created from various combinations of three colors of light emitting elements (red, green, and blue). Given that these differently colored, light-emitting elements can have dramatically different efficacies, power consumption can be significantly influenced by the proportions of light produced by each of these elements. White color typically represents the worst-case power scenario. Well-defined targets for the efficiencies of red, green, and blue microLEDs to achieve low power consumption are lacking in the literature. In this work, we address this issue

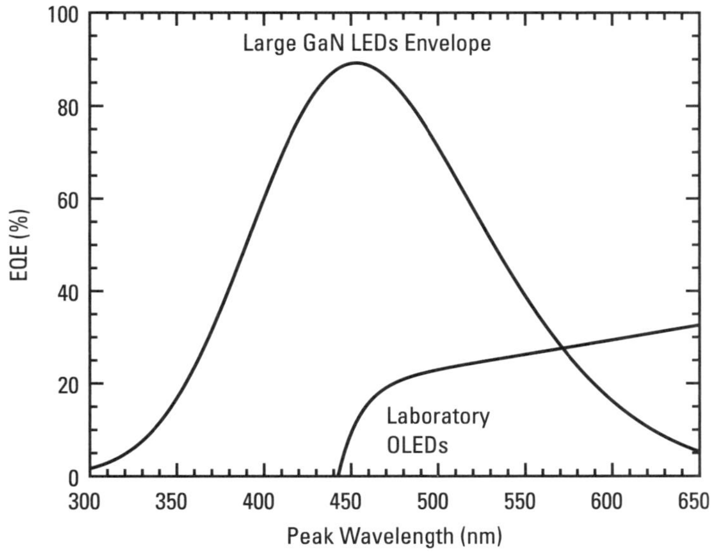


**Figure 5.4** Envelope curves for EQE versus wavelength for OLEDs and GaN microLEDs. Data used to construct the envelope curves is shown in [2].

and discuss the prospects of microLED displays for mobile display applications through physics-based simulations of emissive display power consumption, and measured display emitter power consumption on state-of-the-art OLED displays.

### 5.3.1 Model Assumptions

A model is a description of natural phenomenon that scientists and engineers can use to make predictions. A good model is both as accurate as possible and as simple as possible, which makes it not only powerful but also easy to understand. However, no matter how good they are, models will almost always have limitations. Like most models, our model includes some approximations as a convenient way to describe the display power consumption as a function of the characteristics of the display constituent (i.e., microLEDs). These approximations are not exact, so predictions based on them tend to be slightly different from what is actually observed. In our model, we assumed that red, green, and blue LEDs have the same far-field radiation patterns and same subpixel per inch density. We also assumed that microLED efficiencies are not dependent on the far-field radiation pattern. Finally, we assumed that the microLEDs are driven using pulse width modulation scheme where the microLED current will correspond to the peak efficiency. With these simplifying assumptions, our predictions will deviate slightly from experimental measurements, but the observed trends will still be accurate with some small errors.

### 5.3.2 The Model

The display emitter power consumption is a function of brightness, the information content of a display, the viewing angle (defined as the angle at which the viewer has to be positioned in relation to the screen in order to clearly see the image on a display), and size of the display. The viewing angle is a function of the radiation pattern of the microLED devices. The emitter power consumption is estimated by a sequence of calculations. First, a few specifications of the display panel must be defined such as panel size, number of pixels, desired brightness, and the polarizer efficiency (a circular polarizer is used in OLED or microLED displays to reduce glare due to ambient light). We derived an expression for the luminous flux (a measure of the total quantity of visible light emitted by a source) that must be emitted by each microLED pixel to achieve a given on-axis brightness:

$$L_W = B_0\, 2\pi \left( \int_0^{\theta_{1/2}} f(\theta) \sin\theta \; d\theta \right) A_P / T_P \tag{5.1}$$

For a Lambertian radiation pattern, $f(\theta) = \cos\theta$, (5.1) reduces to the well-known analytical formula [5, 6]:

$$L_w = B_0 \times \pi \times A_P \left(1 - \cos\theta_{1/2}\right) / T_P \tag{5.2}$$

where $\theta_{1/2}$ is half of the total viewing angle, $L_W$ is the pixel luminous flux (lumens), $B_0$ is the on-axis brightness (cd/m$^2$ or nits), $\theta$ is the angle measured from normal to display plane, $f(\theta)$ is the normalized radiation pattern, $A_p$ is the pixel area, and $T_P$ is the polarizer transmittance. The relative luminous flux requirement for each of the *R*, *G*, and *B* subpixels ($L_R$, $L_G$, $L_B$) within each pixel is determined to produce *D*65 white color point or any other color point ($L_W = L_R + L_G + L_B$). Applying color mixing principles [5, 6], the following two equations can be written:

$$x_{D65} = \frac{x_R L_R / y_R + x_G L_G / y_G + x_B L_B / y_B}{L_R / y_R + L_G / y_G + L_R / y_R} \tag{5.3}$$

$$y_{D65} = \frac{L_R + L_G + L_B}{L_R / y_R + L_G / y_G + L_B / y_B} \tag{5.4}$$

where $L_R$, $L_G$, and $L_B$ are the luminous fluxes for red, green, and blue microLEDs, respectively, needed to produce a white color of coordinates $x_{D65} = 0.31271$ and $y_{D65} = 0.32901$. The values of $x_R$, $y_R$, $x_G$, $y_G$, $x_B$, and $y_B$ are calculated given the measured power spectra for the red, green, and blue curves. By solving the (5.1)–(5.3) system of equations we can determine three values of the light fluxes $L_R$, $L_G$, and $L_B$ that are needed to produce the specified brightness of the $D65$ white color (or any other color). The solution can be found using the following matrix equation:

$$\begin{bmatrix} (x_R - x_{D65}) & (x_G - x_{D65}) & (x_B - x_{D65}) \\ (y_R - y_{D65}) & (y_G - y_{D65}) & (y_B - y_{D65}) \\ y_R & y_G & y_B \end{bmatrix} \begin{bmatrix} L_R / y_R \\ L_G / y_G \\ L_B / y_B \end{bmatrix} = \begin{bmatrix} 0 \\ 0 \\ L_W \end{bmatrix} \tag{5.5}$$

Now, one calculates luminous efficacy of radiation (LER) for each subpixel using the definition [5, 6]:

$$LER_j = \int_{380}^{825} V(\lambda)\ S_j(\lambda)\ d\lambda \Big/ \int_{380}^{825} S_j(\lambda)\ d\lambda \tag{5.6}$$

where $j = R$, $G$, or $B$, $V(\lambda)$ is the spectral luminous efficiency of photopic vision (eye sensitivity curve) defined by CIE, which is defined in the visible range of 380 to 780 nm [5], $\lambda$ is wavelength, and $S_j(\lambda)$ is the microLED emission spectrum, which can be measured experimentally for each microLED color. Using $LER$ and light fluxes calculated from (5.1)–(5.5), the optical power ($P_o$) emitted from each subpixel can be calculated using the following equation:

$$P_{o,j} = L_j / LER_j \tag{5.7}$$

Now one can determine the photon flux (photons/second) ($\Phi$) for each microLED using the equations

$$\Phi_j = P_{o,j} / E_{ph,j} \tag{5.8}$$

$$E_{ph,j} = \int_{380}^{825} \frac{hc}{\lambda} S_j(\lambda)\ d\lambda \Big/ \int_{380}^{825} S_j(\lambda)\ d\lambda \tag{5.9}$$

where $h$ is Planck's constant, $c$ is the speed of light, and $E_{ph}$ is the average photon energy, and $j = R$, $G$, or $B$.

If the external quantum efficiency (*EQE*) is measured for each microLED, one can calculate the electric current though each microLED to achieve the above calculated photon flux. The following equation may be used:

$$I_j = q\,\Phi_j \,/\, EQE_j \tag{5.10}$$

The electrical power consumptions by red (*R*), green (*G*), and blue (*B*) can be calculated using

$$P_j\ (\mathrm{W}) = I_j\ (\mathrm{A}) \times V_j\ (\mathrm{V}) \tag{5.11}$$

The total emitter power consumption by all RGB pixels in a display is given by

$$P_e\ (\mathrm{W}) = N_P \times \left(P_R + P_G + P_B\right) \tag{5.12}$$

where $N_P$ is the total number of pixels on the display.

A relationship between the power efficacy of a microLED ($\eta_p$) and its *EQE* may be easily derived as

$$\eta_p\,(\mathrm{lm/W}) = LER \times EQE \times \frac{E_{ph}}{qV_F} \tag{5.13}$$

The system of (5.1)–(5.12) may be used to calculate emitter power consumption for a given display size, on-axis brightness level, and resolution under a white color condition.

Shown in Table 5.1 are the assumed parameters used to simulate the emitter power consumption of microLED displays: peak emission wavelength ($\lambda_p$), full-width-half-maximum of the emission spectra (FWHM), power efficacy ($\eta_p$), forward voltage ($V_F$), and CIE color coordinates ($x$, $y$). The polarizer transmission factor was fixed at 42% and the aperture ratio was fixed at 0.7 for all calculations.

The FWHM of a MicroLED emission spectrum was calculated using the equation [7]

$$FWHM \approx \left(3k_BT \,/\, hc\right) \lambda_p^2 \tag{5.14}$$

The microLED emission spectrum was described by the following equation [8]:

$$S(\lambda) = \frac{g\left(\lambda, \lambda_p, FWHM\right) + 2g^5\left(\lambda, \lambda_p, FWHM\right)}{3} \tag{5.15}$$

**Table 5.1**
Assumed Parameters Used to Simulate the Emitter Power Consumption in MicroLED Displays

| | Red | Green | Blue |
|---|---|---|---|
| $\lambda_p$ (nm) | 630 | 532 | 467 |
| FWHM (nm) | 25 | 20 | 15 |
| $V_F$ (V) | 2.22 | 2.58 | 2.90 |
| CIE Coordinate $x$ | 0.6969 | 0.1817 | 0.1313 |
| CIE Coordinate $y$ | 0.3031 | 0.7800 | 0.0498 |
| Power Efficacy (lm/W) | 10–100 | 100–200 | 10–30 |
| $\theta_{1/2}$ | 45° | 45° | 45° |
| Display Diagonal | 5.8″ | | |
| Display Resolution | 2436 × 1125 | | |
| Aperture Ratio | 100% | | |
| Polarizer Efficiency | 42% | | |
| Pixel Side | 54.9 × 54.9 $\mu$m | | |
| Display Brightness | 200 cd/m$^2$ | | |
| Displayed Color | D65 white | | |

$$g\left(\lambda,\lambda_p,FWHM\right)=\exp\left[-\left(\frac{\lambda-\lambda_p}{FWHM}\right)^2\right] \tag{5.16}$$

Example spectra are shown in Figure 5.5.

### 5.3.3 Required Efficiencies for 25-lm/W White Power Efficiency Displays

As seen in Figure 5.6, fix blue and then calculate green EQE versus red EQE to produce 25 lm/W. Repeat for different blue EQE (5%, 10%, 15%, 20%, and 25%). Sweep red EQE from 1% to 20%.

## 5.4 Manufacturing of MicroLED Displays

In Figure 5.7 a manufacturing flow diagram of microLED displays on glass backplane is shown. Three microLED wafers (one for red microLEDs, one for green microLEDs, and one for blue microLEDs) are fed to microLED transfer equipment that will transfer microLEDs onto a display backplane. The display backplane includes pixel driving circuits (according to the architecture shown in Figure 5.1) that are made of thin film transistors (TFTs) on glass substrate. After transfer, an insulating layer is deposited, exposing the top electrode (e.g.,

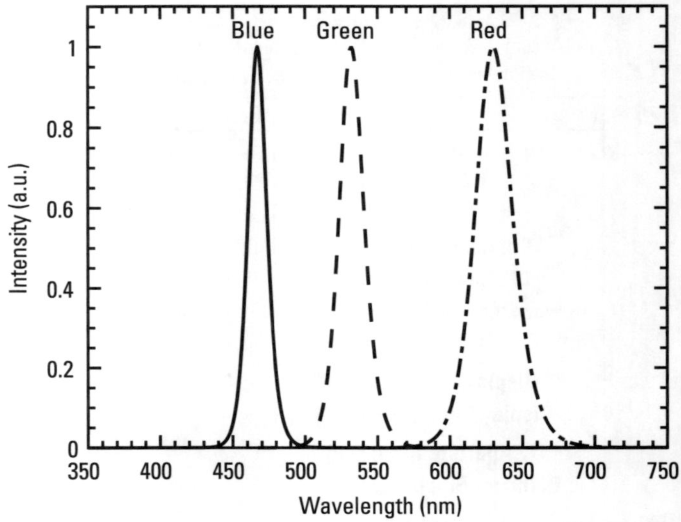


**Figure 5.5** Example source spectra for red, green, and blue microLEDs based on (5.15) and (5.16) with the aid of (5.14).

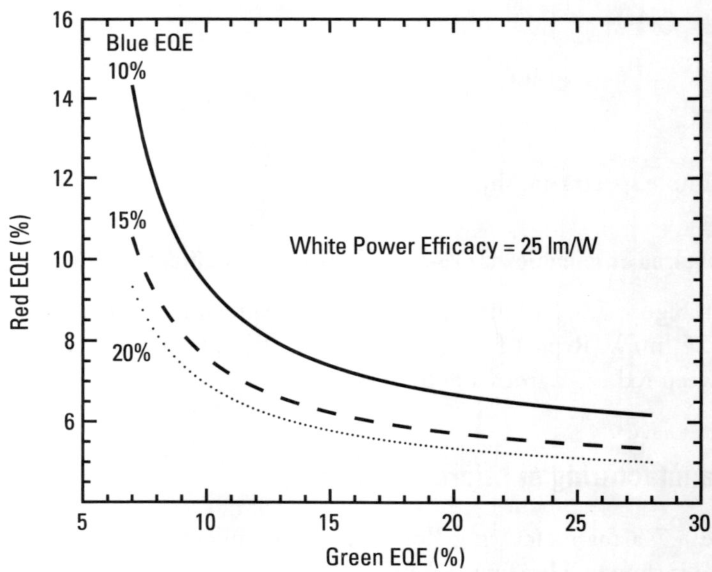


**Figure 5.6** Required red, green, and blue microLED external quantum efficiencies to achieve a display power efficacy of 25 lm/W under an all-white condition. The curves are labeled by the EQE values for blue microLEDs.

cathode) of the microLEDs. A transparent conducting oxide is then deposited to act as a common cathode. Finally, a top glass protection is attached.

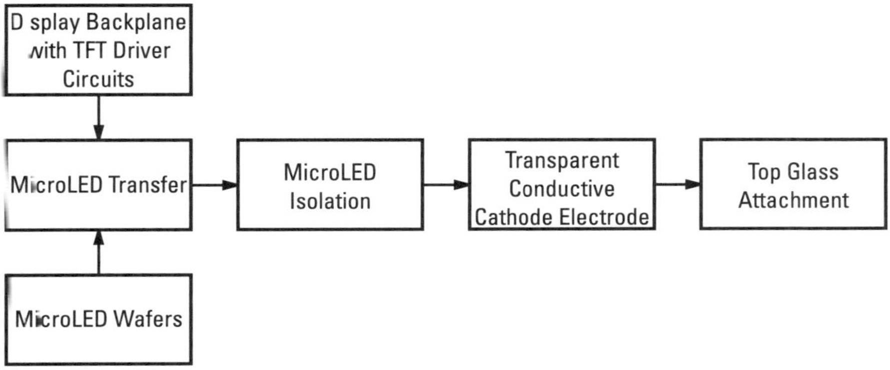


**Figure 5.7** Block diagram of the key steps used to manufacture a microLED display.

### 5.4.1 MicroLED Transfer

The viability of transferring microLEDs from mother wafers to a display backplane to meet target production cost requires that microLEDs have a much smaller pitch on the wafer compared to the pitch on the display backplane. Any transfer method must optimize (maximize) the number of displays per microLED wafer. The concept of pitch scaling is demonstrated schematically in Figure 5.8.

A number of transfer methods have been proposed [9–25]. Two transfer methods bracket the multitude of transfer methods investigated by multiple research and development organizations across the world: (1) pick and place (PnP) with a stamp, and (2) direct transfer method (DTM).

#### 5.4.1.1 Pick and Place—PnP Transfer

Schematics demonstrating the working of PnP transfer are shown in Figure 5.9. In Figure 5.9(a), three wafers for red, green, and blue emitting microLEDs are provided. A stamp that is equipped to pick up the microLEDs from each wafer then place it on the backplane is used to transfer the microLEDs. Sequential movement of the stamp to/from the wafer and the backplane is used to populate large displays. In Figure 5.9(b), the stamp is aligned to the donor wafer, then attached to the microLEDs on the donor wafers to pick up the microLEDs, the stamp is then moved and aligned to where the microLEDs are to be placed on the backplane, the microLEDs are bonded to the backplane, and finally the stamp is detached from the microLED top surface. In Figure 5.9(c), a sacrificial layer (release layer) is used during the growth of the microLEDs on the growth wafer as shown in (1). In (2) a tether (e.g., photoresist) is deposited on the structure as shown. In (3), chemical liftoff is used to etch the release layer. In (4), a stamp is attached to the top surface of the microLED. By pulling

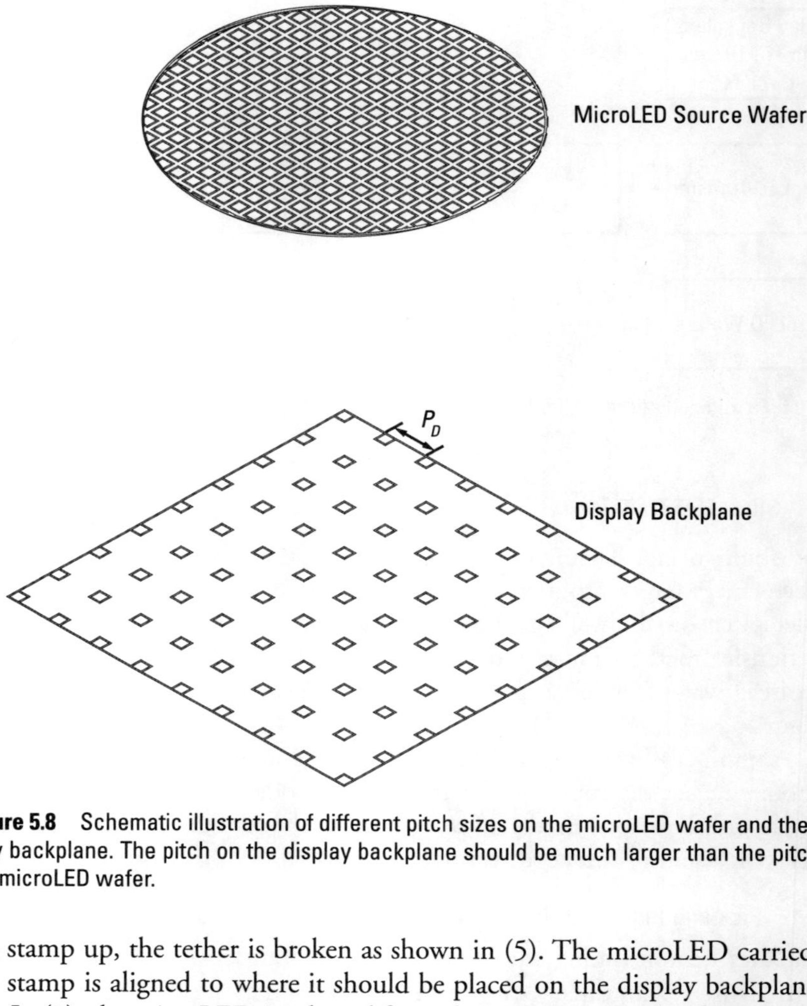


**Figure 5.8** Schematic illustration of different pitch sizes on the microLED wafer and the display backplane. The pitch on the display backplane should be much larger than the pitch on the microLED wafer.

the stamp up, the tether is broken as shown in (5). The microLED carried by the stamp is aligned to where it should be placed on the display backplane in (6). In (7), the microLED is released from the stamp. In (8), the final state of a transferred microLED on the display backplane is illustrated.

#### 5.4.1.2 Direct Transfer Method

Low-cost production of microLED displays for smartphones or laptops require a low cost of the microLED donor wafer and low cost of transferring microLEDs to the display backplane. Both can be addressed by using 300-mm silicon wafers to grow the GaN-based microLEDs. However, silicon's mismatch in coefficient of thermal expansion with the III-nitrides results in cracking of the III-nitride layers if additional engineering is not employed. One approach to eliminate the cracking of the III-nitride films/devices is to compressively strain the film as it grows so that when it cools to room temperature the film is

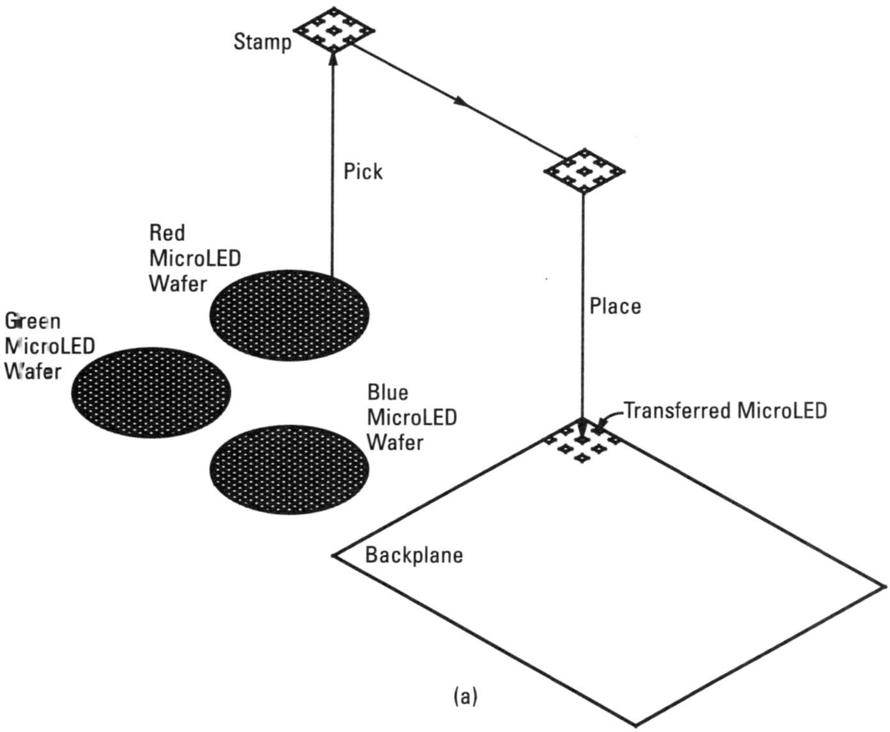


**Figure 5.9** (a) Schematic illustration of PnP transfer. (b) Schematic illustration of the detailed process steps used to perform PnP transfer of microLEDs. (c) Schematic illustration of PnP transfer illustrating the details of how microLEDs are picked up from the wafer then placed on the display backplane using a tether layer (e.g., photoresist).

relaxed. This is typically done with intermediate AlN and AlGaN films when growing GaN on silicon. The disadvantage of this technique is that during growth the substrate is not flat, but instead is bowed, which leads to poor quality and nonuniformity of quantum well growth, and difficulty transferring the microLEDs directly from the silicon wafer to the display backplane. An alternative way of eliminating the cracking of the III-nitride film without causing a bow in the wafer during growth is to use patterned silicon substrates. With this technique, only small areas of the silicon substrate seed GaN, and these regions are small enough that the GaN films do not crack due to the stresses induced from the mismatch in the coefficient of thermal expansion. Selective area epitaxy may be used to grow nanowires or nanopyramids out of a patterned seed layer that had been deposited on the silicon substrate. The patterned seed layer can have patches of size $1 \times 1\ \mu m$ to $10 \times 10\ \mu m$, for example, separated by streets of 0.1 to 1 $\mu m$, for example. The seed layer may be made of a thin

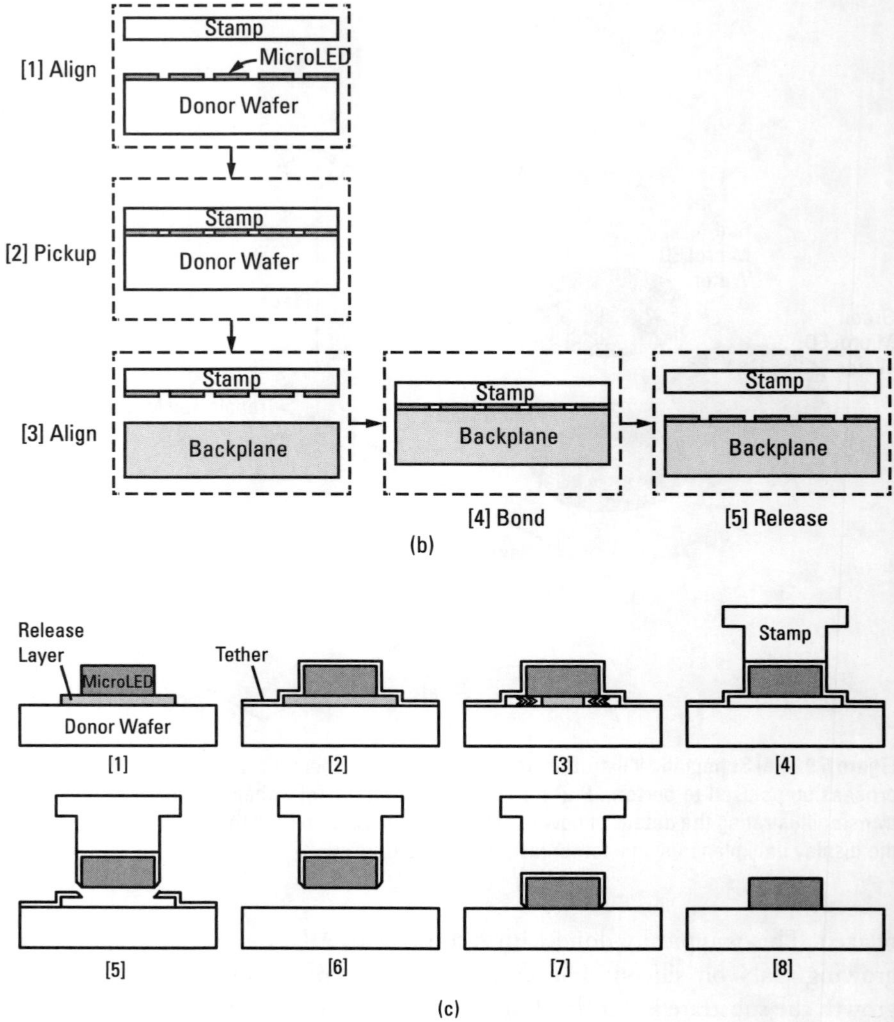


**Figure 5.9** (continued)

transition metal nitride that has crystal structure similar to GaN. To prevent interdiffusion between metal nitride and silicon, a thin AlN buffer (e.g., 25 nm in thickness) may be first grown on Si wafer that is preferably Si (111). When transferring the microLEDs from the silicon wafer to a display backplane, the seed layer can be utilized as a release layer by ablating or vaporizing it by infrared irradiation through the silicon substrate. The infrared light, which can have a wavelength of ~2000 nm, will not be absorbed by the silicon wafer. The release of microLEDs, *selectively*, from the silicon wafer will enable low cost and mass direct transfer of microLEDs from the silicon wafer to the display backplane. A simple schematic illustrating the DTM working principle is shown in Figure 5.10. First, the donor wafer is aligned to the display backplane so that the microLEDs are facing interconnect metal pads on the display backplane. These metal pads are connected to the driving circuits that are made of thin film transistors. Next, selective bonding is performed of the microLEDs to the metal pads on the backplane. In this case, the surface of the microLED is coated with a metal pad as well and metal-to-metal bonding can be done without using solder. Finally, a laser beam is used to selectively release the already-bonded microLEDs from the donor wafer to the display backplane. In this step, the laser beam is steered through the backside of the donor wafer toward the release layer holding the microLEDs to the donor wafer. Upon exposure to pulsed laser beam, the release layer is vaporized/disintegrated and the microLED is released to the display backplane [22, 23, 25].

## 5.5 Defect Management

In the manufacturing process of the microLED displays, the microLED chips are generally transferred to substrates by a mass transfer method, and after the mass transfer is completed, the microLED chips are detected for defective pixels. When a defective pixel is detected, the defective pixel is usually repaired by a repairing method of removing the defective pixel and placing a single pixel in a designated position. That is, each defective pixel is removed and a new microLED chip is placed at the defective pixel position. However, the repairing method needs to repeatedly remove defective pixels and repeatedly place new microLED chips, resulting in an extremely low repair efficiency. Alternatively, redundant microLED chips can be used to avoid the high repair cost. In microLED displays, a fault means that a microLED does not emit light due to defects during the semiconductor process steps of making the microLEDs on the donor wafers, or due to poor or no bonding to the display backplane when

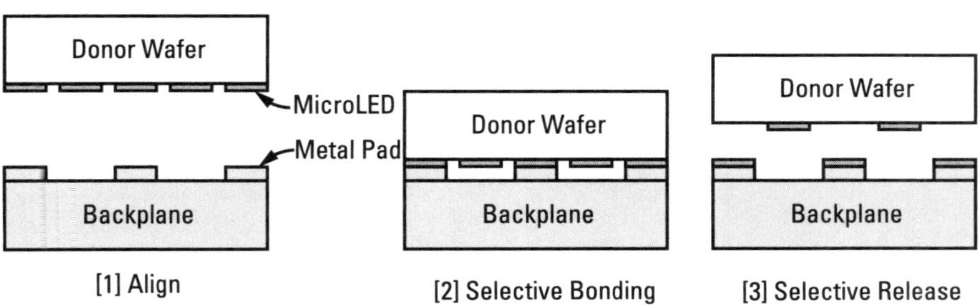


**Figure 5.10** Schematic illustration of the DTM where the donor wafer is used instead of a stamp to donate its microLEDs directly to the display backplane.

the microLEDs are transferred from the donor wafer to the display backplane. A display failure means that the display has more than a specified maximum number of faulty (e.g., dark) pixels. This number in many cases is zero. The main question is how much redundancy is required to achieve defect-free microLED displays. Here, a statistical yield model is derived for RGB microLED displays to quantify the required level of redundancy given a microLED wafer with specific functional yield, and a transfer process that is characterized by a specific transfer yield.

Figure 5.11 illustrates an example of a display architecture with a redundancy level of three (i.e., two additional microLEDs are used per color per pixel). As can be seen in Figure 5.11, three red microLEDs, three green microLEDs, and three blue microLEDs are used for each pixel. For red, one pixel control circuit is used to control the luminance of the working microLEDs. If one or two fail to operate (due to epi process, transfer process, etc.) the third one will compensate for the faulty microLEDs and the target defect count per display can be met. If all three microLEDs per color per pixel are dark, then the pixel is counted as a defective pixel.

The production yield model was derived from first principles statistical theory and is based on the binomial statistics. The model is described by the following equations:

$$p = \exp(-\lambda_w) \times \exp(-\lambda_t) \tag{5.17}$$

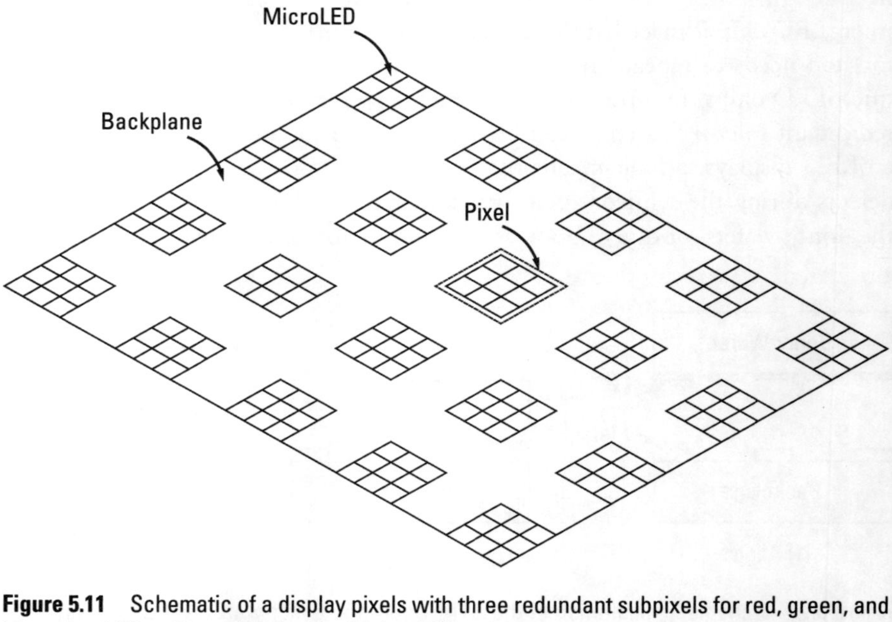


**Figure 5.11** Schematic of a display pixels with three redundant subpixels for red, green, and blue microLED emitters, forming 3 × 3 microLED array.

$$q = 1 - p \tag{5.18}$$

$$p_p = 1 - \left( \sum_{k=0}^{R-1} \binom{R}{k} q^k (1-q)^{R-k} \right)^3 \tag{5.19}$$

$$Y = \sum_{i=0}^{m} \binom{N}{i} p_p^i (1 - p_p)^{N-i} \tag{5.20}$$

Equation (5.20) provides the probability that a microLED is defect-free after transfer; $\lambda_w = A_c D_w$ and $\lambda_t = A_c D_t$, with $A_c$ being the area of a microLED, $D_w$ is the defect density (#/cm$^2$) on the microLED donor wafer, and $D_t$ is the defect density on the display due to transfer issues. The term $\exp(-\lambda_t)$ represents the Poisson-based estimation of transfer yield, and the term $\exp(-\lambda_w)$ represents the Poisson-based estimation of the wafer die yield. Equation (5.17) provides the probability that a microLED is defective. Equation (5.18) provides the probability of defective *pixel* on the display. The exponent of three corresponds to the number of colors (red, green, and blue) per pixel. Equation (5.20) provides the display yield given the definition a display is considered defect-free if there are only up to *m* defective pixels out of *N* total pixels. In (5.18) *R* represents the redundancy level (i.e., the number of microLEDs per color per pixel).

In the above model, *R* subpixels are used per color per pixel, and three colors are used to form a display pixel. For the pixel to be considered defective, *R* subpixels of the same color are defective (i.e., either always dark or always bright). The always dark microLED situation can result in a dark microLED from the donor wafer that gets transferred properly to the backplane, or a functional microLED on the donor wafer that was not properly bonded to the interconnect pad on the display backplane where it was intended, as a way of example. In other words, the production yield of microLED displays is a function of die yield of donor wafers and transfer yield. The die wafer yield does not need to have a Poisson distribution. Several die yield distributions have been considered for semiconductor device wafer manufacturing [26]. The transfer yield distribution will depend on the specifics of the transfer technology. In this work, we use a Poisson distribution for the sake of simplicity. However, the model equations above can accept any yield distribution model for the transfer process. The other assumptions used to formulate the above model include the assumption that the probability of failure of a microLED is independent of the emission color of the microLED, and the assumption that the failure probability of transferring a microLED does not depend on its color. These assumptions are reasonable for the purpose of this study, which is to gain a directional (as opposed to precise) insight about the effectiveness of redundancy in achieving high display production yield. We have assumed that defects are not clustered. For a more accurate yield model one will have to relax these assumptions. The

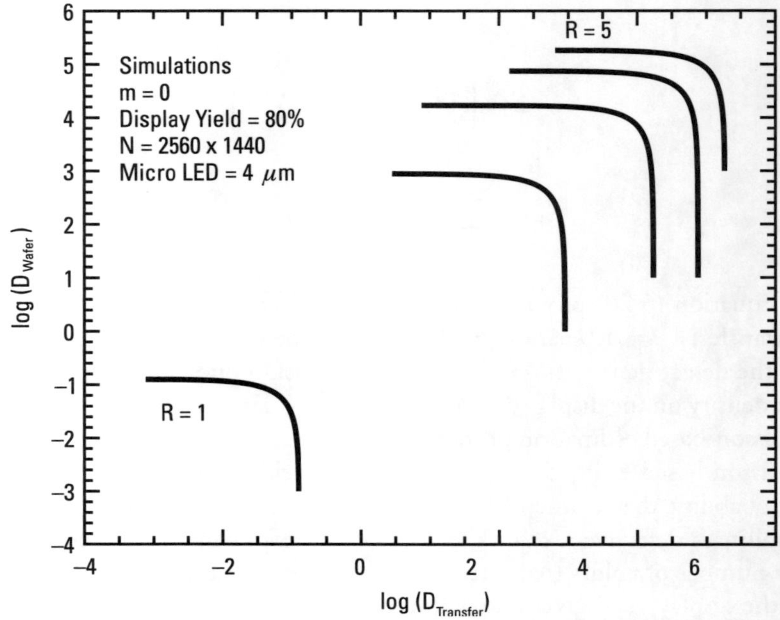


**Figure 5.12** Calculated defect density for wafer and transfer process required to achieve a display line yield of 80% with various redundancy values (R = 1 – 5).

yield model derived above is not computationally intensive and can quickly evaluate the required minimum redundancy needed to hit a specific display production yield target.

The system of (5.17) to (5.20) was used to calculate the display yield for a given set of parameters including microLED wafer die yield, microLED transfer yield, redundancy level (*R*), and maximum number of allowed defective pixels (*m*) on a display with a specific resolution. Large-number binomial coefficients multiplied by the failure probability factors are calculated using well-established recursive methods [27].

The impact of redundancy level on required defect densities on wafer and post transfer are shown in Figure 5.12. Significant relaxation of required defectivity values is seen when redundancy is used.

# References

[1] Jiang, H., X. S. X. Jin, J. Li, J. Shakya, and J. Y. Lin, "III-Nitride Blue Microdisplays," *Applied Physics Letters*, Vol. 78, No. 9, 2001, p. 1303.

[2] Ahmed, K., "Heuristics of OLED and Micro LED Efficiencies," in *SID Symposium Digest of Technical Papers*, Vol. 65, 2021, pp. 864–867.

[3] Ahmed, K., "Micro LEDs Efficiency Targets for Displays," in *SID Symposium Digest of Technical Papers*, 2019, pp. 125–128.

[4] Ahmed, K., "High Performance Light Emitting Diode and Monolithic Multi-color Pixel," US Patent 10957818B2, March 23, 2021.

[5] McCluney, W., *Introduction to Radiometry and Photometry*, Norwood, MA: Artech House, 1994.

[6] Schubert, E. F., *Light-Emitting Diodes*, Cambridge, UK: Cambridge University Press, 2003.

[7] Khanna, V. K., *Fundamentals of Solid-State Lighting*, Boca Raton, FL: CRC Press, 2014.

[8] Ohno, Y., "Spectral Design Considerations for White LED Color Rendering," *Optical Engineering*, Vol. 44, No. 11, 2005, p. 111302.

[9] Virey, E. H., and Z. Bouhamri, "Status of MicroLED Mass-Transfer Processes and Equipment," *SID Symposium Digest of Technical Papers*, Vol. 53, No. 1, 2022, pp. 650–653.

[10] Bower, C. A., Bonafede, S., Pearson, A., et al., "Mass Transfer Throughput and Yield Using Elastomer Stamps," *SID Symposium Digest of Technical Papers*, Vol. 52, No. 1, 2021, pp. 849–852.

[11] Chen, F., et al., "Mass Transfer Techniques for Large-Scale and High-Density MicroLED Arrays," *International Journal of Extreme Manufacturing*, Vol. 4, No. 4, 2022, p. 042005.

[12] Templier, F., and J. Bernard, "A New Approach for Fabricating High-Performance MicroLED Displays," *SID Symposium Digest of Technical Papers*, Vol. 50, No. 1, 2019, pp. 240–243.

[13] Li, S., and O. Haupt, "Laser Processes for MicroLED Display Manufacturing," *SID Symposium Digest of Technical Papers*, Vol. 53, No. 1, 2022, pp. 465–466.

[14] Linghu, C., S. Zhang, C. Wang, H. Luo, and J. Song, "Mass Transfer for Micro-LED Display: Transfer Printing Techniques," *Semiconductors and Semimetals*, Vol. 106, 2021, pp. 253–280.

[15] Kajiyama, K., et al., "Manufacturing Process for Mass Production of Micro-LED Displays and High-Speed and High-Yield Laser Lift-Off Systems," *SID Symposium Digest of Technical Papers*, Vol. 51, No. 1, 2020, pp. 100–103.

[16] Rupp, B. B., L. S. Crawford, J. P. Lu, et al., "Directed Electrostatic Microassembly for MicroLED Display," *SID Symposium Digest of Technical Papers*, Vol. 52, No. 1, 2021, pp. 845–848.

[17] Ezhilarasu, G., A. Hanna, A. Paranjpe, and S. S. Iyer, "High Yield Precision Transfer and Assembly of GaN $\mu$LEDs Using Laser Assisted Micro Transfer Printing," *2019 IEEE 69th Electronic Components and Technology Conference (ECTC)*, 2019, pp. 1470–1474.

[18] Chang, P. L., "MicroLED Display and Assembly," US Patent 10,128,307, 2018.

[19] Ahmed, K., A. Pancholi, and A. Khakifirooz, "Micro Light-Emitting Diode (LED) Display and Fluidic Self-Assembly of Same," U.S. Patent 10,361,337, 2019.

[20] Ahmed, K., K. Parikh, and P. L. Chang, "Micro-LED Displays," US Patent 10,177,195, 2019.

[21] Ahmed, K., K.S. Parikh, and P. Chang, "Apparatus for Micro Pick and Bond," US Patent 10,217,729, 2019.

[22] Ahmed, K., A. Pancholi, S. Dasgupta, and C. Mair, "Micro Light-Emitting Diode Display Fabrication and Assembly," US Patent 11,637,093, 2023.

[23] Ahmed, K., and A. Pancholi, "Laser Transfer Printing for Making Micro LED Display Devices and Method," US Patent Application 16/053,559, 2020.

[24] Sounart, T. L., K. Ahmed, A. Pancholi, and S.M. Liff, "Micro-LED Displays Including Solder Structures and Methods," US Patent Application 16/946,166, 2020.

[25] Ahmed, K., "Micro Light-Emitting Diode Display Fabrication and Assembly Apparatus," US Patent Application 16/235,831, 2020.

[26] Stapper, C. H., F. M. Armstrong, and K. Saji, "Integrated Circuit Yield Statistics," *Proceedings of the IEEE*, Vol. 71, 1983, p. 470.

[27] Rolfe, T., "Binomial Coefficient Recursion: The Good, and the Bad and Ugly," *ACM SIGCSE Bulletin Inroads*, Vol. 33, No. 2, 2001, pp. 35–36.

# 6

# MicroLED Data Communication Systems

## 6.1 Introduction

Photonic interconnects are being quickly developed and adopted to be an indispensable large-bandwidth data transmission venue in high-performance computing (HPC) and data center (i.e., datacom) applications. The distinct emphasis on power, operational robustness, volume manufacturability, and system cost posts a number of challenges in photonic material platform choice, device design, integration scheme, packaging, and so forth.

The concept of optical communication was developed several decades ago, and large data transmission bandwidth is always ideal. But compared with the conventional long-haul fiber optics, the system catering to the datacom applications has a distinctly different emphasis on power efficiency, reliable operation at a temperature-fluctuating environment (e.g., 30°C–110°C), volume manufacturability, and overall system cost in order to be technically and economically competitive.

As the major roadblock to realize a fully integrated Si-based photonic interconnect system, light sources have attracted significant research and development effort and driven great innovation in the past two decades. Generally speaking, laser sources currently dominate the overall power consumption and component cost in the total optical link and largely affect another critical aspects like packaging, which eventually determines the total system cost and overall performance. Thermal management, from either internal joule heating or external environmental heating, is a long-term inevitable challenge against the diode laser operation. It drastically reduces the device efficiency, shifts the wavelength, and shortens the lifetime. The cost constraint, physical size limit, and photonic integration with the driver chip further complicates the laser source implementation.

Lasers with quantum dot (QD) active regions have shown superior performance over traditional QW designs in their ability to maintain large optical gain at elevated temperatures [1]. Due to the three-dimensional confinement of carriers, QD lasers promise higher temperature stability and lower threshold current densities when compared to quantum well lasers. In addition, due to the size distribution of the dots, QD lasers have a wide gain bandwidth, which allows for a larger channel count in a wavelength-division multiplexing (WDM) link. It has also been found that QD lasers have a low relative intensity noise (RIN). These advantages make QD lasers particularly attractive for on-chip, multiwavelength sources in datacom applications. But before these devices can be adopted at a large scale, a commercially viable solution must be found. Using a pure III-V approach limits a foundry to using relatively small wafers ~150 mm in diameter at relatively old processing nodes of ~250 nm. The integration on Si substrates, on the other hand, would potentially allow the use of widely available CMOS foundries, which would result in high-volume, low-cost integrated III-V lasers with high-quality and reliable Si photonics. Furthermore, the integration of the laser source directly on Si would reduce coupling losses, subsequentially reducing the link budget and packaging costs inherent in multichip solutions. The most promising integration scheme will take advantage of high-performance active devices while also taking advantage of the excellent optical properties of low optical losses in Si. Typical integration schemes include growth, flip-chip bonding, and wafer bonding.

Alternatively, arrayed microscopic emitters such as microLEDs are promising for achieving low-cost parallel optical interconnections for high bandwidth, low-power, and short reach (<10m) applications [2–9]. The advantages of using microLEDs for short-reach datacom include leveraging the developing ecosystem for microLED displays, wider operating temperature range (allowing the possibility of bringing the optical chip closer to the electronics), and compatibility with large silicon wafers and advanced CMOS technology nodes. The architecture of such a system is shown in Figure 6.1, where, in a serial optical interconnect architecture, data is fed into an array of vertical cavity surface emitting laser (VCSELs) emitting light at different wavelengths. The lights are multiplexed and fed into an optical fiber. At the receiver's end, light is multiplexed and fed into an array of photodetectors to recover the electrical data. In a parallel optical interconnect architecture, data is fed into an array of microLEDs. Light emitted by each microLED is fed into a multimode fiber (for example). Data at the receiver's end is detected using an array of microphotodetectors, with one photodetector per one transmitting microLED/fiber.

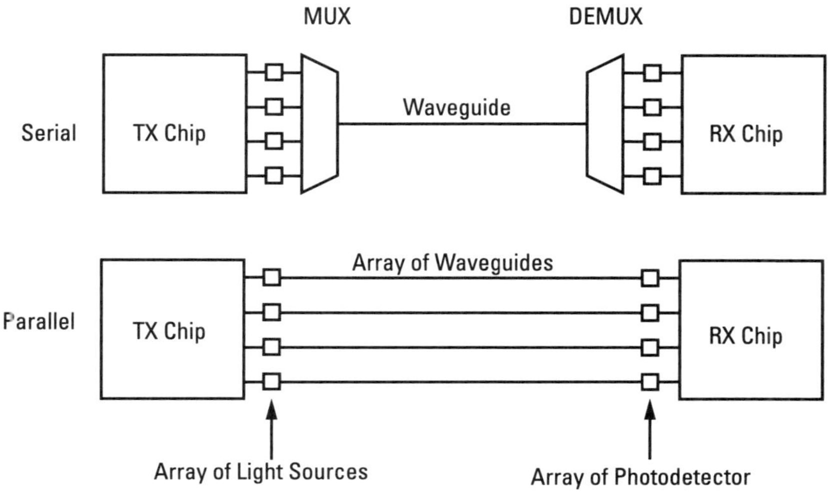


**Figure 6.1** Serial versus parallel interconnect architectures.

In other words, multiplexing and demultiplexing are eliminated in a parallel optical interconnect architecture.

In this chapter, bandwidth and power possibilities are analyzed for optical interconnect links shorter than 10m.

## 6.2 Space Division Multiplexing

Space division multiplexing (SDM) is the only currently known technique to cope with the forecasted demand for capacity. A natural way of scaling bandwidth is dedicating one fiber core per lane along with parallel microscopic scale light emitter (e.g., microLEDs) and microscopic scale photodetector arrays and multicore-multimode optical fibers. Within a single multicore fiber (MCF), multiple cores share one cladding as shown in Figure 6.2. The interconnect density is thus increased by placing more bandwidth within a single strand of fiber cable.

Many technical capabilities of space division multiplexed systems like low loss and crosstalk have been established in numerous long-haul system experiments. Recently more attention has been given to applications of space division multiplexing for short-reach systems, including data center transmission applications. In addition to higher bandwidth density, space division multiplexed systems offer potential advantages in lower power consumption and cost.

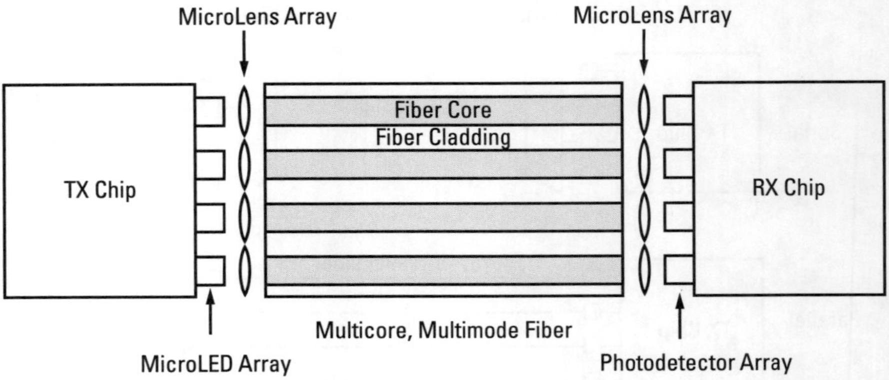


**Figure 6.2** Architecture of a parallel data transmission system using an array of microLEDs, multicore optical fiber, and an array of micro photodetectors (microPDs).

### 6.2.1 MicroLED Light Source

The electro-optical bandwidth of microLEDs can be increased by using high current density and higher radiative recombination coefficient as described by

$$f_{3dB} \approx \frac{\sqrt{3}}{2\pi}\sqrt{\frac{J \bullet B}{q \bullet d}} \tag{6.1}$$

where $J$ is the current density, $B$ is the radiative recombination coefficient, $q$ is the electronic charge, and $d$ is the width of the quantum well. The reduction of microLED chip size results in higher current density and higher frequency $f_{3dB}$ at a given power consumption. Higher values for $B$ is a function of the material and structure properties of the microLED device. Commercially available GaN microLEDs are usually grown on polar c-plane sapphire substrates, which can result in a QCSE leading to reduced efficiency (i.e., efficiency droop) under high injected current density conditions. The QCSE is caused by the natural structure of GaN, a hexagonal crystal with wurtzite structure. Meanwhile, the quantum wells sustain a large piezoelectric field due to the strain-induced polarization from the lattice mismatch between $In_xGa_{1-x}N$ and GaN [10, 11]. These internal polarization fields along the c-plane cause charge to accumulate at the heterojunction in quantum wells, leading to the tilt of the energy band as shown in Figure 6.3. The wave function distribution of electrons and holes will be spatially separated, resulting in a low carrier radiative recombination rate ($B$) and low internal quantum efficiency. QCSE also leads to wavelength-shift and efficiency droop with increasing injected current density.

It is preferrable to use short wavelengths (e.g., blue or violet) to minimize stronger polarization, larger lattice mismatch, high defect density, and stronger

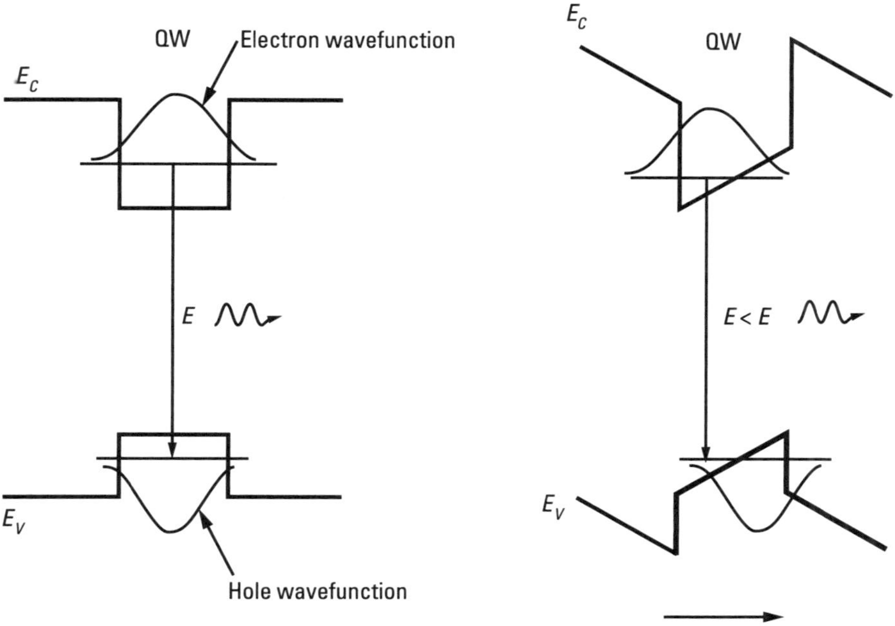


**Figure 6.3** Illustration of the QCSE with (polar, e.g., c-plane) and without (nonpolar, e.g., m-plane) built-in field. The built-in field in the quantum well results in electron and hole wavefunction separation, which is more pronounced at high current injection. This effect results in lower internal quantum efficiency of the microLED and less efficient electron-hole radiative recombination.

strain caused by the increase in indium (In) composition necessary for longer wavelength emission (e.g., green and red).

The use of semipolar or nonpolar substrates to grow the quantum wells has been found to help increase the modulation frequency $f_{3dB}$ at a given current density, or to achieve a given modulation frequency at lower current density as shown in Figure 6.4. Nonpolar (e.g., m-plane) microLEDs have 2× higher $f_{3dB}$ compared to semipolar (e.g., r-plane) microLEDs, and 5× higher $f_{3dB}$ compared to polar (c-plane) microLEDs. Nanowires provide m-plane type microLEDs.

### 6.2.2 Photodetectors for Visible Light

The primary purpose of a photodetector is conversion of an input optical signal into an electrical signal for further processing. Like microLEDs, photodetectors used in fiber optic communication are also based on semiconductors. Detectors for optical communications in the visible regime may be based on silicon. When light falls on a detector current is generated, its magnitude depending on the power falling on the detector. The detector converts the optical pulse stream

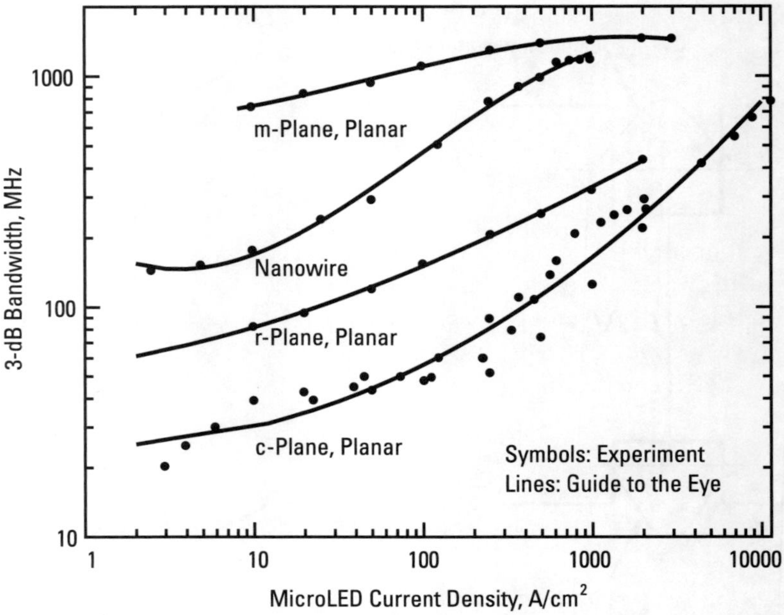


**Figure 6.4** Survey of 3-dB modulation bandwidth for III-nitride LEDs of various crystal orientations and nanowires [12, 13].

into an electrical pulse stream, which can be processed using electronic circuits. Photodetection takes place by generating in the semiconducting material electrons and holes which then flow in the circuit to generate current. This generation is random, which introduces noise in the electrical signal being detected. If the noise becomes comparable to the signal-generated current, this may lead to errors in detection. There are two primary noise-generating mechanisms in the detection process: shot noise and thermal noise [14]. The ratio of the current produced to the input optical power is referred to as responsivity.

There are primarily two types of semiconductor detectors: p-type–intrinsic–n-type (PIN) [15–17] and avalanche photodiodes (APDs) [18–21]. In the former there is no amplification within the detector, whereas in the latter case there is an avalanche multiplication of electrons within the detector itself, brought about by high electric fields within the detector. Another important aspect of photodetectors is the speed of response. This is determined primarily by three factors: the transit time of the photo-generated carriers through the detector, the electrical frequency response as determined by the resistance and capacitance in the circuit (including that of the photodetector itself), and slow diffusion of the current carriers within the detector. To achieve high bandwidth, photodetectors should have a small capacitance, which in turn implies that they must have a small area. In APDs an internal current gain by multiplication of the current carriers is achieved by providing a large reverse bias. The large electric field within the detection area results in rapid acceleration of the charges, which then collide and create more charge carriers. These in turn accelerate and create further charge carriers. This results in an avalanche effect and leads to much higher currents in the output for the same input optical power.

#### 6.2.2.1 Responsivity

As mentioned above, the responsivity measures the gain in measured current per incident optical power. Example responsivity versus wavelength curves for silicon and InGaN/GaN MQW photodetectors is shown in Figure 6.5. InGaN/GaN MQW photodetectors promise higher speed for similar responsivity to silicon. The theoretical curves were based on the definition of responsibility

$$\mathcal{R} = \frac{\lambda}{1240}(1-R)\left[1-\exp(-\alpha \bullet d)\right]$$

where $\lambda$ is the wavelength of incident light in nanometers, $R$ is the reflection coefficient of the light by the detector surface, $\alpha(\lambda)$ is the absorption coefficient of the photodetector active layer, and $d$ is the detector thickness. In the calculations shown in Figure 6.5, the absorption coefficient for $In_xGa_{1-x}N$ with indium mole fraction $x$ is given by [22]

$$\alpha(\lambda) \approx \frac{10^5\sqrt{a\left(1240/\lambda - 1240/\lambda_g\right) + b\left(1240/\lambda - 1240/\lambda_g\right)^2}}{1+\exp\left(\dfrac{1240/\lambda - 1240/\lambda_g}{\delta\lambda}\right)}$$

where $\dfrac{1240}{\lambda_g} \approx 0.7x - 1.43x(1-x) + 3.42(1-x)$, $a(x) \approx 12.87x^4 - 37.79x^3 + 40.43x^2 - 18.35x + 3.52$ [23, 24], $b(x) \approx -2.92x^2 + 4.05x - 0.66$ [23, 24], $\delta\lambda \in [100, 300 \text{ nm}]$, and $0 \leq x \leq 1$. In the case of using an antireflective coating, $R \approx 0$.

The performance of InGaN-GaN MQW photodetectors has been explored experimentally by many authors [25–34]. The reported performance is consistent with the theoretical predictions.

#### 6.2.2.2 Shot Noise

Shot noise arises from the fact that an electric current is made up of a stream of discrete charges—namely, electrons—which are randomly generated. Thus, even when a photodetector is illuminated by constant optical power $P$, due to the random generation of e–h pairs, the current will fluctuate randomly around

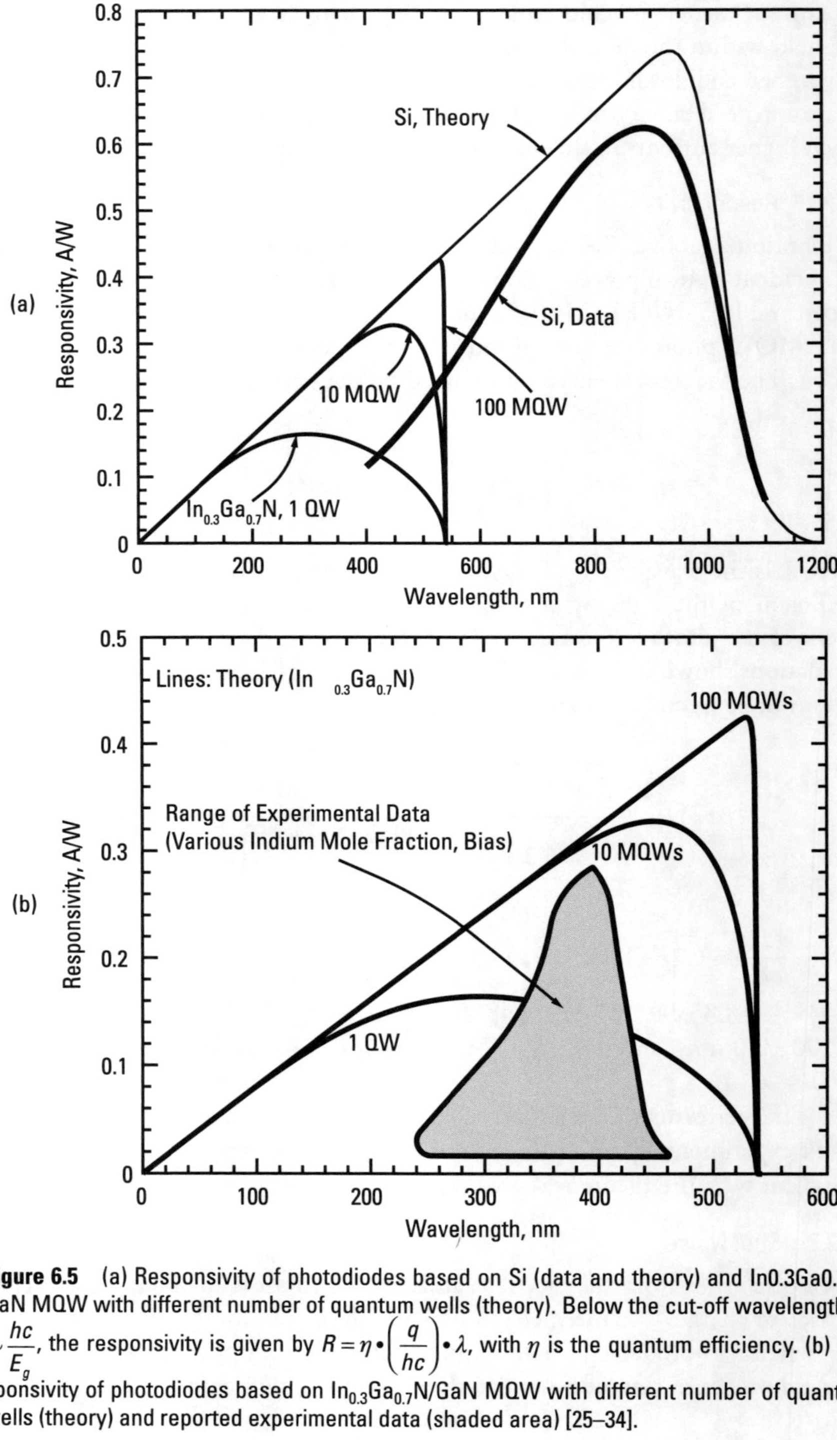


**Figure 6.5** (a) Responsivity of photodiodes based on Si (data and theory) and In0.3Ga0.7N/GaN MQW with different number of quantum wells (theory). Below the cut-off wavelength of $\sim\frac{hc}{E_g}$, the responsivity is given by $R=\eta\bullet\left(\frac{q}{hc}\right)\bullet\lambda$, with $\eta$ is the quantum efficiency. (b) Responsivity of photodiodes based on $In_{0.3}Ga_{0.7}N$/GaN MQW with different number of quantum wells (theory) and reported experimental data (shaded area) [25–34].

an average value determined by the average optical power $P$. From Poisson statistics, the mean square shot noise current is given by

$$\overline{i_{SN}^2} = 2q \bullet (I + I_d) \bullet \Delta f \qquad (6.2)$$

where $q$ is the electron charge, $I$ is the average current generated by the detector, $I_d$ is the dark current, and $\Delta f$ is the bandwidth over which the noise is being considered. The current $I$ is proportional to the incident optical power using the relationship

$$I = \mathcal{R} \bullet P_D \qquad (6.3)$$

where $\mathcal{R}$ for PIN photodetectors, and $P_D$ is the incident light power on the detector.

#### 6.2.2.3 Thermal Noise

Thermal noise arises in the load resistor of the photodiode circuit due to random thermal motion of the electrons. The mean square thermal noise current in a load resistor $R_L$ is given by

$$\overline{i_{TN}^2} = \frac{4q \bullet k_B T / q}{R_L} \bullet \Delta f \qquad (6.4)$$

where $k_B = 1.3805 \times 10^{-23} \frac{J}{K}$ is the Boltzmann constant, $T$ is the absolute temperature in Kelvin, and $\Delta f$ is the bandwidth of detection. The signal-to-noise ratio is given by

$$SNR = \frac{\mathcal{R}^2 \bullet P^2}{2q(\mathcal{R} \bullet P_D + I_d)\Delta f + (4k_B T / R_L)\Delta f} \qquad (6.5)$$

#### 6.2.2.4 Noise Equivalent Power

A detector is specified by its responsivity $\mathcal{R}$ and a parameter called noise equivalent power (NEP). NEP is expressed by

$$NEP = \frac{1}{\mathcal{R}}\left(2q \bullet I_d + \frac{4k_B T}{R_L}\right)^{1/2} \quad \left(\mathrm{W} / \sqrt{\mathrm{Hz}}\right) \qquad (6.6)$$

Typical good detectors have NEP in the range 1–10 $\frac{pW}{\sqrt{Hz}}$.

For an APD with gain $M$, the SNR is given by [35]

$$SNR = \frac{\mathcal{R}^2 \bullet P_D^2}{M^x \bullet 2q \bullet \left(\mathcal{R} \bullet P_D + I_d\right) \bullet \Delta f + \left(1/M^2\right)\left(4k_B T / R_L\right) \bullet \Delta f} \tag{6.7}$$

where $0.25 \leq x \leq 0.35$. The optimal APD gain is given by

$$\left(M_{\text{opt}}\right)^{x+2} = \frac{4k_B T}{x \bullet q \bullet R_L \times \left(\mathcal{R} \bullet P_D + I_d\right)} \tag{6.8}$$

For example, when $T = 300\text{K}$, $R_L = 1000\Omega$, $P_D = 100$ nW, $\mathcal{R} = 0.65\frac{A}{W}$, $x = 0.3$, the optimal gain is $M_{op} = 42$.

### 6.2.3 Optical Fibers

The simplest optical fiber is a dielectric cylindrical waveguide consisting of a central core with a higher refractive index that is surrounded by a cladding with lower refractive index. The cladding is usually enclosed in a protective jacket. As other waveguides, optical fibers can be single-mode and multimode. The important parameter that defines a number of modes is the parameter, given by $v = \frac{2\pi a}{\lambda} \bullet n_1 \bullet \sqrt{2\Delta}$ with $\Delta = \frac{\left(n_1 - n_2\right)}{n_2}$. Here, $a$ is the radius of the core, $\lambda$ is a free space wavelength of light, $n_1$ is the refractive index of the core, $n_2$ is the refractive index of the cladding, and $\Delta$ is the relative difference of the refractive indices. The fiber supports only one mode if $v < 2.405$. In standard telecom fibers, the difference between $n_1$ and $n_2$ is typically small, so that $\Delta << 1$. Optical fibers satisfying this condition are called weakly guiding. The typical value for a single-mode fiber (SMF) is $\Delta$ approximately 0.003.

#### 6.2.3.1 Multimode Fiber

If the microLED emits a light pulse with peak power of $P_{microLED}$, the microLED-to-fiber efficiency is $\eta_c$, the fiber attenuation factor is $\alpha\left(\frac{dB}{km}\right)$, and the fiber length is $L(km)$, then the optical power arriving at the photodetector at the receiver end of the link is given by

$$P_D = P_{\text{LED}} \times \eta_c \times 10^{-\alpha \bullet L/10} \tag{6.9}$$

To meet a bit error rate (BER) target for a given photodetector, the coupling efficiency needs to meet a minimum requirement (e.g., < –3 dB coupling loss).

Unlike lasers, microLEDs are incoherent sources. The implication of this is that the coupling efficiency from a microLED to a single mode fiber is limited to [36]

$$\eta_c\,(\mathrm{SMF}) \approx 4\pi \times \left(\frac{\lambda}{2\pi D}\right)^2 \text{ with } \frac{\lambda}{2\pi D} \ll 1 \tag{6.10}$$

For a microLED with diameter $D = 7\ \mu$m and for $\lambda = 0.45\ \mu$m, we calculate that $\eta_c(SMF) \approx 0.13\%$ (–28 dB). This means that for microLEDs to work in the system shown in Figure 6.2, a multimode fiber must be used. This translates into $\eta_c$ (multimode fiber (MMF)) ≈ 4% (–14 dB) for a direct butt coupling configuration and a Lambertian-type microLED. This implies that an optical element (e.g., a microlens) that helps increase the coupling efficiency is necessary.

In order to appreciate the operation of multimode fibers with a microLED that emits light with a finite (e.g., 25 nm) linewidth, it is necessary to take a closer look at the details of wave propagation into a multimode fiber from an incoherent light source. One can determine the propagating modes for a light with wavelength $\lambda$ and a fiber with core radius $a$, core refractive index $n_1$, and cladding refractive index $n_2$ by solving Maxwell's equations. Rigorous analyses for the transverse electric (TE), transverse magnetic (TM), and hybrid modes in a step index fiber can be described mathematically. For practical optical fibers, the refractive-index difference is of the order of 1%. Then we can approximate as $\frac{n_1}{n_2} \approx 1$. This approximation allows us to simplify the analysis of optical fibers drastically and enables us to obtain quite clear results. Such mode groups with the approximation $\frac{n_1}{n_2} \approx 1$ are designated as linearly polarized (LP) modes. Since an LP mode is derived by the approximation of $\frac{n_1}{n_2} \approx 1$, it means that the light confinement in the core is not so tight. Therefore, this approximation is called weakly guiding approximation. Determination of the propagating optical modes can be done by solving (6.11), (6.12), and (6.13) with the help of (6.14)–(6.16). The modes are found by solving the following equations [37, 38]:

$$\mathrm{LP}_{0m} \quad \frac{J_0(u)}{u\,J_1(u)} = \frac{K_0(w)}{w\,K_1(w)} \tag{6.11}$$

$$\mathrm{LP}_{1m} \quad \frac{J_1(u)}{u\,J_0(u)} = -\frac{K_1(w)}{w\,K_0(w)} \tag{6.12}$$

$$\mathrm{LP}_{\ell m}\ (\ell \geq 2) \quad \frac{J_\ell(u)}{u\, J_{\ell-1}(u)} = -\frac{K_\ell(w)}{w\, K_{\ell-1}(w)} \tag{6.13}$$

$$b_{\ell m} = \frac{\left(\beta_{b_{\ell m}} / k\right)^2 - n_2^2}{n_1^2 - n_2^2} \tag{6.14}$$

$$w = 2\pi\left(\frac{a}{\lambda}\right)\sqrt{b_{\ell m}\left(n_1^2 - n_2^2\right)} \tag{6.15}$$

$$u = 2\pi\left(\frac{a}{\lambda}\right)\sqrt{\left(1 - b_{\ell m}\right)\times n_1^2 + \left(1 + b_{\ell m}\right)\times n_2^2} \tag{6.16}$$

The fractional power propagating in the fiber core with respect to total power in cladding and core for a given mode is given by

$$\frac{P_{\ell m,\mathrm{core}}}{P_{\ell m}} = 1 - \frac{w^2}{v^2}\left[1 - \xi_\ell(w)\right] \tag{6.17}$$

$$\xi_\ell(w) = \frac{K_\ell^2(w)}{K_{\ell-1}(w)\times K_{\ell+1}(w)} \tag{6.18}$$

$$v = 2\pi\left(\frac{a}{\lambda}\right)\sqrt{n_1^2 - n_2^2} \tag{6.19}$$

A light with a wavelength shorter than a cutoff value $\lambda_{c,lm}$ will not propagate in the core of an optical fiber as an $LP_{lm}$ mode. Since a microLED emits light with wavelengths in the range $\lambda_0 - \Delta \leq \lambda_0 \leq \lambda_0 + \Delta$, only wavelengths with $\lambda > \lambda_{c,lm}$ will excite an $LP_{lm}$ propagating mode. For a given $LP_{lm}$ mode, $\lambda_{c,lm}$ can be found by solving (6.11), (6.12), and (6.13) for the $b_{lm} = 0$. Then one can calculate the percentage of power that will be coupled into the core by integrating the source spectra $S(\lambda)$ for one mode with cutoff wavelength $\lambda_{c,lm}$

$$\eta_c = \eta_{01} + \sum_{m=1}^{N}\sum_{l=1}^{N}\eta_{lm} \tag{6.20}$$

where $\eta_{lm}$ is given by

$$\eta_{lm} = \int_{\lambda_{c,lm}}^{\infty} S(\lambda)\,d\lambda \Big/ \int_{0}^{\infty} S(\lambda)\,d\lambda \tag{6.21}$$

Equation (6.20) is valid for large value of normalized frequency $v$ (given by (6.19)).

If $\eta_c$ is calculated for a given microLED with spectrum $S(\lambda)$ at various values of fiber core radius $a$, then one can determine the minimum core radius that guarantees at least 95% of the power emitted by the microLED is available for coupling into the optical fiber core.

#### 6.2.3.2 Pulse Dispersion

In digital communication systems, information is encoded in the form of pulses and then these light pulses are transmitted from the transmitter to the receiver. The larger the number of pulses that can be sent per unit time and still be resolvable at the receiver end, the larger is the capacity of the system. However, when the light pulses travel down the fiber, the pulses spread out, and this phenomenon is called pulse dispersion. The concept of pulse dispersion is illustrated in Figure 6.6. This dispersion is caused by the wave confinement in the fiber core and its magnitude is proportional to fiber length, fiber design (i.e., refractive index profile), and fiber material. There are two types of pulse dispersion: (1) model dispersion, and (2) chromatic dispersion. If the pulse broadening due to model dispersion is $\sigma_m$ and the pulse broadening due to chromatic dispersion is $\sigma_c$, then a Gaussian pulse with RMS width of $\sigma_0$ will propagate through the fiber and the output pulse will have an RMS width of $\sigma$ that is given by [39]:

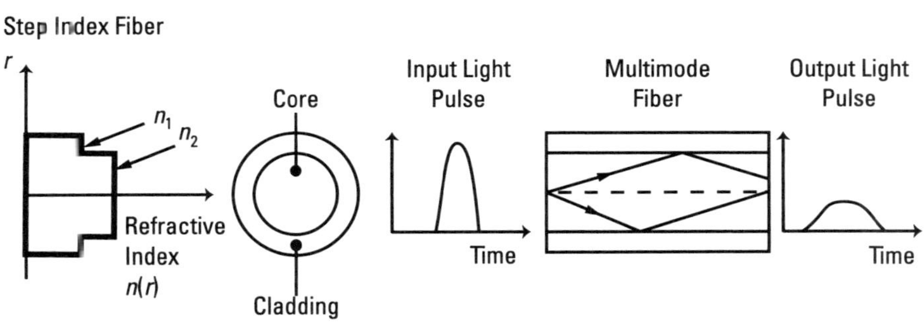


**Figure 6.6** Schematic diagram showing a fiber, illustrating the concept of pulse broadening.

$$\sigma = \left[\sigma_0^2 + \sigma_m^2 + \sigma_c^2\right]^{1/2} \quad (6.22)$$

#### 6.2.3.2.1 Modal Dispersion

Modal dispersion is only important in multimode fibers. Many different modes propagate in a multimode fiber. Each of these modes takes a different path and thus different length when traveling down the fiber. Another factor is the differing propagation constants associated with each mode (each mode's group velocity). Both factors contribute to modal dispersion. The time pulse broadening due to modal dispersion in a step-index multimode fiber can be expressed by the simple equation [40]

$$\sigma_{m(\text{step-index})} = \frac{L}{c} \bullet (n_1 - n_2) \bullet \left(1 - \frac{\pi}{V}\right) \quad (6.23)$$

$$V = \frac{2\pi a}{\lambda} \bullet \sqrt{n_1^2 - n_2^2} = \frac{2\pi a}{\lambda} \bullet n_1 \bullet \sqrt{2\Delta} \quad (6.24)$$

$$\Delta = \frac{1}{2} - \frac{1}{2}\left(\frac{n_2}{n_1}\right)^2 \quad (6.25)$$

The number of modes propagating through the fiber is given by

$$M = \frac{1}{2}\left(\frac{2\pi a}{\lambda}\right)^2 \left(n_1^2 - n_2^2\right) \quad (6.26)$$

Here $L(m)$ the fiber length, $c$ is the free-space speed of light, $n_1(\lambda)$ is the refractive index of the core, $n_2(\lambda)$ is the refractive index of the cladding, and $\lambda$ is the peak emission wavelength of the microLED. The refractive index as function of wavelength depends on the material used to fabricate the fiber. An example is shown in Figure 6.7.

Intermodal dispersion in multimode fibers can be minimized with the use of graded-index fibers. Hence, multimode graded-index fibers show substantial bandwidth improvement over multimode step-index fibers. For instance, a

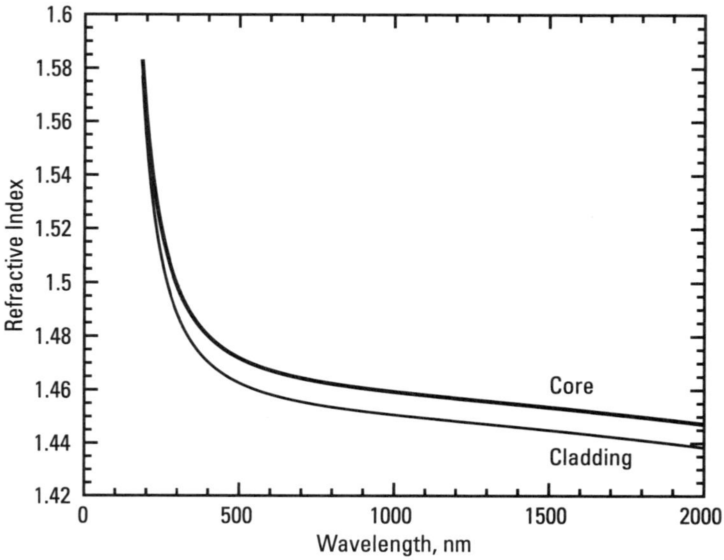


**Figure 6.7** Refractive index as function of wavelength for cladding (fused silica) and core ($GeO_2$-doped fused silica) [41].

nearly parabolic index of refraction profile has been observed to give a minimal amount of intermodal dispersion and to reduce pulse distortion by an order of magnitude in comparison with step-index fibers [42]. To illustrate the potential of graded-index fibers, we consider the class of circular-symmetric fibers described by the refractive index profile

$$n(r) = \begin{cases} n_1 \bullet \sqrt{1 - 2\Delta \bullet (r / a)^{\alpha}}, & 0 \le r < a \\ n_1 \bullet \sqrt{1 - 2\Delta}, & r \ge a \end{cases} \tag{6.27}$$

where $r$ is an offset distance from the core center, $\alpha$ is the core index exponent, $n_1$ is the refractive index in the center of the core, $\Delta$ is the refractive index contrast, and $a$ is the core radius.

Multimode optical fibers described by (6.25) potentially support a large but finite number of modes that are particular solutions of Maxwell's equations. Each guided mode has its own propagation constant and therefore propagates at its own particular velocity. From the Wentzel-Kramers-Brillouin (WKB) analysis it was shown that propagated modes are actually clustered within groups in which each mode has nearly the same propagation constant.

The pulse broadening is given by [43, 44]

$$\sigma_{m(\text{graded-index})} \approx \begin{cases} \dfrac{L}{c} \bullet n_1 \bullet \Delta \bullet \dfrac{\alpha - \alpha_{\text{opt}}}{\alpha + 2}, & \alpha \neq \alpha_{\text{opt}} \\ \dfrac{L}{c} \bullet \dfrac{n_1 \bullet \Delta^2}{2}, & \alpha = \alpha_{\text{opt}} \end{cases} \tag{6.28}$$

where $\alpha_{\text{opt}}$ is given by

$$\alpha_{\text{opt}} \approx 2 - 2 \bullet \frac{n_1}{\xi} \bullet \frac{\lambda}{\Delta} \bullet \frac{\partial \Delta}{\partial \lambda} \tag{6.29}$$

$$\xi = n_1 - \lambda \bullet \frac{\partial n_1}{\partial \lambda} \tag{6.30}$$

Note when $\alpha$>>2 then we have a step-index fiber. In (6.28), negative value for $\sigma_{m(\text{graded index})}$ means that higher-order modes arrive before the lower-order modes. The calculated modal dispersion is shown in Figure 6.8 for step-index and graded-index fibers.

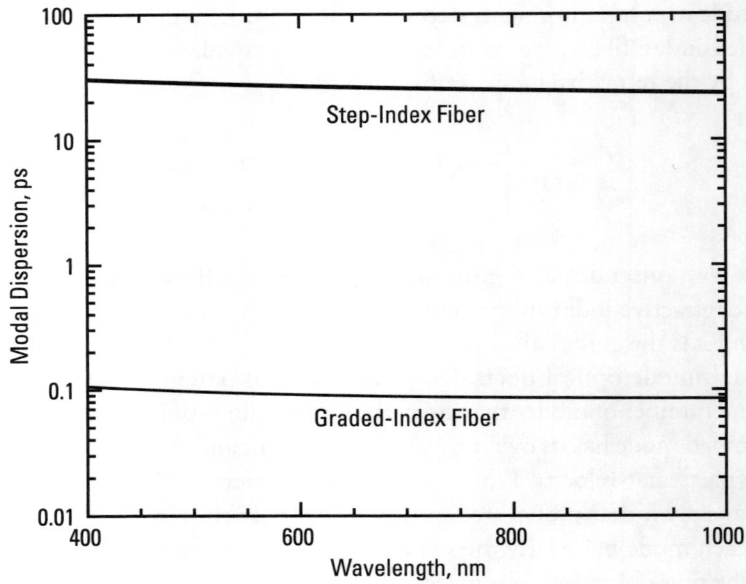


**Figure 6.8** Modal dispersion in step-index and graded-index fibers versus wavelength. Optimal refractive index profile is used for the graded-index case. The link length was assumed to be 1m and the fiber diameter was assumed to be 32 $\mu$m.

The refractive index of silica-based fiber is well approximated by the Sellmeier polynomial [41]:

$$n(\lambda)=\left[1+\sum_{i=1}^{3}\frac{a_i\lambda^2}{\lambda^2-b_i}\right]^{1/2} \tag{6.31}$$

where the $a_i$ and $b_i$ are Sellmeier coefficients, which for pure silica are given by: $a_1 = 0.6965325$, $a_2 = 0.4083099$, $a_3 = 0.8968766$, $b_1 = 4.368309 \times 10^{-3}$, $b_2 = 1.394999 \times 10^{-2}$, $b_3 = 97.93399$. The Sellmeier coefficients of $GeO_2$-doped glass with 6.3 mol% concentration may be represented by the following coefficients: $a_1 = 0.7083952$, $a_2 = 0.4203993$, $a_3 = 0.8663412$, $b_1 = 7.290465 \times 10^{-3}$, $b_2 = 1.050294 \times 10^{-2}$, $b_3 = 97.93428$.

#### 6.2.3.2.2 Chromatic Dispersion

Chromatic dispersion is caused by the velocity of light (or refractive index) being a function of wavelength. All light sources (even a laser source) have some degree of spectral width. This means that even in a single-mode fiber (since a laser source also has some spectral linewidth), longer wavelengths travel faster and arrive earlier than shorter wavelengths at the receiver, and this causes pulse spreading. The nonzero spectral width in microLED can have an important effect on the communication system bandwidth. The chromatic pulse broadening due to material dispersion is defined by [40]

$$\sigma_c=\frac{L}{c}\bullet\Delta\lambda\bullet\lambda\bullet\frac{d^2n}{d\lambda^2} \tag{6.32}$$

Here $\Delta\lambda$(nm) is the spectral width of the microLED, $\lambda$(nm) is the peak wavelength of the microLED, and $L$(m) the fiber length, $n(\lambda)$ is given by (6.32). The calculated chromatic and modal dispersions are shown in Figure 6.9.

### 6.2.3.3 Optical Fiber Attenuation

As light travels through a medium such as an optical fiber, its intensity is reduced through effects such as absorption or scattering of photons. Attenuation (dB/km), by definition, is the ratio of the light intensity at a distance ($L$) to the light intensity at the source. Fiber losses depend on the wavelength, $\lambda$, and are considerably higher at visible wavelengths. In the visible light regime (400–700 nm), the attenuation is dominated by Rayleigh scattering. This scattering is a fundamental loss mechanism arising from density fluctuations frozen in the material matrix during manufacturing. These density fluctuations cause local fluctuations in the refractive index, acting as light scattering centers in all direc-

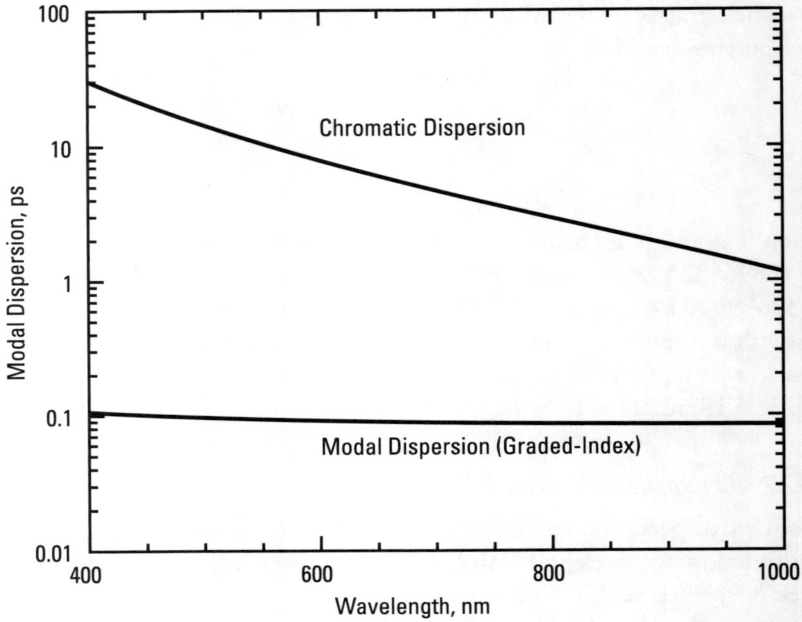


**Figure 6.9** Calculated pulse dispersion due to chromatic dispersion and modal dispersion as a function of wavelength. At a wavelength of 450 nm, chromatic dispersion is 20 ps and modal dispersion is 0.1 ps for a link length of 1m.

tions. The subsequent scattering due to the density fluctuations, which is in almost all directions, produces an attenuation proportional to $1/\lambda^4$ following the Rayleigh scattering formula. For silica-based fiber with length $L(m)$, the power attenuation is given by (with $\lambda$ is given in $\mu$m):

$$\alpha = \frac{0.822988}{\lambda^4} \text{ dB / km} \tag{6.33}$$

For wavelength of 0.45 $\mu$m, $\alpha \approx 20$ dB/km. For a 1m link, we calculate attenuation loss as $20 \times 0.001 = 0.02$ dB.

### 6.2.4 Light Coupling into Optical Fibers

Figure 6.11 illustrates five different microLED-to-fiber coupling configurations: (1) butt coupling, (2) a lensed fiber end, (3) a small sphere lens in contact with both the fiber and the source, (4) a truncated aspherical $\mu$lens (e.g., comprised of a drop of cured silicone on the source), and (5) floating hyperbolic lens integrated with the microLED.

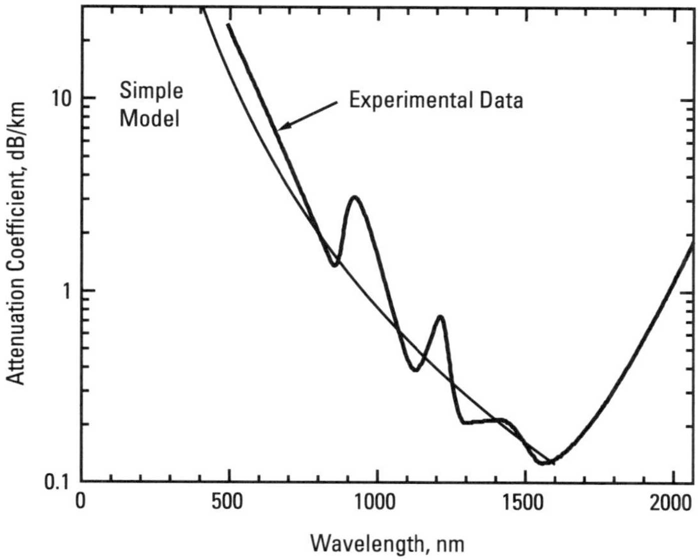


**Figure 6.10** Example fiber attenuation versus wavelength [45].

Improving the coupling efficiency between a semiconductor light source and optical fiber is generally achieved by using of a $\mu$lens formed on the end of the fiber, as shown in Figure 6.12, by using a microlens integrated on the microLED emitting surface, or by using resonant-cavity LED structure to produce directional light with a small divergence angle.

#### 6.2.4.1 Hyperbolic-Lensed Fiber

The lens serves to match the modes of the microLED and the fiber. The most common way to fabricate $\mu$lenses is by tapering the fiber down to a point and melting the end. The resulting $\mu$lenses are hemispherical in shape and typically collect approximately 50% (–3 dB) of the available light source radiation [46]. The ideal lens was found to be hyperbolic [47, 46], with a measured coupling efficiency of about 90%. A hyperbolic lens shape is free of spherical aberration and does not suffer from a limited aperture for typical lasers when matching the laser and fiber modes [46].

The same conclusion had been reached [47] with the polar surface of the lens given by

$$\rho(\theta) = \frac{f \times (n - n_0)}{n \times \cos\theta - n_0} \tag{6.34}$$

where $f$ is the focal length and $n$ is the refractive index of the lens material. If the microLED radiation pattern is given by $I(\theta)$, the coupling efficiency is given by:

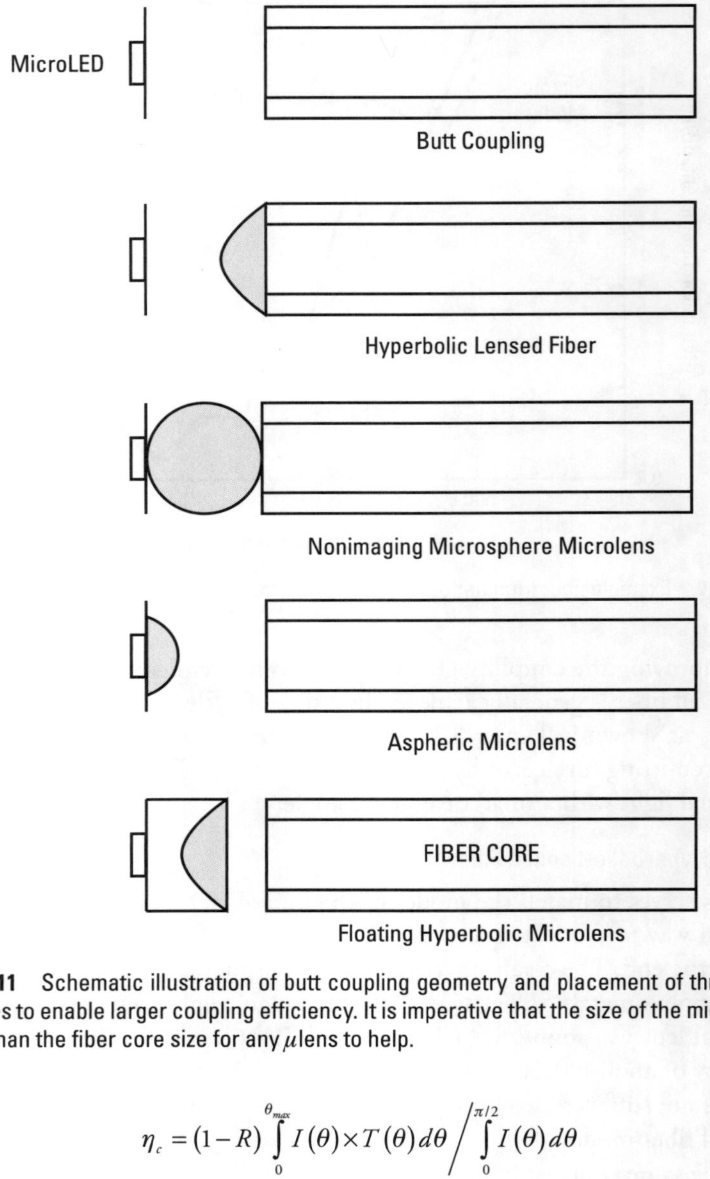


**Figure 6.11** Schematic illustration of butt coupling geometry and placement of three types of $\mu$lenses to enable larger coupling efficiency. It is imperative that the size of the microLED is smaller than the fiber core size for any $\mu$lens to help.

$$\eta_c = (1-R)\int_0^{\theta_{max}} I(\theta)\times T(\theta)\,d\theta \Big/ \int_0^{\pi/2} I(\theta)\,d\theta \tag{6.35}$$

where $\theta_{max}$ is imposed by the size of the lens (i.e., radius $r_0 > r_f$). Based on the geometry shown in Figure 6.12, $\theta_{max}$ can be calculated from

$$r_0 = \frac{f\times(n-n_0)}{n\times\cos\theta_{max} - n_0}\times\sin\theta_{max} \tag{6.36}$$

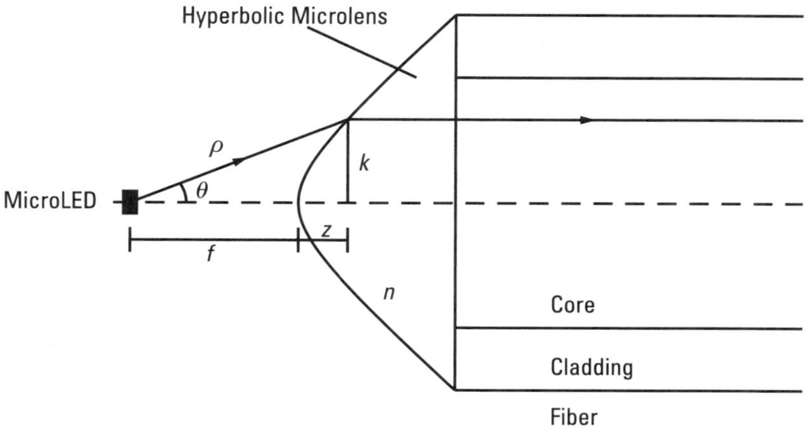


**Figure 6.12** Illustration of a lensed fiber configuration with a hyperbolic $\mu$lens integrated on the fiber end. This is an aberration free lens that has all rays converging at the focus in phase; all optical path lengths from a given wave front to the focus are equal (i.e., $\rho = f + n \times z$, with $\rho = \sqrt{r^2 + (z+f)^2}$).

The lens thickness $t$ is given by

$$t = \frac{n_0 - \cos\theta_{max}}{n \times \cos\theta_{max} - n_0} f \tag{6.37}$$

The exit angle ($\theta_2$) and the entrance angle ($\theta_1$) are related though Snell's law and geometry as follows:

$$n_0 \sin\theta_1 = n \sin\theta_2 \tag{6.38}$$

$$\sin\theta_2 = \sin(\theta - \theta_1) \tag{6.39}$$

For the *p*-polarization, the transmission coefficient is given by (assuming a medium with refractive index $n_0$ between the microLED surface and the lens)

$$T_p(\theta) = \left( \frac{2 \times n_0 \times \cos\theta_1}{n_0 \cos\theta_1 + n \cos\theta_2} \right)^2 \tag{6.40}$$

For the *s*-polarization, the transmission coefficient is given by

$$T_s(\theta)=\left(\frac{2\times n_0\times\cos\theta_1}{n_0\cos\theta_2+n\cos\theta_1}\right)^2 \tag{6.41}$$

For each value of $\theta$, (6.39) and (6.40) are solved to find $\theta_1$ and $\theta_2$ as a function of $\theta$. Then either (6.41) or (6.42) is used to find the transmission coefficient as a function of $\theta$. This is necessary for calculating the coupling efficiency using (6.36).

It is useful to calculate the coupling efficiency as a function of the lens radius of curvature. The radius of curvature is calculated from (6.35) and the definition of radius of curvature given by

$$R_c\equiv\left|\left.\frac{\left(\rho^2+\rho'^2\right)^{3/2}}{\rho^2+2\rho'^2-\rho\rho''}\right|_{\theta=0}\right| \tag{6.42}$$

where $\rho'\equiv\partial\rho/\partial\theta$ and $\rho''\equiv\partial^2\rho/\partial\theta^2$. This leads to the following simple equation:

$$R_c=\left(n-n_0\right)\times f \tag{6.43}$$

The calculated coupling efficiency is shown versus the lens radius of curvature in Figure 6.13, with the assumption of a Lambertian source: $I(\theta)=\cos\theta$ or a super-Lambertian source (i.e., $I(\theta)=\cos^4\theta$).

#### 6.2.4.2 MicroLED-Integrated Hyperbolic Lens

Here we propose the configuration shown in Figure 6.14 with an upside-down hyperbolic $\mu$lens integrated on the surface of the microLED to achieve near 100% coupling efficiency to fibers. The $\mu$lens may be implemented with metasurface technology [48].

Metasurface technology utilizes the fabrication of subwavelength dielectric structures to passively modulate the phase of incoming light. Constructed from high-index dielectric materials, the shape and size of structures can create a desired phase shift at any specific location on the metasurface structure. When carefully designed, this phase shift can bend or refract light at an angle that is desirable for a given application. Metasurface structures have the additional advantages of being planar, and subwavelength in thickness, making them relatively simple to integrate with on-chip photonic devices [48].

To create a hyperbolic $\mu$lens, the metasurface can be designed in such a way as to recreate the same phase shift at each location along the lens as shown in Figure 6.15. Because metasurfaces lenses are planar, they have the additional advantage of being placed closer to the microLED, which keeps the outcoupled beam size significantly smaller than the fiber core.

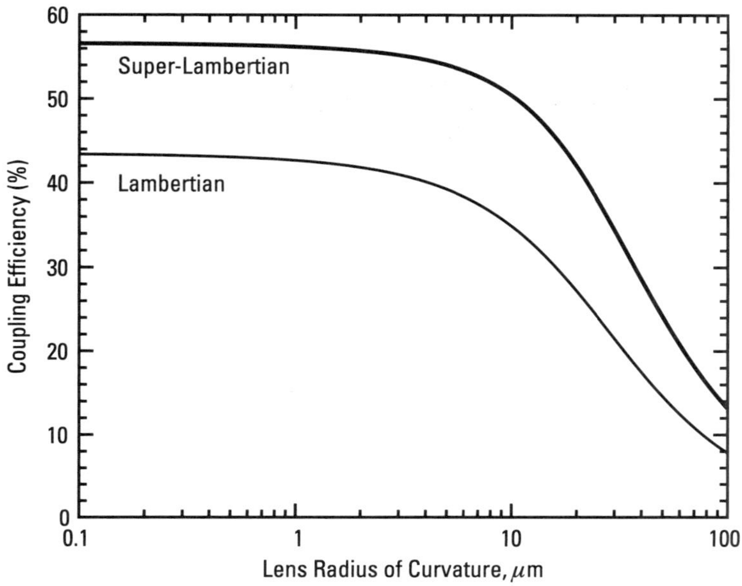


**Figure 6.13** Simulated coupling efficiency versus lens radius of curvature ($n = 1.5$, $r_f = 25\ \mu$m, $n_0 =$ ˙, $r_0 = r_f$). A lens with a smaller radius of curvature results in higher coupling efficiency, as expected. A super-Lambertian source outperforms a Lambertian source at a given lens radius of curvature. The coupling efficiency without a lens (i.e., butt coupling) is approximately 3% in the case of a Lambertian source.

### 6.2.4.3 Directional Radiation with Resonant Cavity MicroLEDs

Now that it was demonstrated above that super-Lambertian LEDs can be of great value for coupling more power to an optical fiber, we discuss how a super-Lambertian radiation pattern is realized. A resonant cavity LED structure can produce super-Lambertian radiation patterns; even sharper than the $\cos^m(\theta)$ pattern. Compared with conventional LEDs, the resonant cavity LEDs (RCLEDs) reveal inherent advantages including narrower spectrum linewidth, larger modulation bandwidth, superior directionality of the emitted light (i.e., smaller angular dispersion), and higher light extraction efficiency. In general, the RCLEDs consist of an active region containing MQWs sandwiched in a Fabry-Perot (FP) resonator of two reflectors: front and back [49–51]. A schematic of a typical RCLED is shown in Figure 6.16.

If the reflectivity of the front mirror is $R_F$ the reflectivity of the back mirror is $R_B$, the cavity length is $d$, and the refractive index of the cavity material is $n$, then the FWHM ($\Delta\lambda$) of the emission spectrum is given by [50]

$$\frac{\Delta\lambda}{\lambda} \approx \frac{1}{\pi} \bullet \frac{1-(R_F \bullet R_B)^{1/2}}{(R_F \bullet R_B)^{1/4}} \bullet \frac{1}{\mathrm{Int}(2n \bullet d/\lambda)} \tag{6.44}$$

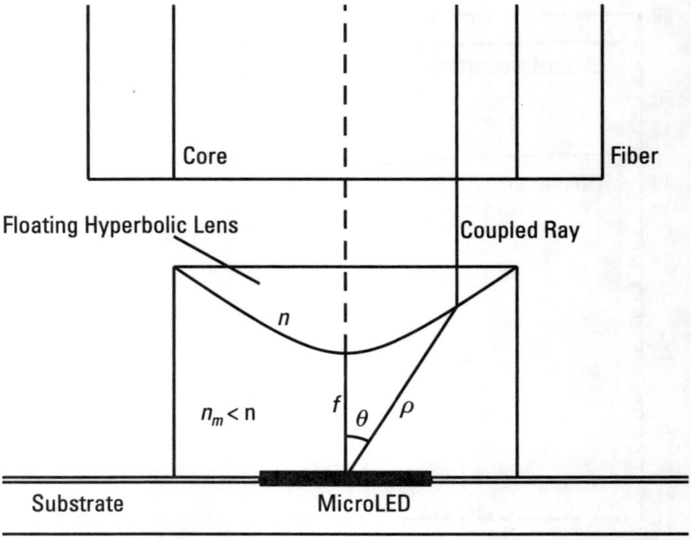


**Figure 6.14** Illustration of an integrated floating hyperbolic $\mu$lens on the microLED for efficient coupling of light into an optical fiber.

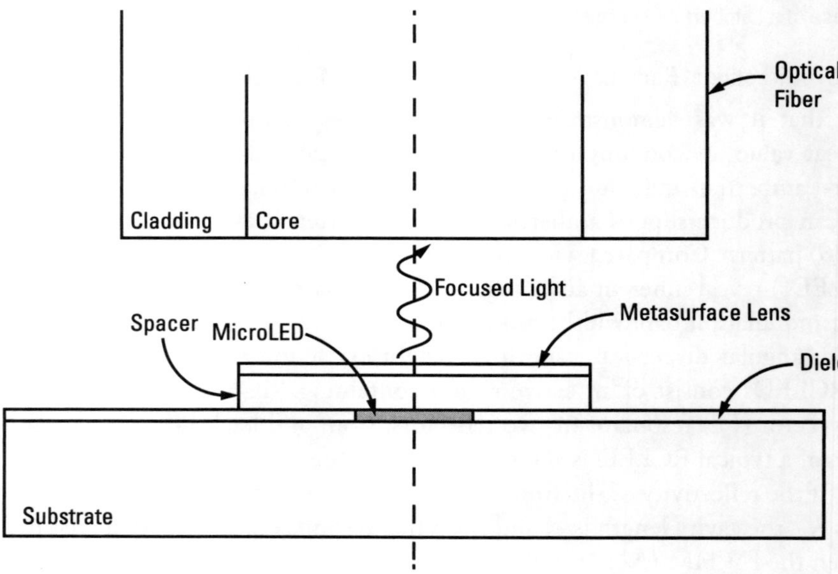


**Figure 6.15** Illustration of an integrated floating metasurface lens above the microLED for efficient coupling of light into an optical fiber.

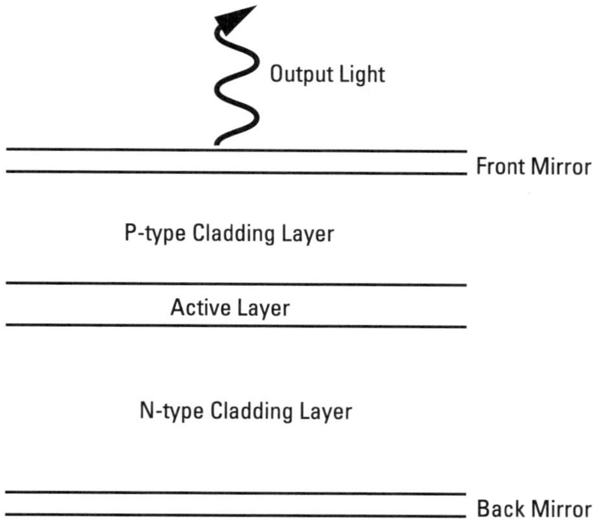


**Figure 6.16** Schematic illustration of the RCLED structure of two mirrors with reflectivity $R_F$ for the front mirror (where light exits) and $R_B$ for the back mirror. The cavity length (distance between front and back mirrors) is equal to $\lambda/2$, where $\lambda$ is the emission wavelength.

The FWHM ($\Delta\theta$) if the radiation pattern is given by [50]

$$\Delta\theta \approx 2 \bullet \cos^{-1}\left[1 - \frac{1}{2} \bullet \left(\frac{\Delta\lambda}{\lambda}\right)\right] \tag{6.45}$$

The resonant-cavity LED also promises an enhanced extraction efficiency versus the conventional LED. The enhancement factor is a function of $R_F$, $R_B$, $n$, $d$, and $\lambda$ according to the approximation [49]

$$\xi \approx \frac{16}{\pi} \bullet \frac{1 - R_F}{\left(1 - \left(R_F \bullet R_B\right)^{1/2}\right)\left(R_F \bullet R_B\right)^{1/4}} \bullet \tan^{-1}\varphi \tag{6.46a}$$

$$\varphi \approx \frac{\pi}{2n^2} \bullet \frac{\left(R_F \bullet R_B\right)^{1/4}}{\left(1 - \left(R_F \bullet R_B\right)^{1/2}\right)} \mathrm{Int}\left(2n \bullet d / \lambda\right) \tag{6.46b}$$

The spectral and angular full-width-half-maxima $\Delta\lambda$ and $\Delta\theta$ are calculated for blue ($\lambda = 450$ nm) emissions using the above equations and reasonable values for $R_F$, $R_B$, $n$, and $d$. The spectral width was calculated to be <5 nm and the divergence angle was around <10°. Indeed, significant reductions of $\Delta\lambda$ and

$\Delta\theta$ are predicted from (6.45) to (6.47) compared to conventional LEDs ($\Delta\lambda$ = 30 – 60 nm and $\Delta\theta$ = 120° (i.e., ±60°).

## 6.3 System Design Framework

### 6.3.1 Maximum Data Rate

Dispersion of the transmitted optical signal causes distortion for digital transmission along optical fibers. When considering the major implementation of optical fiber transmission that involves some form of digital modulation, then dispersion mechanisms within the fiber cause broadening of the transmitted light pulses as they travel along the channel. The phenomenon is illustrated in Figure 6.17, where it may be observed that each pulse broadens and overlaps with its neighbors, eventually becoming indistinguishable at the receiver input. The effect is known as intersymbol interference (ISI) [39]. Thus, an increasing number of errors may be encountered on the digital optical channel as the ISI becomes more pronounced. The error rate is also a function of the signal attenuation on the link and the subsequent signal-to-noise ratio (SNR) at the receiver. This factor is considered in the next section. However, signal dispersion alone limits the maximum possible bandwidth attainable with a particular optical fiber to the point where individual symbols can no longer be distinguished.

A good estimate of the maximum bit rate for an optical channel with dispersion may be obtained by considering the light pulses at the output to have a Gaussian shape with an RMS width of $\sigma$. When employing a nonreturn-to-zero pulse, the maximum bit rate is equal to 2 × $B_{opt}$, then [52]

$$B_{T,max} \approx \frac{2 \bullet 0.187}{\sigma} \ (\text{bit/s}) \tag{6.47}$$

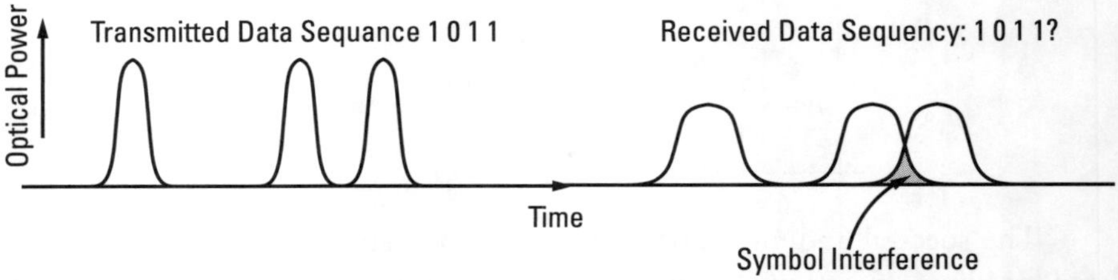


**Figure 6.17** An illustration using the digital bit pattern 1011 of the broadening of light pulses as they are transmitted along a fiber: (left) fiber input, and (right) fiber output.

This analysis allows for the existence of a certain amount of signal overlap on the channel while avoiding any SNR penalty that occurs when ISI becomes pronounced. Using (6.22), we can then write

$$B_{T,max} \approx \frac{2 \bullet 0.187}{\left[\left(0.187 / f_{3dB}\right)^2 + \sigma_m^2 + \sigma_c^2\right]^{1/2}} \text{ (bit / s)} \tag{6.48}$$

where $f_{3dB}$ is the 3-dB modulation bandwidth of the microLED as reported in Figure 6.4.

The calculated system bandwidth is shown in Figure 6.18 as a function of fiber length for fixed 3-dB modulation bandwidth of 1 GHz and two different values for the emission linewidth.

### 6.3.2 Bit Error Rate

The quality of a digital communication system is specified by its BER, which essentially specifies the average probability of incorrect bit identification. Thus, a BER of $10^{-9}$ means that 1 bit out of every $10^9$ bits is, on average, read incorrectly. If the system is operating at 100 Mb/s—that is, $10^8$ pulses per second—

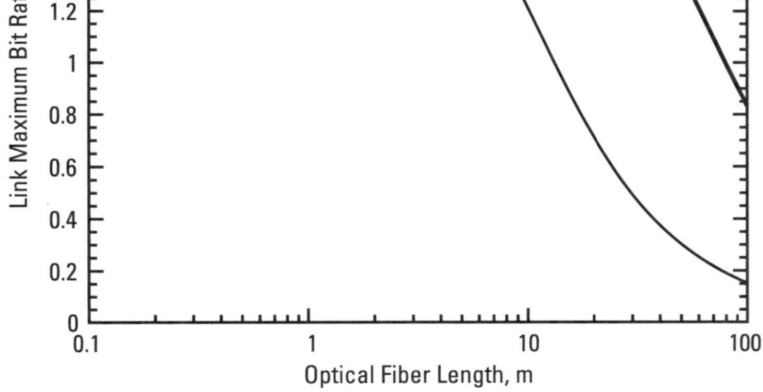


**Figure 6.18** Projected link maximum bit rate as function of fiber length for 3-dB modulation frequency of 1 GHz, wavelength = 450 nm, and two cases with linewidth = 5 and 30 nm. It is observed that the reach can be extended from 1 to 10m by reducing the emission linewidth and using graded-index optical fiber.

then to receive $10^9$ pulses, the time taken would be $10^9/10^8 = 10$s, which is the average time for an error to occur. On the other hand, if the BER is $10^{-6}$, then on average, an error would occur every 0.01s, which is unacceptable. The BER is related to the noise components using the simple approximation [35, 53–55]

$$BER = \frac{1}{4}\left[\text{erfc}\left(\frac{I_{TH} - I_0}{\sqrt{2}\sigma_0}\right) + \text{erfc}\left(\frac{I_1 - I_{TH}}{\sqrt{2}\sigma_1}\right)\right] \tag{6.49}$$

where $I_{TH}$ is the detection threshold current, $I_0$ is the mean of the peak pulse for ZERO bit, $\sigma_0$ is the noise superimposed on the ZERO bit (i.e., thermal noise), $I_1$ is the mean of the peak pulse for ONE bit, and $\sigma_1$ is the noise superimposed on the ONE bit (i.e., thermal noise and shot noise).

For most $P-I-N$ receivers, the noise is dominated by thermal noise, which is independent of the signal current. Thus, the noise in bit 1 and bit 0 is the same (i.e., $\sigma_0 \approx \sigma_1$) and in such a case the optimum setting of the threshold value is at the midpoint of the one and zero levels (i.e., $I_{TH} = (I_0 + I_1)/2$), and the BER is related to SNR through the equation in the case of NRZ scheme

$$BER = \frac{1}{2} \bullet \text{erfc}\left(\frac{\sqrt{SNR}}{2\sqrt{2}}\right) \tag{6.50}$$

Note that the quality factor $Q = \sqrt{SNR}/2\sqrt{2}$ will be degraded by the ISI [53].

If $I_D$ is the dark current, $R_L$ is the load capacitance for the photodetector, $\Delta f$ is the detection bandwidth, and $\mathcal{R}$ is the detector responsivity, the minimum power required at the detector can be expressed by

$$P_{D,min} = SNR \bullet \frac{1 + \sqrt{1 + 2\left(\frac{I_D}{q\Delta f}\right)\left(1 + \frac{2k_B T/q}{I_D R_L}\right)}}{\left(\frac{\mathcal{R}}{q\Delta f}\right)} \tag{6.51}$$

For the *NRZ* system considered above, the bit rate $B$ (bit/s) is related to the detection bandwidth using

$$\Delta f = \frac{B}{2} \tag{6.52}$$

Also, if $C$ represents the photodetector capacitance (farads), then

$$\Delta f = \frac{1}{2\pi \bullet R_L \bullet C} = \frac{B}{2} \tag{6.53}$$

Or

$$R_L = \frac{1}{\pi \bullet C \bullet B} \tag{6.54}$$

In (6.55), $C$ is given in farads, $\mathcal{R}$ is given in A/W, SNR is given in dB, and $B$ is given in Gb/s.

In the case of APD, if thermal noise remains dominant, then the SNR is improved by a factor $M^2$. One can show that $P_{D,min}$ for the case of APDs reduces by a factor by $M$. Since the shot noise also increases with increasing $M$, there is an optimum value of $M$ for achieving maximum improvement.

### 6.3.3 Minimum Energy Consumption

The minimum power of the system is the sum of the emitter power required to achieve a given bit error rate for the data communication system and the switching power at the receiver. If the microLED emits a peak power of $P_{\mu\text{LED}}$, the microLED-to-fiber efficiency is $\eta_c$, the fiber attenuation factor is $\alpha$(dB/km), and the fiber length is $L$(km), then one can write

$$P_{D,\min} = P_{\mu\text{LED},\min} \bullet \eta_c \bullet 10^{-\alpha \bullet L/10} \tag{6.55}$$

The total system power is then given by

$$P_{T,min} = P_{D,\min} + P_{\mu\text{LED},\min} + P_B \tag{6.56}$$

where $P_B$ is the microLED bias power consumption and is given by

$$P_B = V_{LED} \bullet J_{LED} \bullet A_{LED} \tag{6.57}$$

The relationship between the microLED current and voltage is given by

$$V_{LED} = V_F + n\frac{kT}{q}\ln\left(\frac{J_{LED}}{J_0}\right) + \frac{kT}{q}\left(\frac{J_{LED}}{J_0}\right)^{0.5} + J_{LED} \bullet \rho_s \tag{6.58}$$

This equation was derived in Chapter 3 with $J_0 \approx 1\text{A/cm}^2$, $n \approx 2$, $V_F \approx h \cdot c/\lambda$, and $\rho_s \approx 10^{-5}\ \Omega\text{-cm}^2$.

The energy per bit is given by

$$E_T = \frac{P_T}{B_{max}} \tag{6.59}$$

### 6.3.4 Benchmark Against Electrical and Optical Interconnects

In order to calculate the technology curve for microLED optical interconnect, we use the following procedure. From Figure 6.4, identify a data point on the f3 dB versus $J_{LED}$, and find the corresponding $V_{LED}$ from (6.59). The bias power is calculated from (6.58). The bit rate is determined from (6.49) by assuming a reasonable pulse dispersion due to the light propagation through the optical fiber. By setting the BER at $10^{-12}$, for example, one can determine the signal-to-noise ratio (SNR) using (6.51). From (6.55) and the SNR, calculate the minimum required optical power illuminating the photodetector, assuming $C = 20$ fF and $\mathcal{R} = 0.2$ A/W. From (6.56) determine the minimum microLED optical power, assuming $\alpha \approx 0.02$ dB/m and $0.1 \leq L \leq 100$m. The total link power consumption is calculated using (6.57). If the chip shoreline is $S = 10$ mm, then the Keeler's figure of merit (FOM) [56, 57] can be calculated as

$$\text{FOM} = \frac{B_{max}}{E \bullet S} \tag{6.60}$$

Keeler's FOM for microLEDs is compared with the baseline electrical interconnects in Figure 6.19. The benefits of FOM for microLEDs is greatest at a link length of ~10m, but a significant benefit (e.g., 10×) is being projected for links as long as 30m.

## 6.4 Potential System Application

Ever-increasing size and complexity of artificial intelligence (AI) and machine learning (ML) models and datasets has created a vital need for hyperscale data centers distributed over thousands of processing and memory nodes [58, pp. Th1D–3]. These nodes require low-latency and ultralow power multi-Tb/s inter/intrarack optical input/output (I/O) as well as chip-to-chip interconnects. Today, pluggable optics are placed at the motherboard (printed circuit board (PCB)) edge, typically several inches away from the switch application-specific

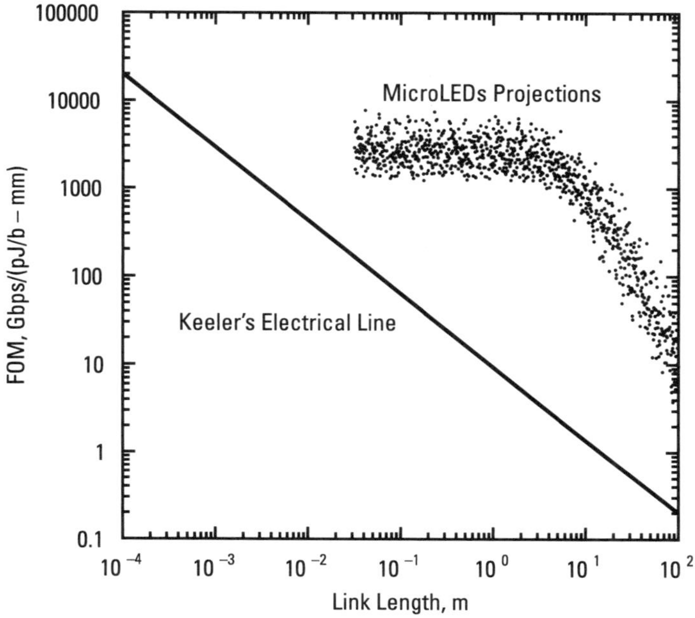


**Figure 6.19** Benchmark plot using Keeler's FOM [56, 57] and the projected performance of microLED links. Significant benefit is projected if microLEDs are used for links as short at 0.1m and as long as 30m. The benefit decreases as the link length increases beyond 30m.

integrated circuit (ASIC). The electronic solution for signal deterioration on the PCB is the addition of retimers but these lead to additional power consumption. In contrast to this, copackaged optics (CPO) are placed on top of the first-level package, in proximity of the ASIC, as shown in Figures 6.20 and 6.21. As such, not only can we overcome the pin density limitations, but we can also have significant energy gains since optics are driven through much shorter wires with significantly lower loss. Demonstrations exist for copackaging a switch ASIC and Si photonics chips and a dozen ribbon optical fiber cables were connected to its package. Such massively parallel optical I/O connections are necessary for high-performance LSIs such as the upcoming high-capacity switch ASICs that are expected to have data transfer rates of over 100 Tbps.

The barriers for optics to penetrate ultrashort reach links (<3m) have been both at generating the light and transmitting it through an appropriate medium.

On the transmission side, lasers are generally unsuitable for use in large numbers for short distance interconnects. Edge emitting lasers are usually relatively large with a length of a few hundred microns. They are typically grown on III-V materials that are incompatible with silicon, with yields that are far below electronic devices in silicon. Semiconductor lasers have high temperature

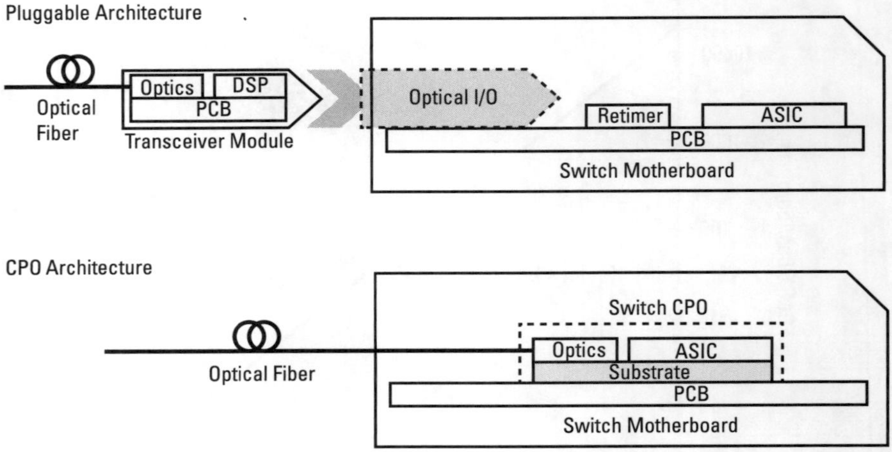


**Figure 6.20** Optical interconnect roadmap illustrating increasing levels of integration of optics and switch ASIC. Today, pluggable optics is used where the optics module is not integrated on the same package as the ASIC switch (top image). Currently, research and development of copackaged optics (bottom image) is underway. CPO promises lower power and cost.

sensitivity, with power and reliability dropping rapidly at the temperatures normal for processor ICs. Lasers also have threshold currents of about a few milliamps, which wastes power. Vertical cavity lasers, rather than waveguide edge-emitting lasers, could be considered more appropriate as they are smaller and have lower threshold currents, but they are even more temperature sensitive. Using an external laser and on-chip modulators has been investigated, but waveguide modulators are lossy, consume a great deal of electrical power and are typically the same size as edge-emitting lasers. Vertical cavity modulators are temperature sensitive and difficult to use. MicroLEDs performance is much less sensitive to temperature and therefore can be brough closer to the CPU/GPU for parallel I/O. As for the optical waveguide, optical interconnects are based on either multimode or single-mode fiber. Historically, multimode optics are lower-cost, due mainly to the relative ease of manufacturing in which large-core diameter multimode fibers are aligned to transmitter or receiver optics. Multimode fibers with large cores do not require tight mechanical tolerances during assembly, which results in negligible losses within the short range between chips. Multimode fibers are perfectly suited for microLEDs, which have finite emission linewidth.

### 6.4.1 Top-of-Rack Switch to Servers Optical Links

The data center network, made of interconnected Ethernet switches arranged in a hierarchical structure, segments, directs, and connects data to and from the

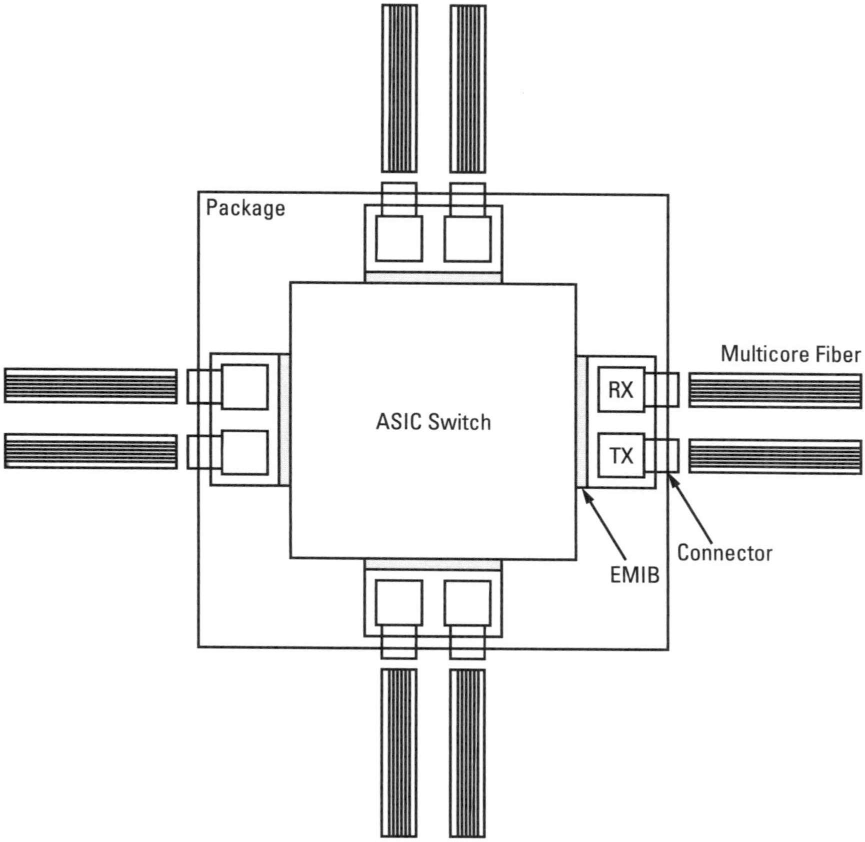


**Figure 6.21** ASIC switch is copackaged with optics modules (TX/RX). The transmitter (TX) and receiver (RX) are made of arrays of microLEDs. The ASIC switch chip is connected with the TX and RX chips via an electrical bridge such as an embedded multilevel interconnect bridge (EMIB).

appropriate server or servers to store data, retrieve data, or to run workloads (see Figure 6.22). As interconnect speed increases to 800G and beyond, copper (machine-to-machine) interconnects will begin to vanish within data centers [59]. The low optical loss of the optical fiber, the intrinsically high bandwidth of light, the lack of interference, and the absence of parasitic inductance and capacitance are all characteristics that favor the modulation of light for interconnects. Starting at long lengths, the advantages of optics has proven itself over shorter distance scales over time.

Figure 6.22 is a schematic illustration of data center network architecture. The data center network is typically hierarchical with a router connecting to the wide area network (WAN) over multiple wavelengths (DWDM) followed by a leaf and spine network of Ethernet switches that aggregate and distribute server

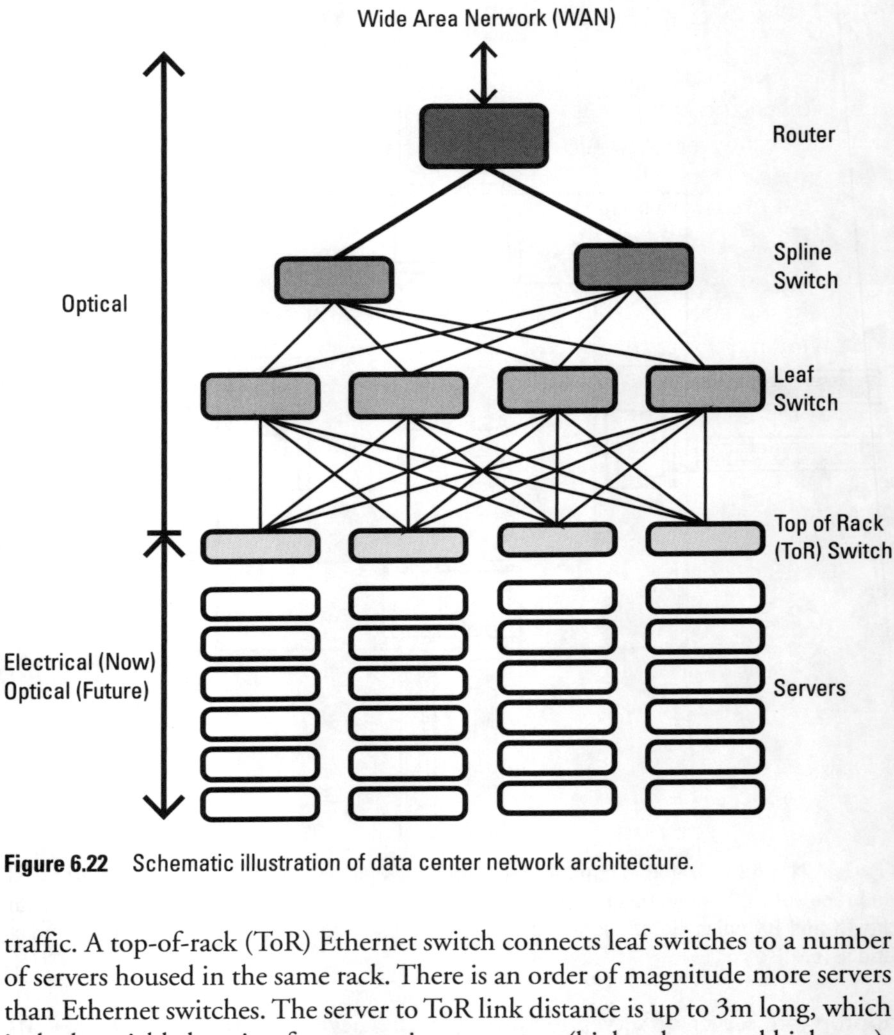


**Figure 6.22** Schematic illustration of data center network architecture.

traffic. A top-of-rack (ToR) Ethernet switch connects leaf switches to a number of servers housed in the same rack. There is an order of magnitude more servers than Ethernet switches. The server to ToR link distance is up to 3m long, which is the last viable location for copper interconnects (high volume and high cost), although there are several trends driving these links toward fiber. Advanced server workloads (artificial intelligence/machine learning) call out for higher bandwidth servers that favor optical solutions.

### 6.4.2 Disaggregated Memory Data Centers

Memory disaggregation is being considered as a strong alternative to traditional architecture to deal with the memory underutilization in data centers [60]. Memory disaggregation decouples memory from compute servers and enables applications to access both local and remote memories. Disaggregated memory expands the memory hierarchy to include a remote level provided by separate memory blades connected over a high-speed backplane, as shown in Figure 6.23.

In a traditional infrastructure model, storage devices are physically connected to specific compute servers. But in a disaggregated architecture, organizations decouple the memory, compute, and storage resources of their data center infrastructure, allowing them to be provisioned and maintained separately. Doing so makes the data center environment more adaptable, with the ability to scale resources as needed, based on application and workload requirements—without interrupting the availability of applications running in the environment. A disaggregated memory system can provide HPC applications with on-demand memory capacity and bandwidth, in contrast to today's monolithic designs, where compute and memory are tightly coupled. In essence, disaggregated memory maintains high performance using fast local memory, while improving capacity and power efficiency using slower remote memory. The use of optical memory channels can provide a low latency and high bandwidth interconnect solution [61]. A photonic solution can potentially be based on microLED-based links.

### 6.4.3 Tiled Supercomputer Architecture

The tile processor architecture consists of a 2D grid of identical compute elements, called tiles [62], as shown in Figure 6.24. Each compute element could include a copackaged optical chip based on microLEDs that facilitate high-speed and low power data transfers with other tiles.

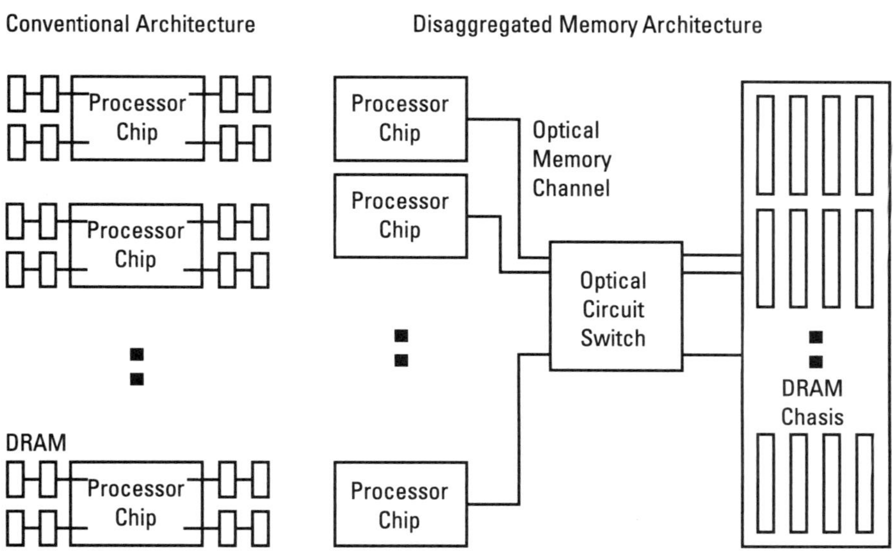


**Figure 6.23** Concept of memory disaggregation.

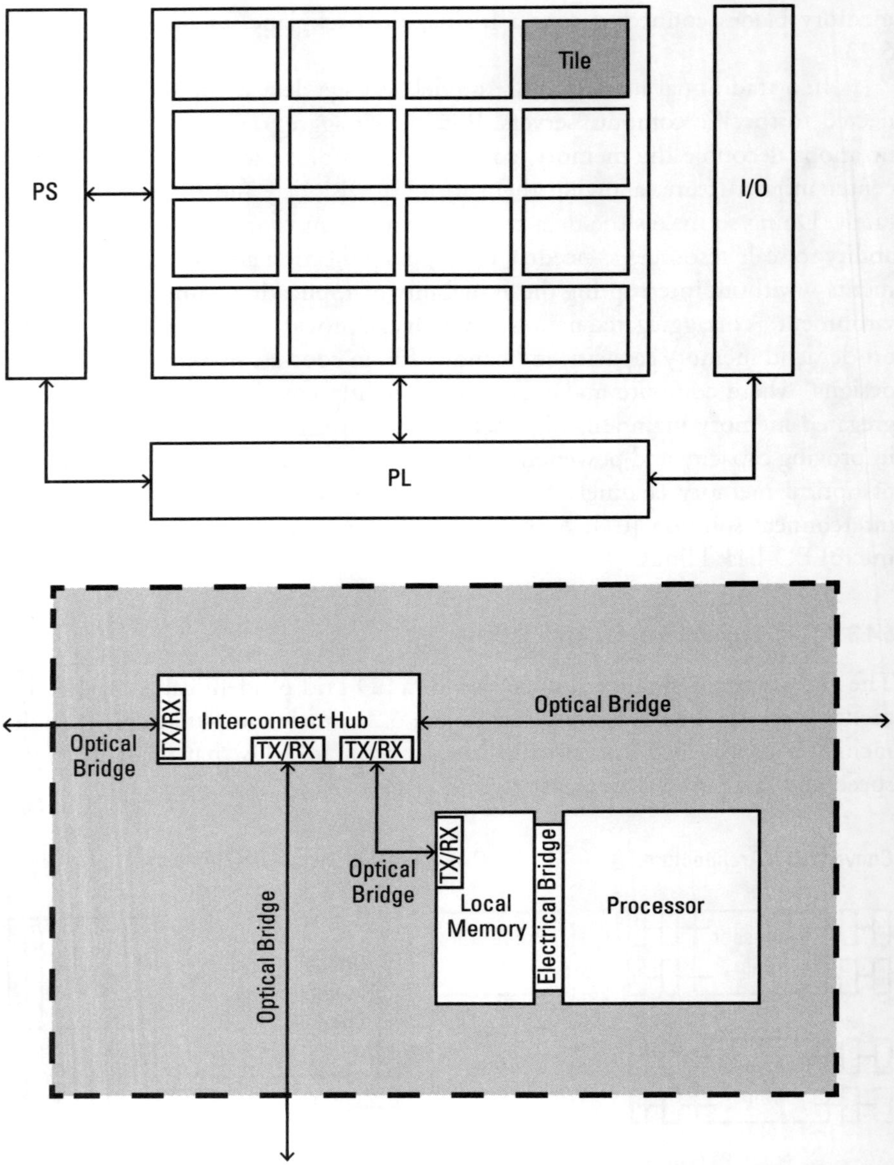


**Figure 6.24** Concept of a tile-based AI engine. MicroLEDs can potentially provide parallel optical links via waveguides in the substrate.

# References

[1] Nishi, K., K. Takemasa, M. Sugawara, and Y. Arakawa, "Development of Quantum Dot Lasers for Data-Com and Silicon Photonics Applications," *IEEE Journal of Selected Topics in Quantum Electronics,* Vol. 23, No. 6, 2017, pp. 1–7.

[2] Lebby, M. S., C. A. Gaw, W. Jiang, et al., "Use of VCSEL Arrays for Parallel Optical Interconnects, Fabrication, Testing, and Reliability of Semiconductor Lasers," *International Society for Optics and Photonics,* Vol. 2683, 1996, pp. 81–91.

[3] Ishak, W. S., K. H. Hahn, B. L. Booth, C. Mueller, A. A. J. Levi, and R. Craig, "Optical Interconnects—The POLO Approach," *Proceedings of SPIE, Optoelectronic Interconnects III,* Vol. 2400, 1995, p. 214–221.

[4] Kosaka, H., M. Kajita, Y. Li, and Y. Sugimoto, "A Two-Dimensional Optical Parallel Transmission Using a Vertical-Cavity Surface-Emitting Laser Array Module and an Image Fiber," *IEEE Photonics Technology Letters,* Vol. 9, No. 2, 1997, pp. 253–255.

[5] Pezeshki, B., A. Tselikov, R. Kalman, and C. Danesh, "Wide and Parallel LED-Based Optical Links Using Multi-Core Fiber for Chip-to-Chip Communications," *Optical Fiber Communication Conference,* 2021, p. F3A1.

[6] Pezeshki, B., R. Kalman, A. Tselikov, and C. Danesh, "High Speed Light MicroLEDs for Visible Wavelength Communication," *Light-Emitting Devices, Materials, and Applications XXV, International Society for Optics and Photonics,* Vol. 11706, 2021, p. 117060N.

[7] Bamiedakis, N., X. Li, J. J. D. McKendry, et al., "Micro-LED-Based Guided-Wave Optical Links for Visible Light Communications," *International Conference on Transparent Optical Networks,* 2015, pp. 1–4.

[8] Maj, T., A. Kirk, D. Plant, et al., "Interconnection of a 2D VCSEL Array to a Receiver Array via a Fiber Image Guide," *Optics in Computing,* Optical Society of America, 1999, p. PD2.

[9] Maj, T., A. G. Kirk, D. V. Plant, et al., "Interconnection of a Two-Dimensional Array of Vertical-Cavity Surface-Emitting Lasers to a Receiver Array by Means of a Fiber Image Guide," *Applied Optics,* Vol. 39, No. 5, 2000, pp. 683–689.

[10] Keller, S., H. Li, M. Laurent, et al., "Recent Progress in Metal-Organic Chemical Vapor Deposition of N-Polar Group-III Nitrides," *Semiconductor Science and Technology,* Vol. 29, No. 11, 2014, p. 113001.

[11] Wong, M. S., S. Nakamura, and S. P. DenBaars, "Progress in High Performance III-Nitride Micro-Light-Emitting Diodes," *ECS Journal of Solid-State Science and Technology,* Vol. 9, No. 1, 2019, p. 015012.

[12] Rashidi, A., M. Monavarian, A. Aragon, A. Rishinaramangalam, and D. Feezell, "GHz-Bandwidth Nonpolar InGaN/GaN Micro-LED Operating at Low Current Density for Visible-Light Communication," in *IEEE International Semiconductor Laser Conference,* 2018.

[13] Feezell, D., A. Rashidi, M. Monavarian, et al., "III-Nitride High-Speed Optoelectronics," in *IEEE Device Research Conference (DRC),* 2019.

[14] Zimmermann, H., *Silicon Optoelectronic Integrated Circuits,* Chapter 1, Berlin: Springer, 2004.

[15] Ciftcioglu, B., L. Zhang, J. Zhang, et al., "Integrated Silicon PIN Photodiodes Using Deep N-Well in a Standard 0.18-$\mu$m CMOS Technology," *Journal of Lightwave Technology,* Vol. 27, No. 15, 2009, pp. 3303–3313.

[16] Schneider-Hornstein, K., B. Goll, and H. Zimmermann, "Ultra-Sensitive PIN-Photodiode Receiver," *IEEE Photonics Journal,* Vol. 15, No. 3, 2023, p. 7201409.

[17] Brandl, P., S. Schidl, and H. Zimmermann, "PIN Photodiode Optoelectronic Integrated Receiver Used for 3-Gb/s Free-Space Optical Communication," *IEEE Journal of Selected Topics in Quantum Electronics,* Vol. 20, No. 6, 2014, pp. 391–400.

[18] Gundlapalli, P., V. Leong, J. Ong, et al., "Visible-Light Integrated PIN Avalanche Photodetectors with High Responsivity and Bandwidth," *Journal of Lightwave Technology,* Vol. 41, No. 8, 2023, pp. 2443–2450.

[19] Xu, H., Y. Yang, J. Tan, L. Chen, H. Zhu, and Q. Sun, "High-Performance Lateral Avalanche Photodiode Based on Silicon-on-Insulator Structure," *IEEE Electron Device Letters,* Vol. 43, No. 7, 2022, pp. 1077–1080.

[20] Yuan, Y., B. Tossoun, Z. Huang, et al., "Avalanche Photodiodes on Silicon Photonics," *Journal of Semiconductors,* Vol. 43, No. 2, 2022, p. 021301.

[21] Huang, M., S. Li, P. Cai, et al., "Germanium on Silicon Avalanche Photodiode," *IEEE Journal of Selected Topics in Quantum Electronics,* Vol. 24, No. 2, 2017, pp. 1–11.

[22] Caria, A., M. Nicoletto, C. De Santi, et al., "Quantum Efficiency of InGaN–GaN Multi-Quantum Well Solar Cells: Experimental Characterization and Modeling," *Journal of Applied Physics,* Vol. 131, No. 22, 2022, p. 224501.

[23] Elbar, M., B. Alshehri, S. Tobbeche, and E. Dogheche, "Design and Simulation of InGaN/GaN p–i–n Photodiodes," *physica status solidi (a),* Vol. 215, No. 9, 2018, p. 1700521.

[24] Saidani, O., and S. Tobbeche, "Numerical Study and Design of High-Efficiency p-In0.1Ga0.9N/i-GaN/n-GaN Heterojunction Photodiode," *Micro and Nanostructures,* Vol. 175, 2023, p. 207490.

[25] Valdueza-Felip, S., A. Mukhtarova, Q. Pan, et al., "Photovoltaic Response of InGaN/GaN Multiple-Quantum Well Solar Cells," *Japanese Journal of Applied Physics,* Vol. 52, No. 8S, 2013, p. 08JH05.

[26] Lee, H., S. Baek, H. Na, and S. Lee, "Effect of a Patterned Sapphire Substrate on InGaN-Based PIN Ultraviolet Photodetectors," *Journal of the Korean Physical Society,* Vol. 75, 2019, pp. 362–366.

[27] Ho, K., R. Chen, G. Liu, et al., "3.2 Gigabit-per-Second Visible Light Communication Link with InGaN/GaN MQW Micro-Photodetector," *Optics Express,* Vol. 26, No. 3, 2018, pp. 3037–3045.

[28] Ohsawa, J., T. Kozawa, H. Hayashi, O. Fujishima, and H. Itoh, "Low-Dark-Current Large-Area Narrow-Band Photodetector using InGaN/GaN Layers on Sapphire," *Japanese Journal of Applied Physics,* Vol. 44, No. 5L, 2005, p. L623.

[29] Pereiro, J., C. Rivera, Á. Navarro, et al., "Optimization of InGaN–GaN MQW Photodetector Structures for High-Responsivity Performance," *IEEE Journal of Quantum Electronics*, Vol. 45, No. 6, 2009, pp. 617–622.

[30] Rivera, C., J. Pau, F. Naranjo, and E. Munoz, "Novel Photodetectors Based on InGaN/GaN Multiple Quantum Wells," *physica status solidi (a)*, Vol. 201, No. 12, 2004, pp. 2658–2662.

[31] Madhusoodhanan, S., A. Sabbar, H. Tran, et al., "High-Temperature Analysis of GaN-Based MQW Photodetector for Optical Galvanic Isolations in High-Density Integrated Power Modules," *IEEE Journal of Emerging and Selected Topics in Power Electronics*, Vol. 9, No. 4, 2020, pp. 3877–3882.

[32] Huang, Y., P. Yeh, Y. Huang, et al., "High-Performance InGaN PIN Photodetectors using LED Structure and Surface Texturing," *IEEE Photonics Technology Letters*, Vol. 28, No. 6, 2015, pp. 605–608.

[33] Chiou, Y., Y. Su, S. Chang, Y. Lin, C. Chang, and C. Chen, "InGaN/GaN MQW P–N Junction Photodetectors," *Solid-State Electronics*, Vol. 46, No. 12, 2002, pp. 2227–2229.

[34] Chiou, Y., Y. Su, S. Chang, et al., "High Detectivity InGaN-GaN Multi-Quantum Well PN Junction Photodiodes," *IEEE Journal of Quantum Electronics*, Vol. 39, No. 5, 2003, pp. 681–685.

[35] Ghatak, A., and K. Thyagarajan, *Introduction to Fiber Optics,* Cambridge, UK: Cambridge University Press, 1998.

[36] Chen, K.-L., and D. Kerps, "Coupling Efficiency of Surface-Emitting LEDs to Single-Mode Fibers," *Journal of Lightwave Technology*, Vol. 5, No. 11, 1987, pp. 1600–1604.

[37] Mukherjee, B., I. Tomkos, M. Tornatore, P. Winzer, and Y. Zhao, eds., *Springer Handbook of Optical Networks,* Cham, Switzerland: Springer, 2020.

[38] Hui, R., *Introduction to Fiber-Optic Communications,* London: Academic Press, 2019.

[39] Senior, J. M., and M. Y. Jamro, *Optical Fiber Communications Principles and Practice,* Third Edition, Harlow, UK: Prentice Hall, 2009, Chapter 3.

[40] Marcatili, E. A. J., "Modal Dispersion in Optical Fibers with Arbitrary Numerical Aperture and Profile Dispersion," *The Bell System Technical Journal*, Vol. 56, No. 1, 1977, pp. 49–63.

[41] Okamoto, K., *Fundamentals of Optical Waveguides,* Second Edition, Amsterdam: Elsevier, Chapter 3, 2006.

[42] Koizumi, K., Y. Ikeda, I. Kitano, M. Furukawa, and T. Sumimoto, "New Light-Focusing Fibers Made by a Continuous Process," *Applied Optics*, Vol. 13, No. 2, 1974, pp. 255–260.

[43] Yabre, G., "Theoretical Investigation on the Dispersion of Graded-Index Polymer Optical Fibers," *Journal of Lightwave Technology*, Vol. 18, No. 6, 2000, p. 869.

[44] Olshansky, R., and D. Keck, "Pulse Broadening in Graded-Index Optical Fibers," *Applied Optics*, Vol. 15, No. 2, 1976, pp. 483–491.

[45] Keiser, G., F. Xiong, Y. Cui, and P. P. Shum, "Review of Diverse Optical Fibers Used in Biomedical Research and Clinical Practice," *Journal of Biomedical Optics*, Vol. 19, No. 8, 2014, p. 080902.

[46] Presby, H. M., and C. A. Edwards, "Near 100% Efficient Fibre Microlenses," *Electronics Letters*, Vol. 28, No. 6, 1992, pp. 582–584.

[47] Kurokawa, K., and E. E. Becker, "Laser Fiber Coupling with a Hyperbolic Lens," *IEEE Transactions on Microwave Theory and Techniques*, Vol. 23, No. 3, 1975, pp. 309–311.

[48] West, P. R., J. L. Stewart, A. V. Kildishev, et al., "All-Dielectric Subwavelength Metasurface Focusing Lens," *Optics Express*, Vol. 22, No. 21, 2014, pp. 26212–26221.

[49] Benisty, H., H. D. Neve, and C. Weisbuch, "Impact of Planar Microcavity Effects on Light Extraction—Part I: Basic Concepts and Analytical Trends," *IEEE Journal of Quantum Electronics*, Vol. 34, No. 9, 1998, pp. 1612–1631.

[50] Baets, R., "Micro-Cavity Light Emitting Diodes," in *Semiconductor Quantum Optoelectronics* (A. Miller, D. Finlayson, M. Ebrahimzadeh, eds.), Boca Raton, FL: CRC Press, 2020, pp. 213–264.

[51] Song, Y.-K., M. Diagne, H. Zhou, A. V. Nurmikko, R. P. S. Jr., and T. Takeuchi, "Resonant-Cavity InGaN Quantum-Well Blue Light-Emitting Diodes," *Applied Physics Letters*, Vol. 77, No. 12, 2000, pp. 1744–1746.

[52] Brown, G., "Bandwidth and Rise Time Calculations for Digital Multimode Fiber-Optic Data Links," *Journal of Lightwave Technology*, Vol. 10, No. 5, 1992, pp. 672–678.

[53] Hui, R., *Introduction to Fiber-Optic Communications*, London: Academic Press, 2020.

[54] Agrawal, G. P., Fiber-Optic Communication Systems, New York: John Wiley & Sons, 1997.

[55] Ong, D. S. G., J. S. Ng, M. M. Hayat, P. Sun, and J. P. R. David, "Optimization of InP APDs for High-Speed Lightwave Systems," *Journal of Lightwave Technology*, Vol. 27, No. 15, 2009, pp. 3294–3302.

[56] R. Mahajan, X. Li, J. Fryman, et al., "Co-Packaged Photonics for High Performance Computing: Status, Challenges and Opportunities," *Journal of Lightwave Technology*, Vol. 40, No. 2, 2021, pp. 379–392.

[57] Rizzo, A., S. Daudlin, A. Novick, et al., "Petabit-Scale Silicon Photonic Interconnects with Integrated Kerr Frequency Combs," *IEEE Journal of Selected Topics in Quantum Electronics*, Vol. 29, No. 1, 2022, pp. 1–20.

[58] Maniotis, P., L. Schares, and D. Kuchta, "How Data Center Networks Can Improve Through Co-Packaged Optics," *in Optical Fiber Communication Conference*, 2023.

[59] Piehler, D., "Optical Interconnects in Enterprise and Hyperscale Datacenters," in *SPIE Optical Interconnects XX* (Volume 11286), 2020.

[60] Shalf, J., G. Michelogiannakis, B. Austin, et al., "Photonic Memory Disaggregation in Datacenters," in *Photonics in Switching and Computing*, Optica Publishing, 2020.

[61] Michelogiannakis, G., M. Glick, J. Shalf, and K. Bergman, "Photonics as a Means to Implement Intra-Rack Resource Disaggregation," in *SPIE Metro and Data Center Optical Networks and Short-Reach Links V*, Vol. 12027, 2022.

[62] Taylor, M., W. Lee, J. Miller, et al., "Tiled Multicore Processors," in *Multicore Processors and Systems* (S. W. Keckler, K. Olukotun, and H. P. Hofsee, eds.), New York: Springer, 2009, pp. 1–33.

# 7

# Techno-Economics of MicroLEDs

## 7.1 Introduction

Economic benefit is found in changes: a new product, a new process, an improved product, an improved process, or combinations of these. The boundary between "new" and "improved" is often blurred but if the changes meet the patent office criteria of "novelty" and "inventiveness," then they may be said to be "new." Techno-economic analysis (TEA) examines costs, benefits, risks, and time frames for introducing a novel product in high-volume manufacturing. While passing a suitable techno-economic assessment of a proposed novel product is no guarantee of success, not doing one is virtually a guarantee of failure in economic terms and possibly technological terms as well. This chapter will present a TEA for microLED displays. First, TEA theory is discussed so similar analysis of other microLED systems can be analyzed by the readers as desired. Then the theory is applied to the microLED display system with some level of depth. The chapter concludes with the results of a should-cost model (SCM) of microLED displays of 6" and 14" diagonal sizes corresponding to smartphone and laptop applications.

## 7.2 Theory

Figure 7.1 shows the four main functions involved in bringing about a beneficial change in one or more of a company's products. The theoretical framework for quantifying these functions and the linkage between them is the techno-economic model (TEM).

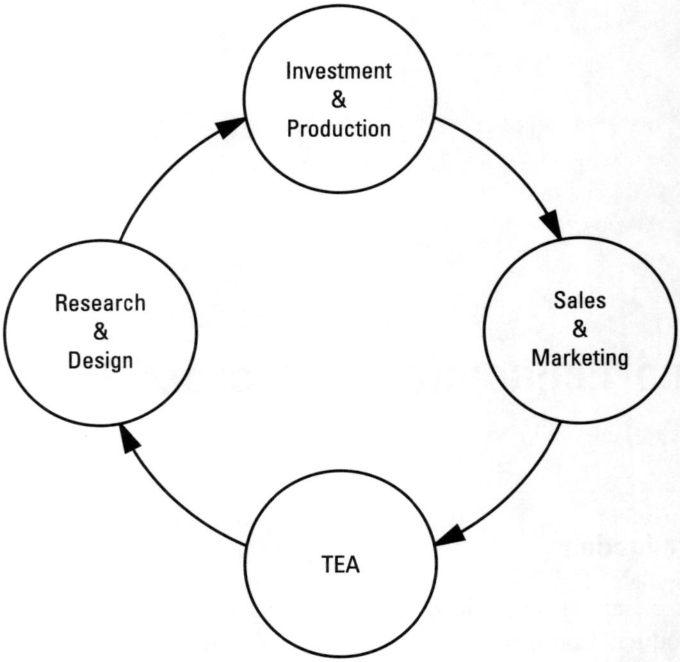


**Figure 7.1** Basic sequences needed to realize a new product. Starting from a TEA, to research and design, to raising investment and moving to production, to executing sales and marketing strategies, a novel product concept can find its way to commercial success (i.e., innovation).

The cyclic form of the sequence in Figure 7.1 emphasizes two points often lost in public discussion of innovation and enterprise: research and design is only one of several elements in the creation of a new product or process, and new ideas can enter at any point of the cycle, which may be traversed several times during their gestation. To be useful, the basic structure of Figure 7.1 must be made quantitative to the point where the management of a company can make decisions to launch a project, to continue with it, or as important, to stop it. In particular, allowances must be made to provide the necessary investment in production and marketing facilities so that sales can reach a self-sustaining level within a set time scale. Matching resources to the research and design to achieve this is what is meant by the stoichiometric principle of innovation. This is the purpose of the TEM as applied to an individual company in competition with other companies.

The introduction of disruptive technologies such as microLEDs into the production of existing products (such as displays) require upfront TEM that captures the interactions between technology design choices and production cost. A good TEM should be based on as much physics as possible and as much initial data as possible to guide technological decisions for a viable product. A mathematical TEM can be used to perform optimization of product performance per product cost given a set of boundary conditions imposed by the existing ecosystem. The model can be fed into a genetic algorithm [1] with objective function being the performance per cost and the output would be different scenarios towards the desired performance per cost targets that are guided by competing products. It also can be used to envision a roadmap of the ecosystem to further optimize performance per cost for future releases of the product. A TEM will also help define different tiers of the product based on the value of performance per cost.

### 7.2.1 Techno-Economic Analysis

TEA examines costs, benefits, risks, uncertainties, and time frames for introducing a product in high-volume manufacturing. A TEA aims at maximizing performance per manufacturing cost, or minimizing cost per a given target performance.

Manufacturing costs can be broken down into two main categories: capital expenses and operating expenses. Capital expenses (CapEx) are nonrecurring costs such as equipment, buildings, and construction. In a TEA, these one-time facility costs are amortized over the assets' useful lifetime to relate CapEx to a specific production volume. Operating expenses (OpEx) are recurring costs such as materials, labor, and energy. These recurring costs can be either fixed or variable. Fixed operating expenses, like labor, do not change with production output, while variable operating expenses, like materials, are directly tied to production volume.

For all cost estimations, we assume that the new technology has been deployed at a full industrial scale—even if its current technology readiness level (TRL) is low. Figure 7.2 illustrates steps to perform a TEA. It starts with constructing a Process Flow Diagram, which includes key steps of process with equipment needed as well as material streams showing inputs and outputs. The second step is Mass Balance, which is used to understand what percentage of feedstocks finalize into desired product and measure how much waste or byproducts will be created. The third step is Capital Cost Estimation, which looks into combined equipment and facility costs derived from the process flow

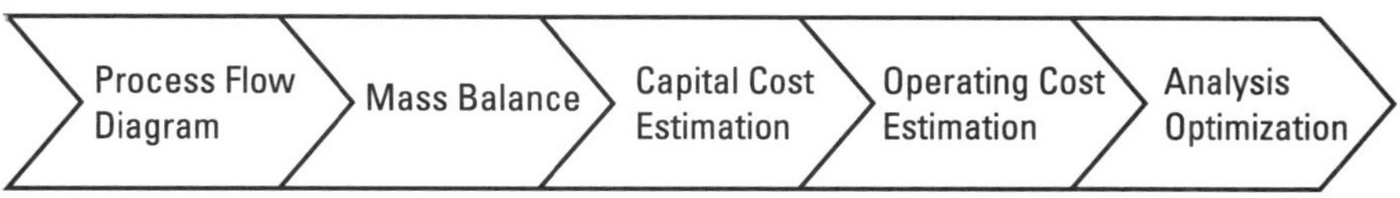


**Figure 7.2** Steps to perform techno-economic analysis.

diagram. The fourth step is Operating Cost Estimation, which considers combination of annual utility, maintenance, and labor costs estimated from process flow diagram and material costs estimated from mass balance and desired production volume. The last step is Analysis/Optimization, which includes analysis of breakeven cost determined for the product and price comparison.

### 7.2.2 Product Cost Evolution

Businesses whose revenues derive from sales of engineered products of their own design and manufacture often suffer from a lack of means to accurately estimate and allocate the costs of product development during the initial design phases of its lifecycle. It is during these early conceptual design phases that decisions are made that dictate the majority (at least 70% [2–5]) of overall costs of the product. These costs are only fully revealed several phases later, however, when they are incurred to put the product into production. Figure 7.3 illustrates how the cost incursion of a product lags behind the cost commitment across its lifecycle phases [2]. During later lifecycle phases, a business has fewer opportunities to revise the product design and optimize for cost. The result is that the final products may generate suboptimal values to the business, its customers, and other stakeholders. Despite the apparent importance of the design phase for controlling value, it is most commonly only at later lifecycle phases, once the product has entered production, where product value is closely scrutinized and metered by means of statistical process control paradigms for quality management such as Taguchi Methods [6], Six Sigma [7], and Lean Manufacturing [8]. These focus on increasing value and reducing costs by reducing manufacturing defects and nonvalue-added expenditures rather than optimizing the product design itself.

### 7.2.3 Generating Best Design

Figure 7.4 describes the process for incorporating design-for-cost and design-to-cost early in the development cycle. Once the conceptual design is complete, the detailed design process is used to ensure that the part design has the highest likelihood of success in meeting all the design requirements. By designing a product in such a way as to minimize the effort required for its manufacture, very often it is possible to reduce costs while improving the quality of the product without loss in functionality or performance.

#### 7.2.3.1 Design for Manufacturability

Design for manufacturability addresses the physical limitations of the manufacturing process in yielding the desired part geometry and topology. Manufacturability addresses a class of defects that will cause a part to be rejected upon

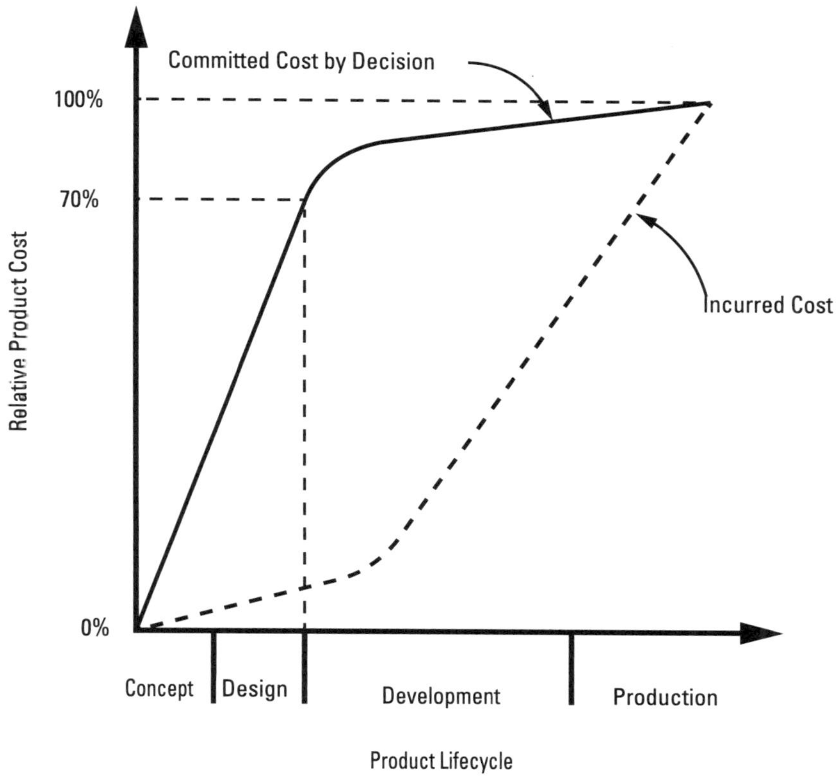


**Figure 7.3** Evolution of committed and incurred costs, adapted from [2]. Surprisingly, >70% of all product costs are determined before production starts (i.e., in the phase of product development). Linking this fact to the idea of product-cost optimization to ensure economic success, it becomes obvious that product development phases offer the most potential to optimize product costs.

immediate inspection. It also involves selecting materials, processes, and equipment that minimize variability during production (see Figure 7.5).

#### 7.2.3.2 Design for Assembly

The design for assembly technique involves two important steps: (1) minimization of the number of separate parts, and (2) improvement in the ability to assemble the remaining parts. By far the most important of these steps is the reduction in part count—a procedure that is convenient to carry out during considerations of the assembly of the various parts of a proposed product. A procedure suggested by Boothroyd et al. [4] involves asking three simple questions with respect to each part as it is added to the assembly. These questions are: (1) During the operation of the product, does this part move bodily with respect to all other parts already assembled? (2) For fundamental reasons, does the part have to be of a different material from all the other parts already assembled? (3)

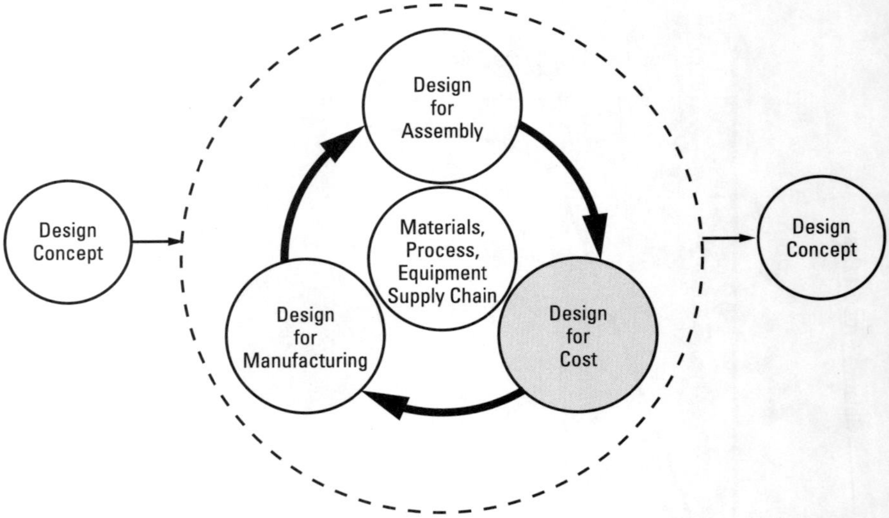


**Figure 7.4** In order to optimize a product design for value, engineering, and manufacturing, businesses need to be able to estimate accurately product lifecycle costs during the early design phases of its development, because this is when the majority of these costs are determined.

Does the part have to be separate from all other parts already assembled because otherwise assembly or disassembly of other separate parts could not be carried out? Figure 7.6 illustrates the concept of design for assembly.

#### 7.2.3.3 Design for Cost

Design for cost (DFC) utilizes cost modeling to address the economic concerns surrounding the manufacture of the part and supports process optimization balancing financial and engineering requirements. DFC uses all organizational and technical possibilities in order to reduce total production costs of the designed product [2]. Design to cost aims at reaching satisfactory parameters of a designed product within the assumed target cost [2].

#### 7.2.3.4 Design to Cost

Design to cost (DTC) is a great methodology to provide a cost model via design decisions. DTC also aims to implement the necessary cost strategy during the development cycle of the project so that cost targets will become independent variables to guide the decision-making. It is prevalent in optimizing costs and increasing system performance. The first stage of applying DTC is to define an acceptable cost for the final product. This can be done by creating multiple standards or tiers for the outcome. The basic standard or lower tier would have only the essential quality and functionality. A tier above this would have some innovation and extra features. The top tier would add even more functionality

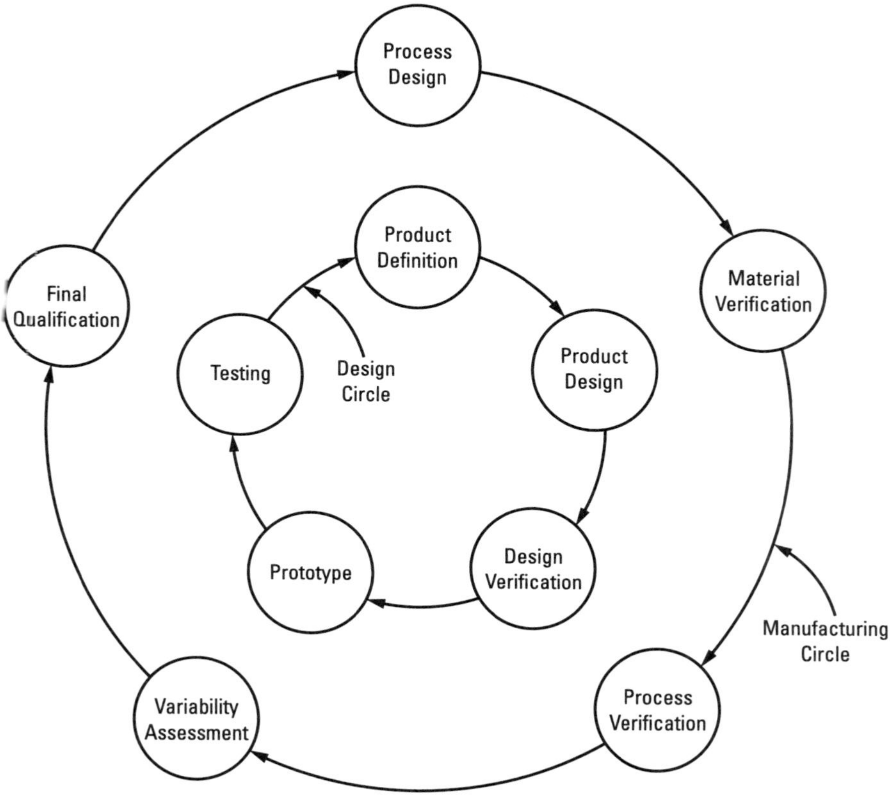


**Figure 7.5** Interaction and relationship of the design and manufacturing components.

and luxury. The latter can also be considered as design to value. Depending on the project type, any of these tiers can be used as a starting point at this stage. This is an essential part of DTC as it will help to understand the needs and scopes of the client and lay out the framework for the following stages. Figure 7.7 illustrates a flow diagram for performing DTC.

The following are the different cost drivers to bear in mind in the product design phase that will influence the final product's price:

- Design standardization;
- Use of standard parts;
- Geographical factors;
- Packaging and transportation;
- Waste minimization;
- Maintenance.

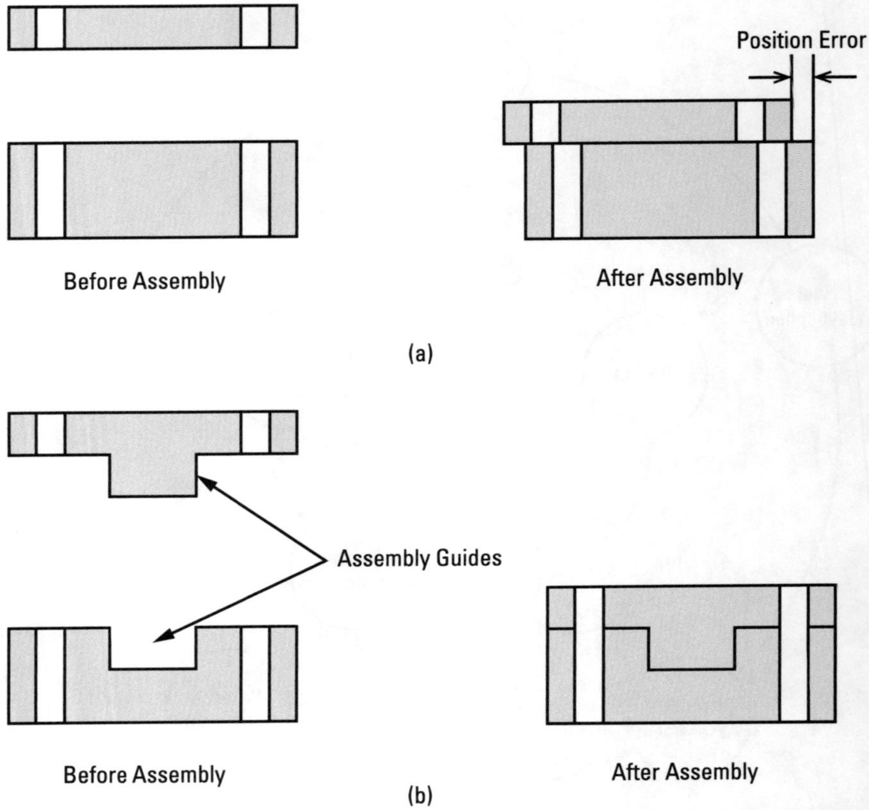


**Figure 7.6** Illustration of the impact of the initial design of components on the assembly: (a) a positional error during assembly results in yield loss and higher manufacturing cost, and (b) assembly guides included in the components led to perfect assembly of the parts, higher yield, and lower product cost.

To implement all of the cost management strategies listed, the design engineering team needs to have component-level knowledge of the manufactured product.

### 7.2.4 Cost Models

Cost models are designed to quantify the component's underlying cost drivers—not precise actual costs—for design decisions. One of the primary benefits of this approach is to focus designers on the one area of the many pricing factors that they can control: the design.

A product (system) incorporates multiple components. Each component may be made by one supplier. It is unlikely that the original equipment manufacturer (OEM), who designs and manufactures a system, will have any control

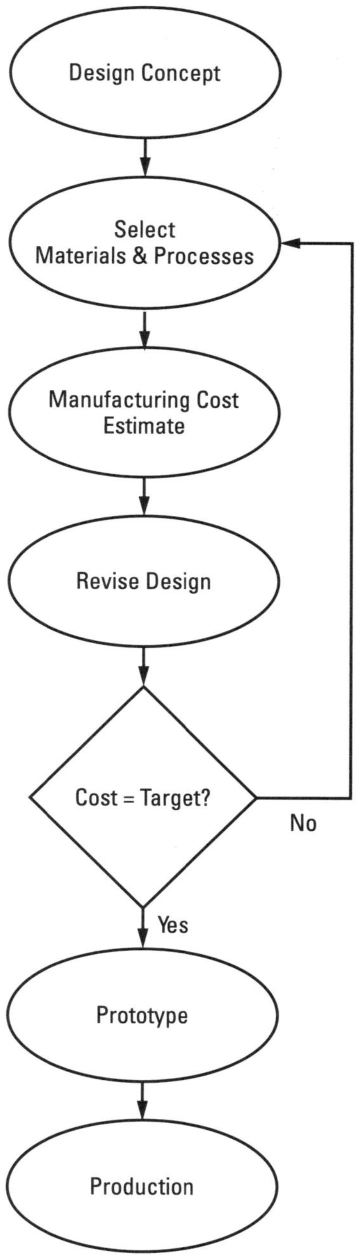


**Figure 7.7** Flow incorporating DTC.

over how a component supplier calculates and distributes overhead, its desired profit margins, or its risk factors. But if the design is optimized for a component supplier's capabilities, everyone benefits because cost is removed from the product instead of reducing a component supplier's profit through unfair pricing negotiations.

In order for a designer to be able to use cost models to make design decisions and technology trade-offs, the cost models require two key features: relative cost accuracy and real supplier cost drivers.

Relative cost accuracy means the models correctly capture the differences between design decisions. The models should answer the question "How much more or less expensive is it if my design is X instead of Y?" The model is not a replacement for the normal quoting and negotiating process because it does not produce either actual supplier costs or formal quotes. The designer uses the cost models to find the technology choices that generate the optimal cost for their design without needing to know supplier confidential details.

The real supplier cost drivers refer to accurately capturing the way a supplier calculates its costs and how those costs are passed on in the pricing.

Components of total cost include direct cost, indirect cost, overhead, profit margin, and risk factors. Of all of these components, most of the cost of the design is captured in either direct or indirect/overhead costs.

The above framework only works if these models incorporate both of these features. A designer can generally determine whether a specific design decision causes the cost to go up or down.

Once the models have been developed, they serve as a source of feedback from the supplier to the designer. It is important to understand what the models are and what they are not in order to receive benefit from them.

For the OEM, the model is a consistent way to evaluate the cost impact of design decisions for different components. The model provides consistency in evaluating a design's cost effectiveness throughout the entire design cycle. It also allows a better design through rapid feedback very early in the design cycle before a majority of the cost has been committed in a specific configuration.

Without the model, each designer/supplier would make different decisions based on a different perceived value, which can lead to surprises later on.

What the model does not do is commit the supplier to any particular pricing or reveal any confidential information about the supplier's costs or margins. The models produce accurate relative costs, but this allows all confidential and sensitive data to remain that way while still providing crucial feedback on how design decisions affect cost. The models are also not designed to be used as negotiation tool to get a better price. The model is fundamentally cooperative and is a vehicle for sharing the best design practices between OEM and supplier.

For the suppliers, the model's benefit is primarily in guiding designers to make better design decisions. If the model is being used as a source of evaluating which design choices are most cost effective, then it also becomes a way for suppliers to provide guidance on which design decisions are best suited for their manufacturing process and capabilities.

Once the models are in use, they require periodic updates. This is especially important with any major technology changes being adopted by either side. By providing the input to create the model, there is an agreement that pricing on different design decisions will be accurate. If subsequent quotes do not seem to follow the relative cost differences originally built, it is reasonable to set up a discussion to find out why and update the models if necessary.

### 7.2.5 Cost Estimate Techniques

A number of techniques may be adapted [2, 9–11]. A hierarchy of cost modeling approaches is shown in Figure 7.8. The approaches shown are defined as follows:

1. Heuristic, which are simple, commonsense rules or sets of rules derived from experience;
2. Parametric, which includes curve fitting to historical cost data;
3. Analytical, which involves closed-form models derived from first principles;

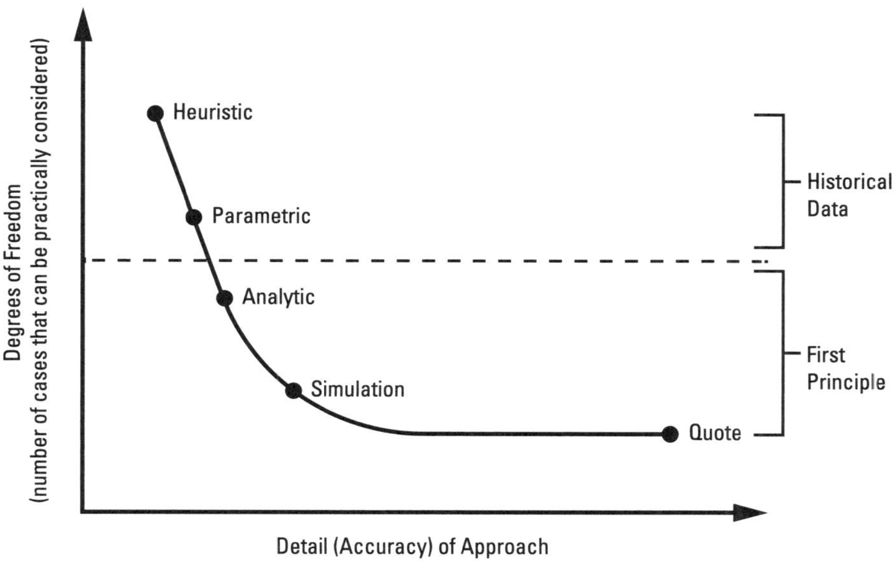


**Figure 7.8** Hierarchy of cost modeling. This illustration indicates that successful manufacturing cost modeling is not necessarily performed using a single methodology or approach, but potentially several approaches.

4. Simulation, which involves nonclosed-form models derived from first principles;
5. Quote, which is a statement from the entity that will perform the manufacturing that constitutes a bid for performing the manufacturing and/or assembly work.

As the accuracy of the modeling approach increases, so does the amount of data necessary to populate the model. Heuristic and parametric modeling approaches may not have any connection to the physics of the manufacturing process; they are purely based on experience and/or historical data. Analytical and simulation are derived from first principles. Heuristics may be the least accurate approach, but it has the advantage of allowing a designer to assess a nearly unlimited number of different cases. As the product development process progresses and more detailed data about the product or system becomes available, more accurate approaches become practical. Finally, the most accurate cost estimation is the actual quote from the organization that will manufacture and/or assemble the item. However, while a quote is absolutely accurate (at least from the customer's perspective, because it represents a contract), the manufacturer is unlikely to be willing to provide quotes for more than a couple of alternatives.

## 7.3 Techno-Economics of MicroLED Displays

Following the procedure illustrated in Figure 7.2, we start with constructing the process flow diagram for making a microLED display. We start with glass and build a TFT backplane. We also start with a silicon or sapphire wafer, build microLED stacks using epitaxial growth using MOCVD technology, and finish with back-end-of-line (BEOL) to provide necessary interconnects and singulation of microLEDs. The finished microLED wafer and the finished TFT backplane are fed into microLED transfer equipment. The microLEDs are transferred from the microLED wafer onto the TFT backplane. Metrology that aims at detecting any transfer defects are used to determine if the transfer yield was acceptable. If an acceptable yield level is achieved, then microLED isolation is implemented followed by a display BEOL process. There is cost associated with each block shown in Figure 7.9. This cost is controlled by a number of independent cost variables.

### 7.3.1 MicroLED Wafer Cost

The process flow for making a planar microLED is shown in Figure 7.10. Starting with a wafer (sapphire or silicon), MOCVD is used to grow a nucleation

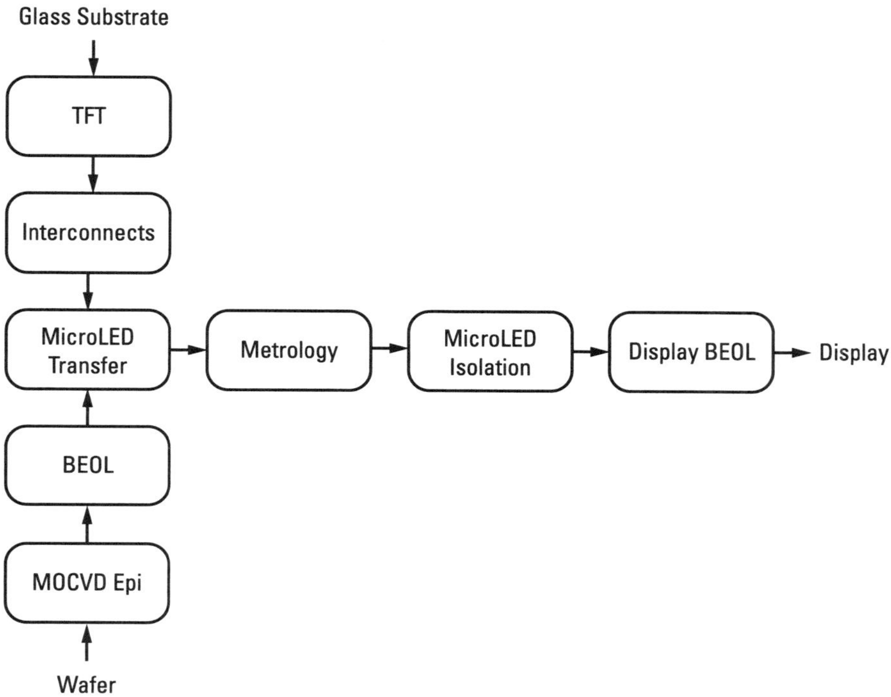


**Figure 7.9** Simplified process flow diagram for making a microLED display.

layer such as AlN. This is followed by the growth of a buffer layer (e.g., GaN) using low-temperature epitaxy. Next, an n-type GaN cladding layer is epitaxially grown with doping $10^{20}$ $cm^{-3}$. The multiple quantum well structure is then grown with undoped GaN and undoped InGaN with the desired indium mole fraction. This is followed by the growth of an EBL made of AlGaN. A p-type GaN is grown epitaxially to provide a source for holes during the operation of the microLED. A transparent metal electrode (e.g., indium-tin-oxide (ITO)) is then deposited using sputtering, for example. A photo mask is used to pattern microLED mesas with the desired dimensions. An inductively couple plasma (ICP) dry etch is used to etch the microLED mesas. This is followed by the deposition (using atomic layer deposition (ALD), for example) of a passivation dielectric such as aluminum oxide. Lithography and etch are then used to singulate the microLED mesas. Figure 7.10 highlights the steps with the most impact on cost including epitaxy, lithography, and ALD. It is therefore necessary to understand the impact of epitaxy growth technology on the cost. Epitaxial growth is the process of depositing materials on a crystalline substrate, often with single atomic layer resolution. The deposited thin film is called an epitaxial film, epitaxial layer, or epilayer, and has a well-defined crystal orientation rela-

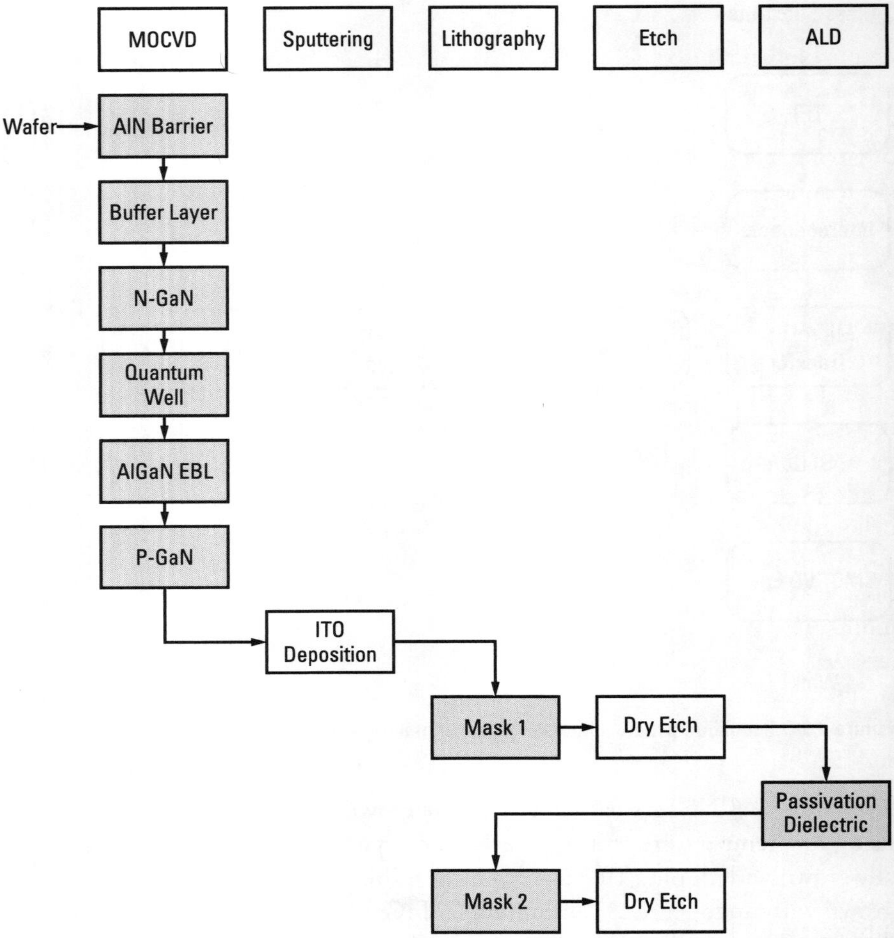


**Figure 7.10** Simplified process flow diagram for making a planar microLED. The steps that contribute the most to the cost of manufacturing are highlighted in gray.

tive to the substrate. As the deposited films and substrate materials may have different lattice constants, the general condition for crystalline epitaxy is that the lattice mismatch must be <1% to facilitate a dislocation-free single crystal film. The thickness of the films must be below the critical thickness limit set by the Matthews and Blakeslee (MB) theory [12], for example. There are two main technologies for epitaxy growth: MOCVD and MBE.

### 7.3.2 Molecular Beam Epitaxy

MBE has played a key role in the demonstration of many new heterostructure device concepts. The inherent features of this technology make it well suited to the research environment and to the demonstration of new device concepts employing thin layers and abrupt interfaces. MBE is growth on a heated substrate in an ultrahigh vacuum (UHV) environment (base pressure ~$10^{-9}$ torr) typically using elemental sources. The UHV environment not only ensures material purity, but it also results in highly directional elemental beams (no carrier gas required) due to the inherently long mean free paths. Layered structures are achieved by shuttering. In addition, valved sources are typically used for group V materials due to their relatively high vapor pressures.

The uniformity of growth rate for a binary compound can be achieved by rotating the substrate at speeds as low as a few rpm, but compositional uniformity of ternary or quaternary alloys requires rotation of the substrate at speeds of up to 120 rpm [13]. The mechanical requirements for a rotating substrate stage in a UHV system are quite demanding, as no conventional lubricants can be used on the bearings or feedthroughs and yet lifetime must exceed several million rotations. Magnetic rotary feedthroughs have largely replaced the earlier bellows type.

The need to rotate the substrate to give uniformity also leads to complications in substrate-temperature measurement. The substrate-preparation techniques used prior to MBE growth are very important, as impurities on the surface provide nucleation sites for defects. Historically, various chemical clean and etch processes were used, but wafers are now usually supplied epi-ready, with a volatile oxide film on the surface that protects the surface from contamination and can be thermally removed within the UHV chamber.

The growth chamber substrate stage is surrounded by a large liquid-nitrogen-cooled cryopanel. This is arranged so that the heated (500°C–700°C) substrate is not directly exposed to thermal sources other than the molecular beams themselves, and impurities emanating from any other source can only reach the substrate after suffering at least one collision with, and probable adsorption by, a surface at liquid-nitrogen temperatures. The cryopanel also reduces contamination arising from outgassing from the walls of the chamber that are exposed to radiation from the effusion cells [13].

Control over the composition and doping levels of the epitaxial layers is achieved by precise temperature control of the effusion cells and the use of fast-acting shutters in front of these cells. In most systems, the growth rate is about 1 monolayer per second (e.g., for GaN a monolayer is approximately 0.59 nm), and the shutter operation time of 0.1s thus corresponds to less than a monolayer of growth.

Commercial MBE systems have increased throughput with multiwafer substrate holders, cassette loading and UHV storage, and preparation chambers linked to the growth chamber with automated transfer, while increased capacity effusion cells have reduced the downtime required for charging.

Gas-source MBE (GSMBE) were developed that combined the advantages of UHV deposition and external gas or metal-organic sources to produce a versatile technique that has some advantages over MBE and MOCVD (discussed below). These techniques utilize the growth chambers developed for MBE and pumping systems with a high continuous throughput, typically liquid-nitrogen-trapped diffusion pumps or turbomolecular pumps. Layers are deposited from molecular beams of the precursor materials introduced via gas-source cells that are essentially very fine leak controllers. As in MBE, there are no interactions within or between beams and the precise control of beams using fast-acting gas-line valves is, therefore, translated into precise control of the species arriving at the substrate. Shutters are not generally required; atomically sharp interfaces and monolayer structures can be defined as a consequence of submonolayer valve switching times. There is, however, a price to pay in system complexity, with the need for gas handling and high-volume pumping arrangements added to the expensive UHV growth chamber.

An advantage of MBE for growing GaN layers is that both N-polarity or Ga-polarity can occur with MBE growth on sapphire substrates. Under typical growth conditions with MOCVD, however, Ga-polarity material is exclusively produced [13].

#### 7.3.2.1 Metal-Organic Chemical Vapor Deposition

The technique of MOCVD was first introduced in the late 1960s for the deposition of compound semiconductors from the vapor phase. It was not until the late 1980s that MOCVD became a production technique of any significance. This success depended on painstaking work with improving the impurity of the organometallic precursors and hydrides. The high-quality epitaxial nature of the films was emphasized by changing the name of the growth method to metalorganic vapor phase epitaxy (MOVPE) or organometallic VPE (OMVPE). All these variants of the name can be found in the literature and, in most cases, they can be used interchangeably.

MOVPE also grows on a heated substrate but in a much different pressure regime than MBE (typically 15 to 750 torr). MOVPE uses complex compound sources, namely metal-organic sources (e.g., trimethyl Ga, In, Al), hydrides (e.g., arsine ($AsH_3$)), and other gas sources (e.g., Di-silane). In MOVPE, the reactants are flowed across the substrate where they react, resulting in epitaxial growth. In contrast to MBE, MOVPE requires the use of a carrier gas (typically hydrogen (H)) to transport reagent materials across the substrate surface. Layered structures are achieved by valve actuation for differing injection ports of a gas manifold.

The characteristics of MOCVD that have taken it from a research curiosity to production have been in the simplicity of delivery of the reactive vapors and the versatility of selecting different alloy compositions, dopants, and layer thickness. Indeed, the success of InGaN in the 1990s for high-brightness blue LEDs has now led to this being the most popular material produced by MOCVD for high-brightness white LEDs for lighting and microLEDs for displays. MOCVD has been employed by a number of manufacturers to fabricate sophisticated multilayer devices employing thin layers and abrupt interfaces such as microLEDs.

The main manufacturing advantages of MOCVD over MBE are the shorter maintenance periods and scaling of overhead cost with run rate.

The precursors used for the nitrides are standard with the methyl alkyls (TMGa and TMIn) for the group III elements and ammonia or hydrazine (not in production today) for the nitrogen. The key technological barriers to obtaining device-quality GaN are in overcoming the problems associated with heteroepitaxy onto the nonlattice-matched substrate such as sapphire, and in controlling the p-type doping [14].

The heteroepitaxial problems have been overcome with a two-stage growth. High-quality GaN requires growth temperatures in excess of 1000°C. At these temperatures, the nucleation onto sapphire is poor and large faceted islands grow before complete coalescence of the film occurs [13]. This not only leads to very poor surface morphology but also a high dislocation density where the islands coalesce. The two-stage growth overcomes this by growing a uniform nucleation (or buffer) layer onto the sapphire at 600°C. This is then heated to the normal growth temperature where a thicker GaN film is then grown. Approximately 50–100 nm of GaN is grown as a smooth layer but during heating, this changes to a rough layer. In some cases, the GaN buffer layer is substituted with an AlN layer, but in all cases a two-stage growth process is required [13]. The growth of device layers is achieved by controlling the bandgap through growth of the alloys InGaN or AlGaN. The bandgap of GaN is 3.4 eV, which is in the UV spectrum, so the color of the LED is determined by the alloy composition, where increasing the In content will reduce the bandgap and push the emission wavelength from blue to green. However, this is not an easy alloy to form due to the different stabilities of the GaN and InN bonds. In fact, it cannot be grown to any useful In content at temperatures above 1000°C, so the temperature has to be reduced to around 700°C. Even with this compromise, the different lattice parameters of GaN and InN result in poor solubility and In content above 40% is not practical. In principle, it is possible to prepare microLEDs of any color by just changing the In content in the alloy, but in practice the high-brightness diodes can only be prepared from nitrides covering the blue to green portion of the spectrum. The growth of different alloy compositions, particularly the growth of higher In content GaInN, has stimulated some research on alternative precursors for nitrogen as ammonia pyrolysis is not very efficient at temperatures below 800°C. One of the candidates is dimethylhydrazine, which reacts readily with trimethylgallium (TMGa), at temperatures down to 400°C.

The dopants used for n-type and p-type GaN are Si from silane and magnesium (Mg) from dicyclopentadienyl magnesium. The n-type doping has proved to be fairly straightforward but Mg doping results in the formation of Mg–H bonds that passivate the acceptor state. This problem was solved by annealing the epitaxial films after growth to remove the hydrogen. This is possible due to the thermal stability of GaN and the high mobility of hydrogen in the lattice. A further problem with p-type doping is that the Mg acceptor has an ionization energy between 160 and 250 meV and only about 10% of the chemically introduced Mg is ionized at room temperature [13].

### 7.3.3 Thin-Film Transistor Backplanes

#### 7.3.3.1 Low-Temperature Poly-Si Thin-Film Backplane

A simplified process flow diagram for making a thin-film transistor (TFT) backplane with polysilicon channel is shown in Figure 7.11. First, a substrate such as a glass substrate is cleaned by using an initial clean process. The glass substrate may have a thickness of 0.3 to 0.7 mm, for example. To prevent deleterious matters such as alkali ions in the glass substrate from influencing the property of later-formed polysilicon layer, a buffer layer is deposited on the glass substrate by using a plasma-enhanced chemical vapor deposition (PECVD) method, and a pre-clean process is conducted before depositing the buffer layer. The buffer layer comprises two portions. First, a layer of silicon nitride (SiNx) film is deposited to a thickness of about 50 to 100 nm, which may effectively inhibit metal ions in the glass substrate from affecting the later formed polysilicon layer. A layer of silicon oxide (SiOx), which matches well with a polysilicon layer, is deposited to a thickness of about 100 to 150 nm on the SiNx film to prevent defects in the SiNx from affecting the crystallization of the later formed polysilicon layer. The completed buffer layer may be annealed to optimize its performance. Next, an amorphous silicon (a-Si) layer is deposited to a thickness of 30 to 100 nm on the buffer layer by using a PECVD method, after which a polysilicon layer is obtained by crystallizing the a-Si. Specifically, after the a-Si layer is deposited on the buffer layer, a dehydrogenating process is performed on the a-Si layer using a high temperature oven so as to prevent occurrence of hydrogen blasting during the later crystallizing process and decrease the defect density within the later crystallized film. After the dehydrogenating process is finished, a low-temperature poly-Si (LTPS) process is performed to crystallize the a-Si layer. Typically, a crystallizing method such as excimer laser anneal (ELA), metal induced crystallization (MIC), or the like is employed to crystallize the a-Si layer. After the crystallizing process, a surface treatment is performed to the resulting polysilicon layer using hydroxyl-oxo-succinic acid

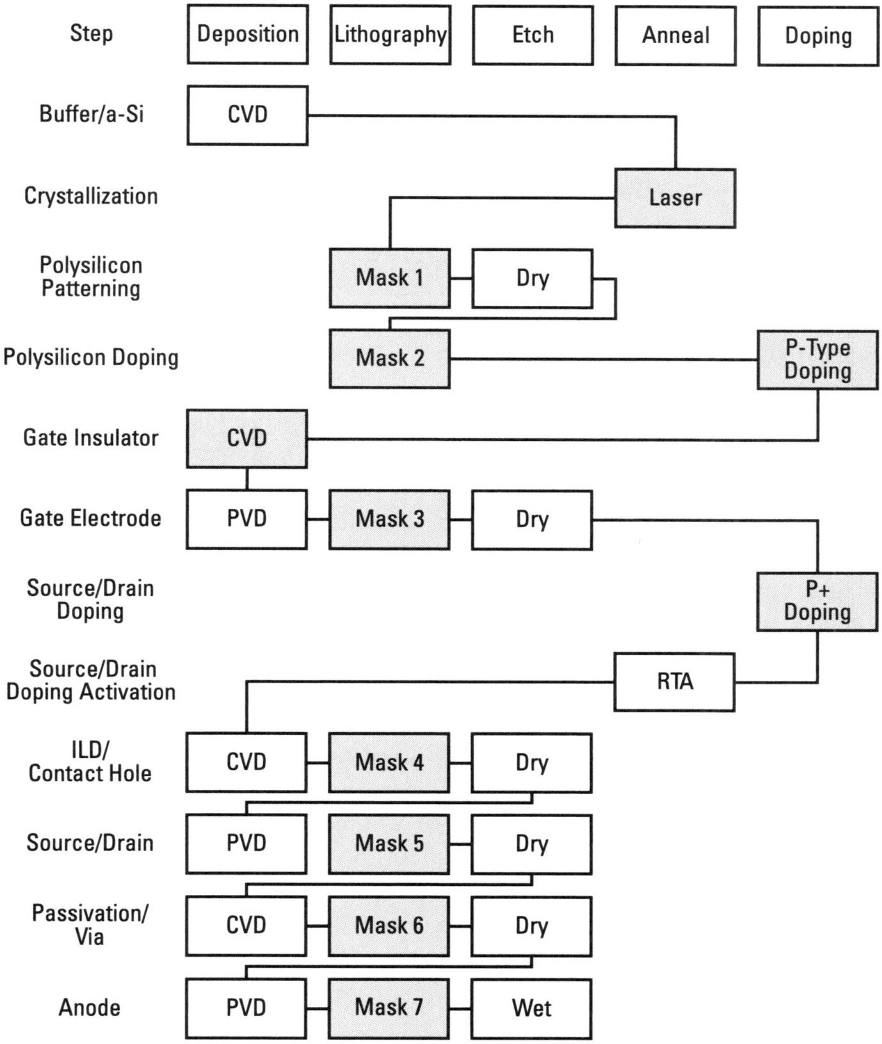


**Figure 7.11** Simplified process flow diagram for making a TFT backplane with polysilicon channel. The steps that contribute most to the cost of manufacturing are highlighted in gray.

dimethyl ester (dihydrofolic acid (DHF), having a purity of 1%–20%) or diluted HF solution, by which the surface roughness of the polysilicon layer is decreased and the wrinkles or tip protrusions resulting from the crystallizing is removed so that the polysilicon layer may come in contact with the later-formed layers more closely and thus the device performance is enhanced. Next, a gate insulating layer is deposited on the treated polysilicon layer using a plasma enhanced chemical vapor deposition (PECVD) method. The gate insulating layer may be a composite silicon oxide (SiOx)/silicon nitride (SiNx) film having a thickness of (30–100 nm)/(60–150 nm). Next, a gate metal layer is formed to a thickness of 250–400 nm using a sputtering method on the gate insulating layer. The material for the gate metal layer may be one selected from a group consisting of aluminum (Al), molybdenum (Mo), composite Al/Mo, and the like.

Next, a layer of photoresist is applied on the substrate having the foresaid structures. Next, an exposure process is performed using the halftone mask (HTM) plate. In a region of the HTM plate corresponding to a TFT, a portion corresponding to the gate electrode region is an opaque region, and a portion of the HTM plate corresponding to the source and drain regions is semi-transparent regions. Next, the gate metal layer in the photoresist-completely removed region is wet etched, after which the gate insulating layer and the polysilicon layer in the photoresist-completely removed region is dry etched. As a result, a polysilicon semiconductor pattern is obtained. Next, the photoresist in the photoresist-partially remained region is removed through a plasma ashing process, with a part of the photoresist in the photoresist-completely remained region remained. The photoresist-completely remained region corresponds to the gate electrode region. Next, the gate metal layer in the photoresist-partially remained region is further etched through a wet etching process. A gate electrode is obtained after the photoresist in the photoresist-completely remained region is removed. BHx (e.g., a mixture of $B_2H_6$ or $BF_3$ with $H_2$, the mole percent of $B_2H_6$ or $BF_3$ is 5%–10%, for example) is doped into the source and drain regions using ion bath or ion implantation through a self-aligning process, with a doping dose of $1 - 2 \times 10^{15}$ $cm^{-2}$ and a doping energy of 5-100 KeV. Next, the doped ions are activated through a rapid thermal annealing (RTA) process. In the meantime, the polysilicon semiconductor pattern is hydrogenated during the RTA activation process by making use of H contained in SiNx of the gate insulating layer. The hydrogenated polysilicon semiconductor pattern refers to the polysilicon semiconductor in total remaining on the substrate, including the source and drain regions formed after the doping process. By the foresaid doping process, a source region and a drain region of the LTPS TFT are formed. Due to the presence of the gate electrode, dopant ions are not doped into a semiconductor layer between the source region and the drain region, which becomes a channel region. Although the present process flow is described with a p-type doping as an example, the process flow is not limited thereto. N-type doping can also be performed in the step with $P_2H_6$ (e.g., a mixture of $P_2H_6$ with $H_2$, the mole percent of $P_2H_6$ is 5%–10%, for example). Next, an interlayer dielectric layer is formed through a PECVD method. The material for the interlayer dielectric may be one selected from a group consisting of composite SiOx/SiNx, SiNx, and SiOx, with a thickness of 100–500 nm. A metal layer of a data line and a power supply (VDD) line is sputtered. The metal layer may be Mo, Al, Al-Mo or the like having a thickness of

300–400 nm. A second patterning process is performed on the metal layer to obtain the data line, the VDD line, and the like. Next, after the data line and the power supply line are formed, a passivation layer having a thickness of 300–500 nm is formed through a PECVD process. The material for the passivation layer may be SiNx or organic coating. Next, via holes are formed through a third patterning process. The via holes expose the source and drain regions of the TFT. In addition, the present step also forms a via hole at a position corresponding to the data line to expose the data line so that the data line can be connected to the source region through subsequent steps. Next, the substrate is cleaned to remove surface particles and some organic remnants. An ultrathin metal layer and a transparent conductive layer (e.g., an indium tin oxide (ITO) layer, or an indium zinc oxide (IZO) layer) are sequentially deposited in a dual electrode manner through a sputtering process, where the metal layer may be a metal selected from a group consisting of Mo, Mo/Al-Nd/Mo, silver (Ag), Al, and the like, and may have a thickness of 1–20 nm. The transparent conductive layer may have a thickness of 50–200 nm. Actually, the electrodes formed in the via holes over the source/drain regions serve as source and drain electrodes to electrically connecting the source/drain regions with the data line and the pixel electrode, respectively. Alternatively, a single transparent conductive layer may be deposited in this step to form a single electrode and a pixel electrode. The transparent conductive layer may have a thickness of 50–200 nm. Lastly, a fourth patterning process is performed to obtain a pixel electrode connected to the drain region through the via hole and make the data line be connected to the source region. A dual electrode may be employed to decrease the resistance of the via hole connection line. If only a transparent conductive layer is used, the resistance of the connection line may be increased; thereby a display delay may be increased to affect the display quality of the panel. Of course, a single transparent conductive layer may be used as a via hole connection line in a small-sized LTPS TFT-LCD. However, for microLEDs, a dual electrode is better be used to decrease the resistance of the via hole connection line.

#### 7.3.3.2 Indium-Gallium Zinc-Oxide TFT Backplane

A simplified process flow diagram for making a TFT backplane with oxide channel is shown in Figure 7.12. An insulating film may be deposited as a base film over a glass substrate. The base film can be formed to have a single-layer structure or a layered structure of a silicon oxide film, a silicon nitride film, a silicon oxynitride film, and/or a silicon nitride oxide film by a CVD method, a sputtering method, or the like. A gate electrode layer is formed using a metal material. As the metal material, aluminum, chromium, titanium, tantalum, molybdenum, copper, or the like is applied. A conductive film which is to be the gate electrode layer is formed to a thickness of from 50 to 300 nm. By forming the gate electrode to a thickness of 300 nm or less, disconnection of a

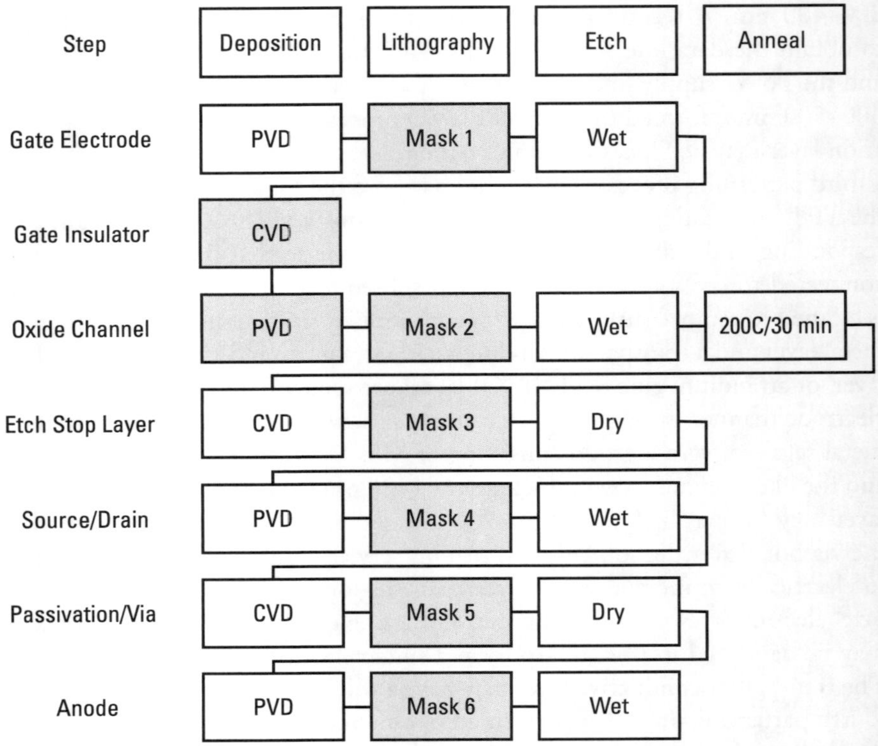


**Figure 7.12** Simplified process flow diagram for making a TFT backplane with oxide channel. The steps that contribute most to the cost of manufacturing are highlighted in gray.

semiconductor film and wirings that are formed later can be prevented. Further, by forming the gate electrode to a thickness of 150 nm or more, resistance of the gate electrode can be reduced and thus the size of the substrate can be increased. Since an oxide semiconductor film and a wiring are to be formed over the gate electrode layer, it is desired that the gate electrode layer be processed to have tapered end portions in order to prevent disconnection. The gate electrode layer can be formed by a sputtering method, a CVD method, a plating method, or a printing method. For example, a molybdenum film is formed as a conductive film over the substrate by a sputtering method and is etched with the use of a resist mask formed using a first photomask so that the gate electrode layer is formed. A gate insulating can be a two-layer structure with two films, and each can be formed using a silicon oxide film, a silicon nitride film, a silicon oxynitride film, or a silicon nitride oxide film with a thickness of from 50 to 150 nm. The gate insulating film can be formed to have a single layer structure of a silicon oxide film, a silicon nitride film, a silicon oxynitride film, or a silicon nitride oxide film, instead of such a two-layer structure. Alternatively, the gate insulating film may be formed to have a three-layer structure. By forming the gate insulating film using a silicon nitride film or a silicon nitride oxide film, adhesiveness between the substrate and the gate insulating film is increased, and in the case where a glass substrate is used as the substrate, an impurity can be prevented from diffusing into the oxide semiconductor layer from the substrate and further, the gate electrode layer can be prevented from being oxidized. That is, film peeling can be prevented, and thus electric characteristics of a thin-film transistor to be completed later can be improved. Further, the gate insulating film preferably has a thickness of 50 nm or more so that it can cover unevenness of the gate electrode layer. In this context, a silicon oxynitride film refers to a film that contains oxygen and nitrogen such that the amount of oxygen is larger than that of nitrogen and contains oxygen, nitrogen, silicon, and hydrogen at concentrations of 55 to 65 at. %, 1 to 20 at. %, 25 to 35 at. %, and 0.1 to 10 at. %, respectively. Further, a silicon nitride oxide film refers to a film that contains oxygen and nitrogen such that the amount of nitrogen is larger than that of oxygen and includes oxygen, nitrogen, silicon, and hydrogen at concentrations of 15 to 30 at. %, 20 to 35 at. %, 25 to 35 at. %, and 15 to 25 at. %, respectively. The gate insulating film can each be formed by a CVD method, a sputtering method, or the like. For example, a silicon nitride film is formed by a plasma CVD method as the gate insulating film.

The oxide semiconductor layer is formed using an amorphous oxide semiconductor film. For the amorphous oxide semiconductor film, a composite oxide of an element such as indium, gallium (Ga), aluminum, zinc (Zn), or tin can be used. In the case of oxide containing indium oxide, gallium oxide, and zinc oxide, the composition ratio of the metal elements is highly flexibly set and the oxide functions as a semiconductor layer at a wide range of mixture ratio. For example, a material in which indium oxide, gallium oxide, and zinc oxide are mixed in an equimolar ratio, and oxide containing In, Ga, and Zn at a ratio of 2.2:2.2:1.0 can be given. The semiconductor film is preferably formed to a thickness of from 2 to 200 nm. Further, when the oxygen vacancy rate in the film is increased, a carrier concentration is increased and thus thin-film transistor characteristics are degraded. Therefore, an indium-gallium zinc-oxide (IGZO) film containing excessive oxygen is formed by performing sputtering by a pulsed DC sputtering method under, for example, an atmosphere containing only oxygen or atmosphere containing oxygen at 90% and Ar at 10%. The amorphous oxide semiconductor film can be formed by a reactive sputtering method. Further, the oxide semiconductor film may be subjected to plasma treatment. By the plasma treatment, damage of the oxide semiconductor film can be repaired. The plasma treatment is preferably performed in an atmosphere of oxygen ($O_2$) or nitrogen dioxide ($N_2O$), or preferably an atmosphere of $N_2$, helium (He), or Ar containing oxygen. The plasma treatment is preferably performed with nonbias. Note that the oxide semiconductor film is formed over the gate insulating film formed in the former step without exposing the gate insulating film to the air by using a multichamber sputtering apparatus provided with a target for an oxide semiconductor film and a silicon target. In the following step, an insulating film to be the channel protective layer is formed over the formed oxide semiconductor film without exposing the oxide semiconductor film to air. The channel protective layer is formed using an insulating film in a region overlapping with a channel formation region of the oxide semiconductor layer. The insulating film to be the channel protective layer can be formed using an inorganic material (such as silicon oxide, silicon nitride, silicon oxynitride, or silicon nitride oxide). The insulating film to be the channel protective layer can be formed by a vapor phase growth method such as a plasma CVD method or a thermal CVD method, or a sputtering method. Next, a resist mask is formed. The insulating film formed over the oxide semiconductor film is selectively etched by using the resist mask so that the channel protective layer is formed. Next, a film having n-type conductivity that functions as a buffer layer is formed over the oxide semiconductor film. The buffer layer functions as an n+ layer and can be called a source region and a drain region. For the buffer layer, metal oxide having n-type conductivity and an oxide semiconductor film containing In, Ga, and Zn can be used. Since the buffer layer formed using the metal oxide has a higher carrier concentration than the IGZO semiconductor layer in which the channel is formed and is superior in conductivity, the contact resistance can be reduced as compared to the case of directly attaching the source and drain electrode layers to the semiconductor layer. The buffer layer can be of thickness larger than 2 nm and smaller than 100 nm. The buffer film can be formed by a sputtering method. Next, a conductive film to be a source electrode layer and a drain electrode layer is formed. The conductive film can be formed using the same material as the gate electrode layer. In particular, a layer in contact with the n-type buffer film is preferably a titanium film. As specific examples of the conductive film, a single titanium film, a layered film including a titanium film and an aluminum film, and a three-layer film in which a titanium film, an aluminum film, and a titanium film are sequentially stacked are given. Next, a resist mask is formed and the conductive film formed over the channel protective layer is etched using the resist mask to be separated, whereby source and drain electrode layers are formed. Further, the buffer film having n-type conductivity is etched using the same resist mask to be separated, whereby two buffer layers are formed for the source and drain contacts. Note that each film may be processed using dry etching or wet etching, or each film may be selectively etched in two separate steps.

Heat treatment may be preferably performed on the semiconductor layer at temperatures of 200°C to 400°C for an hour, for example. The heat treatment may be performed any time after the oxide semiconductor layer is formed. For example, the heat treatment may be performed after a sealing film of the thin-film transistor is formed, or heat curing treatment performed after formation of a planarizing film may also serve as the heat treatment for the semiconductor layer.

#### 7.3.3.3 LTPO TFT Backplane

LTPS TFTs have been widely used as the backplane technology in mobile displays because of their superior driving capability [15]. However, due to the intrinsically higher off-state leakage current, LTPS displays are required to maintain a drive frame frequency at 60 Hz or larger to prevent flicker noise. Compared with LTPS TFTs, metal oxide semiconductors such as IGZO have been shown to enable display frame-rate reduction, owing to the ultralow off-state leakage current. The drawback of metal oxide TFT is its lower mobility, which requires larger circuit size and higher driving voltages. In order to take advantage of both TFT technologies, a new TFT backplane structure, called LTPO, was developed, which embeds metal oxide TFT into an LTPS TFT backplane. With the LTPO architecture, the benefits of low power and slim border with LTPS TFTs can be maintained, and the incorporation of metal oxide switch TFTs in the pixel circuit enables lower refresh rates and reduced power consumption. Moreover, small area CMOS pixel driving circuits may be realized for high-resolution microLED displays [16–24].

In general, LTPS TFT and metal oxide TFT backplane processes are not compatible. LTPS TFTs require significant amounts of hydrogen atoms to passivate the dangling bonds and defects inside poly-Si and at the interface between poly-Si and gate insulator. However, excess amounts of hydrogen will cause an imbalance between oxygen vacancy and metal-oxygen bond that results in oxide TFT device threshold voltage shift during operation. This threshold voltage shift will be more pronounced at low display driving frequency because of the increased negative bias stress that is applied to the metal oxide switching TFT. Therefore, considering the LTPO process integration, it is essential to balance the overall amount and distribution of hydrogen atoms inside the LTPO stack-up. Figure 7.13 shows the LTPO TFT stack-up with top-gate oxide TFT (called top-gate LTPO) [15]. For the top-gate LTPO stack-up, the oxide TFT is fabricated after the completion of the LTPS TFT. In this stack-up, the LTPS TFT and oxide TFT processes can be optimized independently. The process flow for making p-channel TFT and n-channel metal oxide TFT are shown in Figures 7.11 and 7.12, respectively. Utilizing an oxide TFT as a switch transistor demands aggressive device performance requirements, among which is stability of oxide TFT threshold voltage during the lifetime of the display. Such requirements could lead to using special process steps in the process flow, which could increase cost.

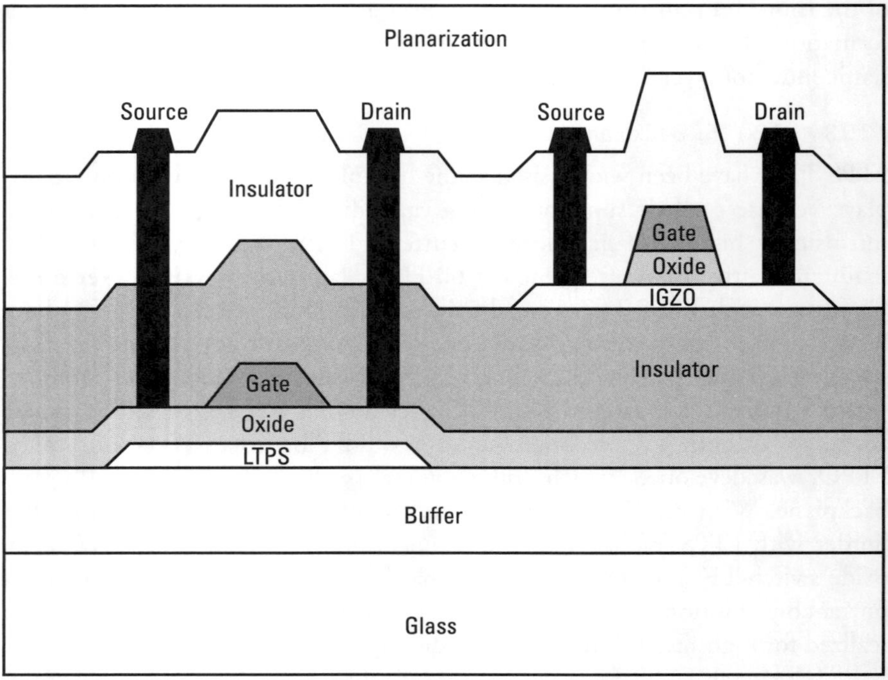


**Figure 7.13** Schematic cross section of LTPO thin-film transistors.

### 7.3.4 Transfer Technology

One state-of-the-art approach to fabricating microLED displays involves direct transfer from source to target. MicroLED devices are fabricated on a source wafer and then transferred directly to a target substrate where the microLED devices are assembled with driving electronics to provide a display [25–29]. This approach, however, lacks compliance, and the associated topography may be problematic for multiple passes associated with transfer of three colors or more from different wafers having red, green, and blue microLEDs. The other approach involves transfer with a stamp [30–32]. For example, a stamp picks from the source wafer and then transfers to a target substrate where microLED devices are assembled with driving electronics to provide a display. This approach, however, requires the need for pick up, bond, and release mechanisms. The approach is typically slow and expensive and requires unique equipment [33–40]. A third approach involves releasing known good microLEDs from the growth wafer to a tank filled with fluid. The fluid is then poured on the surface of a display backplane where microgrooves have been prepared to receive the microLEDs from the fluid along a specific orientation. The third approach is called fluidic self-assembly (FSA) [41, 42].

#### 7.3.4.1 Pick-and-Place

MicroLEDs on a growth wafer are flip-chip transferred to a carrier glass substrate prepared with arrays of patterned solder pads of size similar to the microLED size. The top free surface of the microLED is also coated with solder material. After alignment of the solder pads and microLEDs and their solder bonding layers, the carrier substrate and growth wafer are brought into contact. The assembly is heated to the liquidus temperature of the solder, preferably between 200°C and 300°C. This results in bonding of the two solder layers. The microLEDs can now be donated from the growth substrate to the carrier glass by using laser liftoff or chemical liftoff [43]. One key requirement is sufficiently large bonding interface strength between the microLED and the carrier to provide structural integrity for the system during release of the microLEDs from the growth wafer. Eutectic bonding of the bonding layers can create a strong bonding interface that protects against such delamination during the release process. The microLEDs are now poised to be picked up by a suitable transfer head using electrostatic [1, 2] or Van der Waals force [46], for example. The transfer head may have an area of 1" by 1", for example. The microLEDs are picked up from the carrier by selectively heating the carrier using, for example, a laser beam through the glass carrier over the area of the transfer head, or a heating apparatus attached to the transfer head [44]. Next, the transfer head is moved over the receiving substrate (e.g., display backplane) that has been populated with arrays of solder pads with pitch equal to the microLED pitch on the transfer head. After alignment, the microLEDs' free surface coated with solder layer is brought into contact with the corresponding solder pads on the display backplane. By heating the display backplane to ~200°C, for example, a bond is formed between the two bonding layers on the microLED free surface and the display solder pads. In the case of an electrostatic stamp, the electrostatic force is removed and the microLEDs are now completely transferred to the display backplane.

Solder bonding layers may be sputtered, deposited by electron beam (E-beam) evaporation, or plated with a seed layer to obtain a uniform thickness.

MicroLEDs are described as having a 10 by 10 $\mu$m pitch, 5 by 5 $\mu$m pitch, or the like. At these densities a 6" diameter substrate, for example, can accommodate approximately 150 million microLED structures with a 10 by 10 $\mu$m pitch, or approximately 600 million microLED structures with a 5 by 5 $\mu$m pitch [43]. Thus, a high density of prefabricated microLED structures with a specific functionality may be produced in a manner in which they are poised for pick up and transfer to a receiving substrate.

There is also a possibility of directly picking up microLEDs from donor wafer using the process flow shown in Figure 7.14. In this case, chemical lift-off is used to prepare the microLEDs so that they are poised to be picked up directly by the transfer head. This reduces the number of assembly steps, and

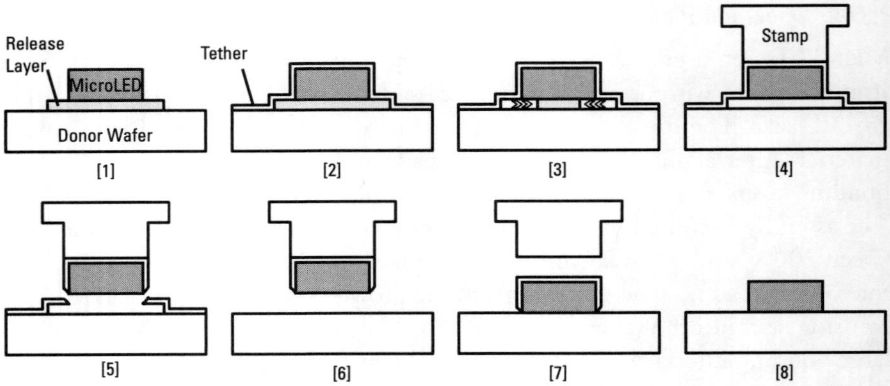


**Figure 7.14** Schematic illustration of PnP transfer illustrating the details of how microLEDs are picked up from the wafer then placed on the display backplane using a tether layer (e.g., photoresist).

thus reduces the cost of manufacturing. The steps are as follows: A sacrificial layer (release layer) is used during the growth of the microLEDs on the growth wafer as shown in (1). In (2) a tether (e.g., photoresist) is deposited on the structure as shown. In (3) chemical liftoff is used to etch the release layer. In (4) a stamp is attached to the top surface of the microLED. By pulling the stamp up, the tether is broken as shown in (5). The microLED carried by the stamp is aligned to where it should be placed on the display backplane in (6). In (7) the microLED is released from the stamp. Lastly, (8) illustrates the final state of a transferred microLED on the display backplane.

#### 7.3.4.2 Direct Transfer Method

Low-cost production of microLED displays for smartphones or laptops require low cost of microLED donor wafer and low cost of transferring microLEDs to the display backplane. Both can be addressed by using 300-mm silicon wafers to grow the GaN-based microLEDs. However, silicon's mismatch in coefficient of thermal expansion with the III-nitrides results in cracking of the III-nitride layers if additional engineering is not employed. One approach to eliminate the cracking of the III-nitride films/devices is to compressively strain the film as it grows so that when it cools to room temperature the film is relaxed. This is typically done with intermediate AlN and AlGaN films when growing GaN on silicon. The disadvantage of this technique is that during growth the substrate is not flat, but instead is bowed, which leads to poor quality and nonuniformity of quantum well growth, and difficulty transferring the microLEDs directly from the silicon wafer to the display backplane. An alternative way of eliminating the cracking of the III-nitride film without causing a bow in the wafer during growth is to use patterned silicon substrates. By this technique, only small areas of the silicon substrate seed GaN, and these regions are small enough that the GaN films do not crack due to the stresses induced from the mismatch in the coefficient of thermal expansion. Selective area epitaxy may be used to grow nanowires or nanopyramids out of a patterned seed layer that had been deposited on the silicon substrate. The patterned seed layer can have patches of size 1 $\mu$m × 1 $\mu$m to 10 $\mu$m × 10 $\mu$m, for example, separated by streets of 1 $\mu$m, for example. The seed layer may be made of a thin transition metal nitride that has crystal structure similar to GaN. To prevent interdiffusion between metal nitride and silicon, a thin AlN buffer (e.g., 20–30 nm in thickness) may be first grown on Si wafer that is preferably Si (111). When transferring the microLEDs from the silicon wafer to a display backplane, the seed layer can be utilized as a release layer by ablating or vaporizing it by infrared irradiation through the silicon substrate. The infrared light, which can have a wavelength of >1,200 nm, will not be absorbed by the silicon wafer. The release of microLEDs, selectively, from the silicon wafer can enable low cost and mass direct transfer of microLEDs from the silicon wafer to the display backplane. A simple schematic illustrating the DTM working principle is shown in Figures 7.15 and 7.16. First, the donor wafer is aligned to the display backplane so that microLEDs are facing interconnect metal pads on the display backplane. These metal pads are connected to the driving circuits that are made of thin-film transistors. Next, selective bonding is performed of the microLEDs to the metal pads on the backplane. In this case, the surface of the microLED is coated with a metal pad as well and metal-to-metal bonding can be done without using solder. Finally, a laser beam is used to selectively release the already-bonded microLEDs from the donor wafer to the display backplane. In this step, the laser beam is steered through the backside of the donor wafer toward the release layer holding the microLEDs to the donor wafer. Upon exposure to the pulsed laser beam, the release layer is vaporized/disintegrated and the microLED is released to the display backplane [47–49].

Details of the process to do selective bonding and selective release is shown in Figure 7.17.

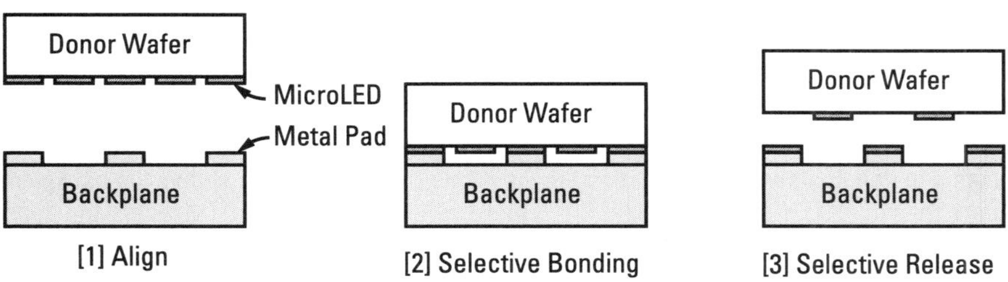


**Figure 7.15** Schematic illustration of the DTM where the donor wafer is used instead of a stamp to donate its microLEDs directly to the display backplane.

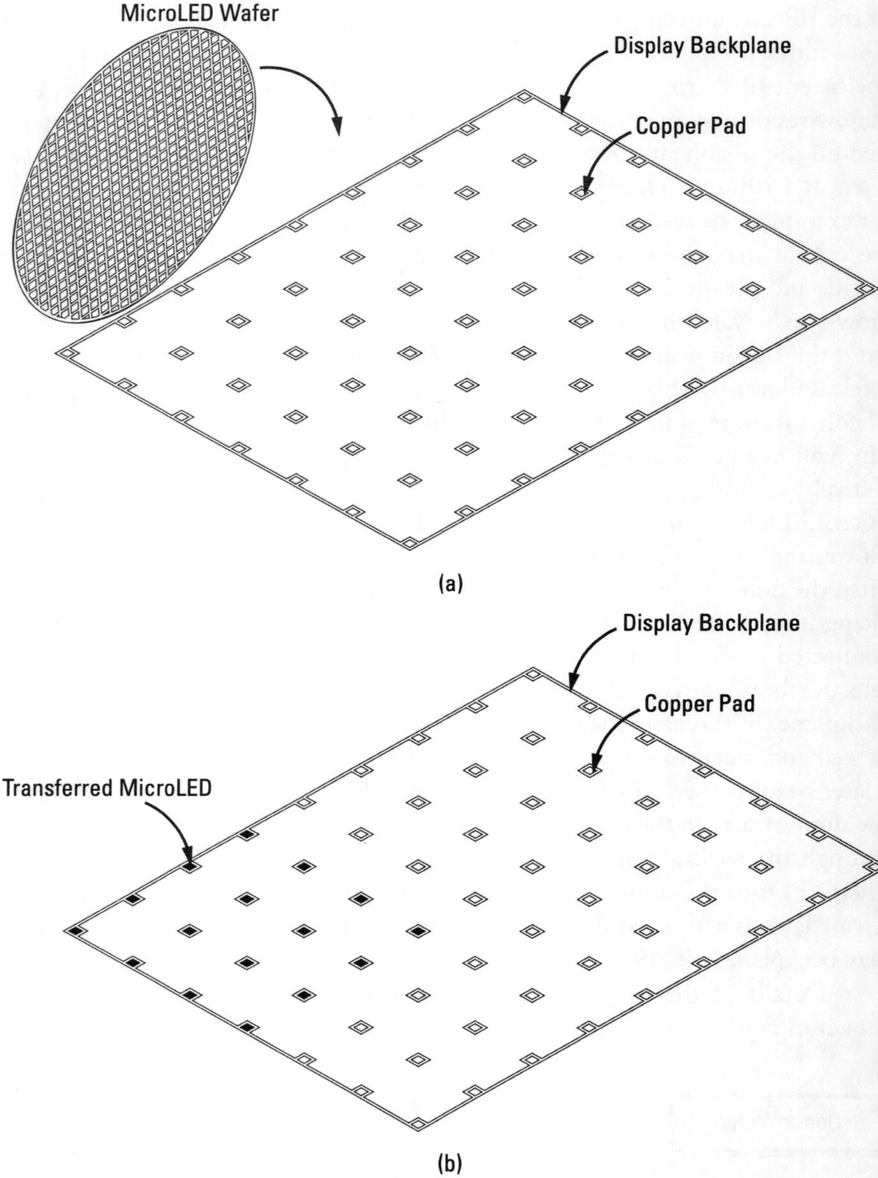


**Figure 7.16** (a) Schematic illustration of the DTM where the donor wafer is used instead of a stamp to donate its microLEDs directly to the display backplane. This shows the backplane before the microLEDs are transferred. (b) Schematic illustration of the DTM where the donor wafer is used instead of a stamp to donate its microLEDs directly to the display backplane. This shows the backplane after the microLEDs have been transferred.

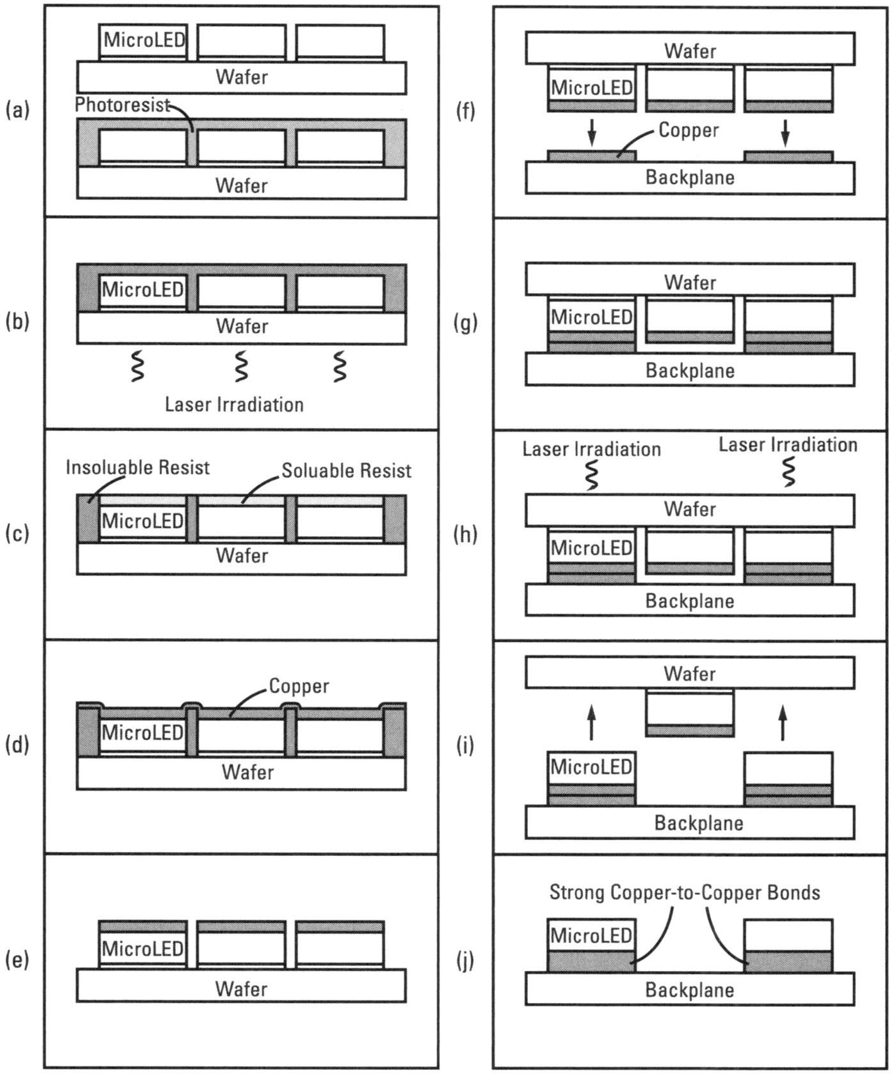


**Figure 7.17** Schematic illustration of the DTM where the donor wafer is used instead of a stamp to donate its microLEDs directly to the display backplane. Shown are the steps to form copper contacts on the microLEDs (steps (a) to (e)), selective bonding (steps (f), (g)), selective release (steps (h) and (i)), and finally annealing bond to form a strong copper bond between the microLEDs and the backplane.

### 7.3.4.3 Fluidic Self-Assembly

The fluidic self-assembly approach involves fabrication of microLEDs on, for example, 150-mm diameter sapphire wafers, 200-mm diameter silicon wafers, or 300-mm diameter silicon wafers, followed by identification of microLEDs that are not working. The nonfunctional microLEDs may be identified according to the following approach: (a) shining UV light (e.g., having a wavelength in the range of 200–400 nm) on microLED wafers, (b) identifying dark spots on the wafer that represent defective microLEDs using appropriate imaging technology (e.g., a CCD RGB camera). The defective microLEDs may then be released from the donor wafers to avoid transferring them onto the display backplane. This is done by using pulsed infrared laser irradiation from the silicon backside of the microLED wafer to selectively detach the defective microLEDs that have been identified, or by using pulsed UV laser irradiation from a sapphire backside of a microLED wafer to selectively detach the defective microLEDs that have been identified. The processing scheme continues with using laser irradiation on the backside of the microLED wafers (e.g., UV for sapphire wafers and infrared for silicon wafers) to detach the good MicroLEDs into a container filled with an appropriate fluid. The processing scheme continues with fabrication or providing of a display backplane with microgrooves of appropriate size (e.g., width, length, and height) to receive microLEDs from a fluid. For example, the microgrooves have a specific shape to selectively receive microLEDs on a specific side where a solder bonding layer has been deposited. A contact metal (solder) is disposed at the bottom of the groove to facilitate bonding of a microLED received from the fluid to the display backplane. The main challenge for this approach is achieving transfer yields higher than 99.9% [42]. This level of transfer yield is required for achieving acceptable target display line yield [50]. The FSA process steps and an example equipment design are shown in Figures 7.18 and 7.19, respectively.

### 7.3.5 Display Should-Cost Modeling

Now that the main building blocks of display manufacturing have been discussed, it is important to understand the sensitivity of the microLED display cost to microLED size, transfer method, wafer size, and epi wafer cost. An SCM has been developed for both DTM and PnP transfer technologies. The model is used to calculate the sensitivity of display manufacturing cost to model parameters for both 6" smartphone display and 14" laptop display with resolution $2560 \times 1440$.

Figure 7.20 shows that estimated production cost of a 6" diagonal display versus microLED size for DTM transfer technology. Different levels of redundancy are used. Larger microLEDs result in larger production cost for a given redundancy level. For a given microLED size, larger redundancy level results in larger production cost. The dependency of production cost on redundancy level and microLED size is quasi-linear. Similar observations were found for 14" diagonal display as shown in Figure 7.21.

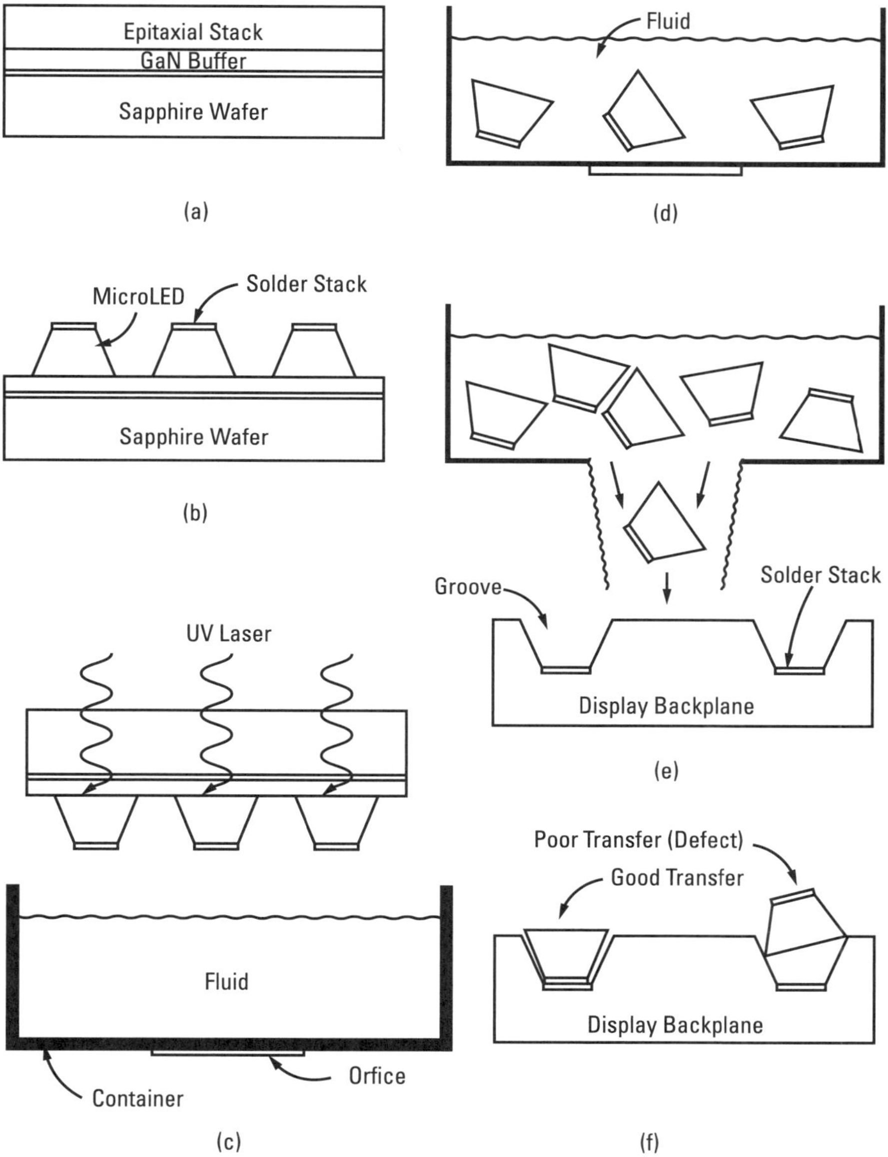


**Figure 7.18** Steps for FSA transfer of microLEDs from a growth wafer to a display backplane. (a) epi stack as grown on growth wafer, (b) after patterning microLEDs and depositing solder bonding layer, (c) and (d) release of microLEDs from growth wafer into a container/tank full of appropriate fluid, (e) pouring suspension of fluid and microLEDs onto the display backplane, and (f) successful and nonsuccessful transfer of microLEDs to the display backplane. Vibrations may be injected into the liquid to induce successful transfer, which could take a long time to reach 100% successful transfer.

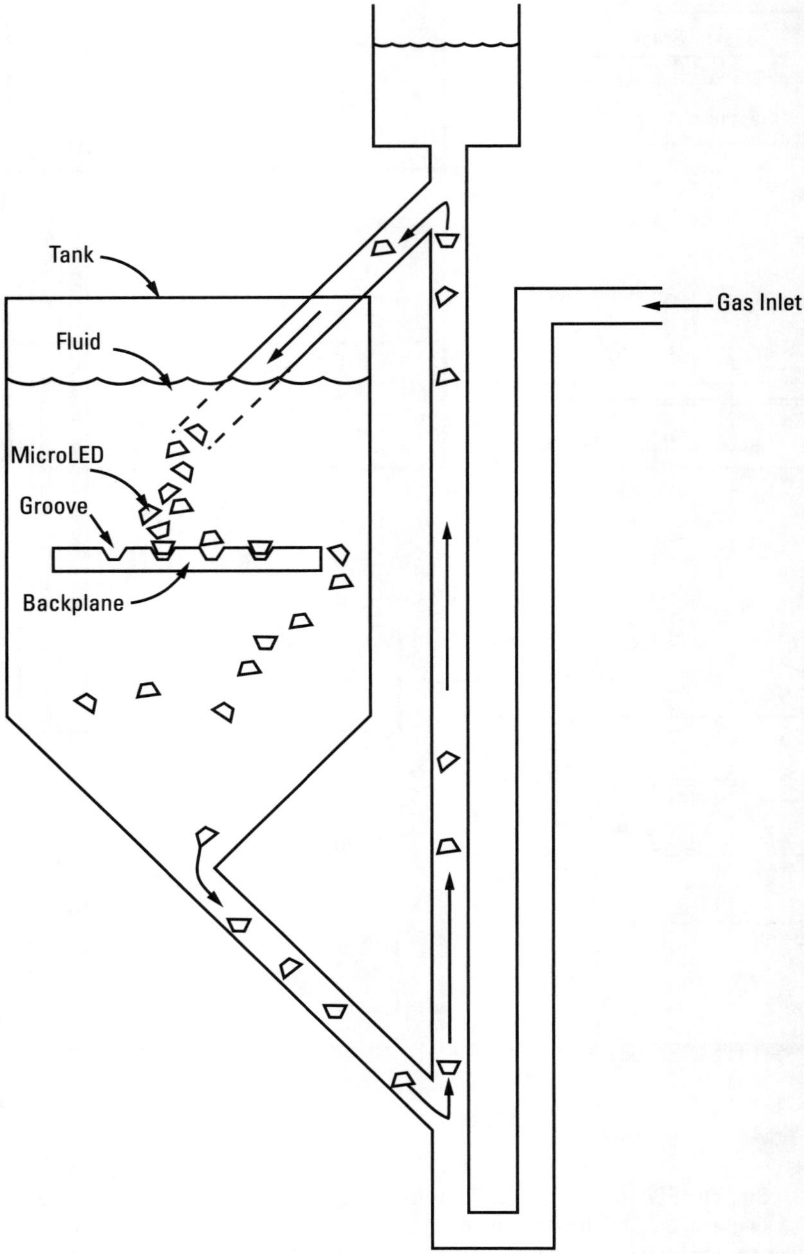


**Figure 7.19** Schematic illustration of an example equipment that may be used for fluidic self-assembly. The equipment design concept is relatively simple, which could result in relatively low cost for the transfer equipment. However, achieving transfer yields more than 99.9% by inducing vibrations of the liquid and/or the backplane may take a long time.

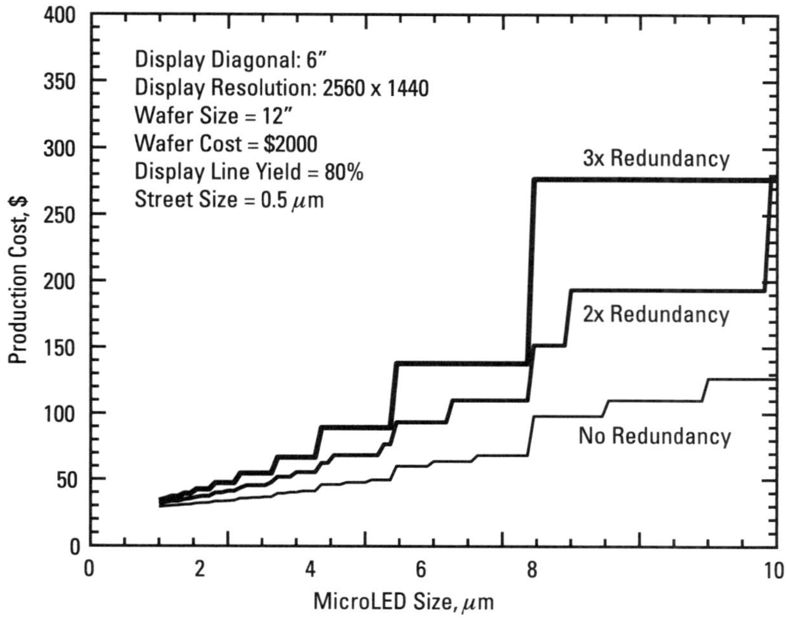


**Figure 7.20** Calculated production cost of a 6″ diagonal display versus microLED size and redundancy level.

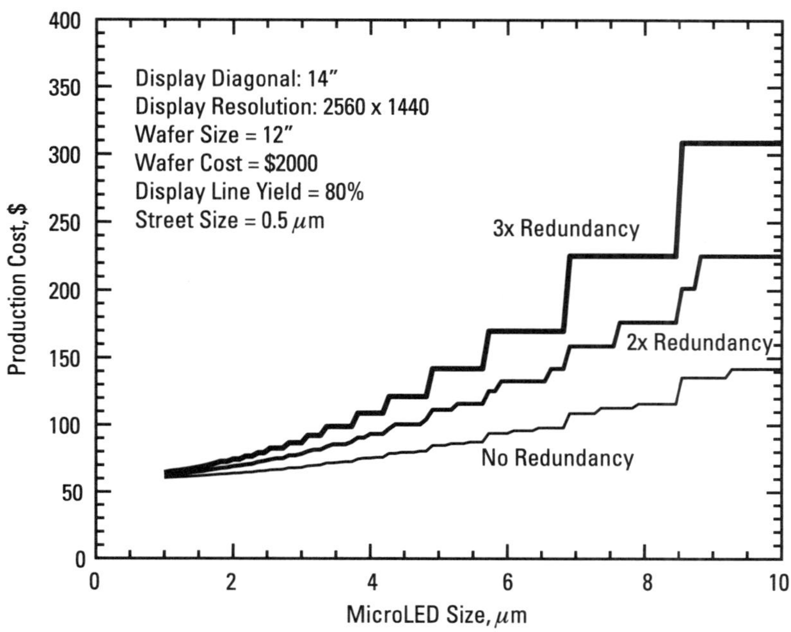


**Figure 7.21** Calculated production cost of a 14″ diagonal display versus microLED size and redundancy level.

Figure 7.22 shows a calculated production cost of 6" diagonal display using DTM. The production cost and microLED size are cross plotted for two different microLED wafer size (8" and 12" diameters). For a given microLED size, smaller microLED wafer results in larger production cost.

The production cost and microLED size are cross plotted in Figure 7.23 for three assumed costs for the microLED wafer. As expected, for a given microLED size the display production cost increases with increasing the microLED wafer cost, with the rate of increase being larger at a larger microLED size. Figure 7.24 is similar to Figure 7.23 but for 14" display diagonal. Figure 7.25 shows a cross plot of the calculated display production cost and microLED wafer cost for three practical sizes of microLEDs. Linear dependence of production cost on microLED wafer cost is observed for these microLED sizes.

From the previous cost sensitivity graphs, it is possible to establish a cost roadmap for microLED displays with an ultimate landing zone characterized by using 12" diameter microLED wafers, using less than 5-$\mu$m pitch microLEDs, lowering the cost of microLED wafers to \$2,000 or below, using 2× redundancy, and having monolithic red, green, and blue microLEDs on the same wafer. This combination should provide the lowest production cost point for microLED displays used in smartphones (6") and laptops (14").

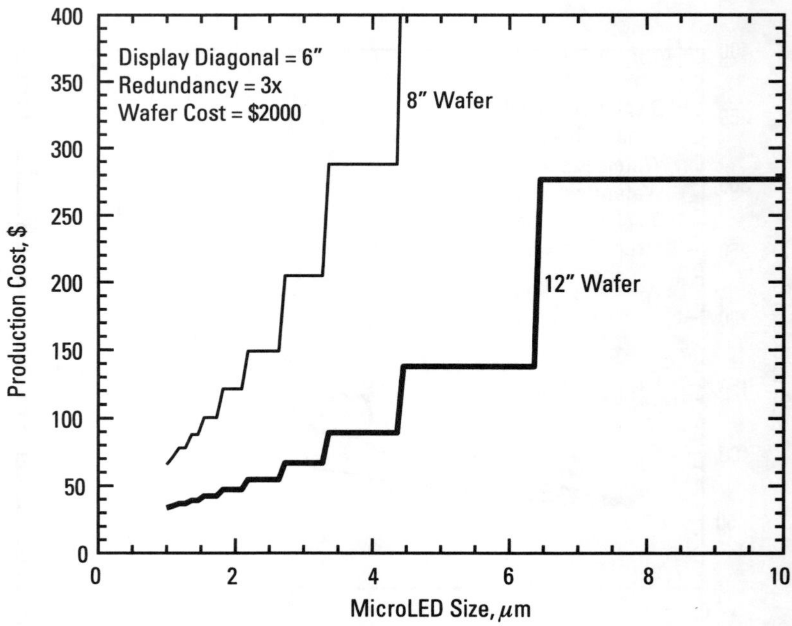


**Figure 7.22** Calculated production cost of a 6" diagonal display versus microLED size and microLED wafer diameter. Larger wafer diameter results in a lower display production cost for a given microLED size.

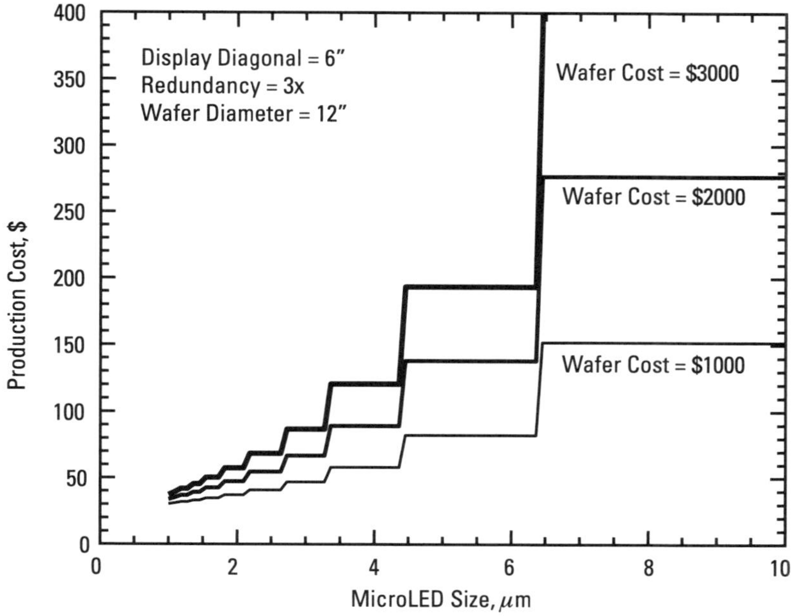


**Figure 7.23** Calculated production cost of a 6″ diagonal display versus microLED size and microLED wafer cost.

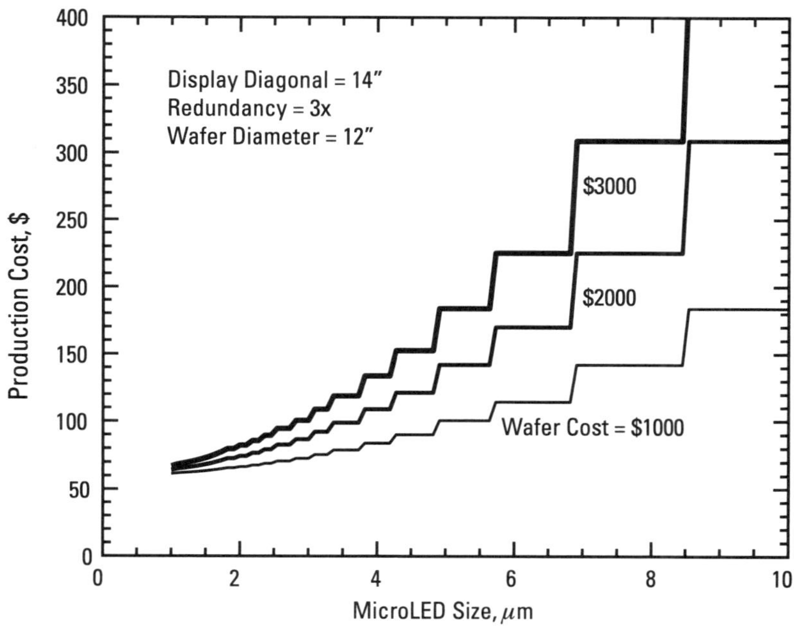


**Figure 7.24** Calculated production cost of a 14″ diagonal display versus microLED size and microLED wafer cost.

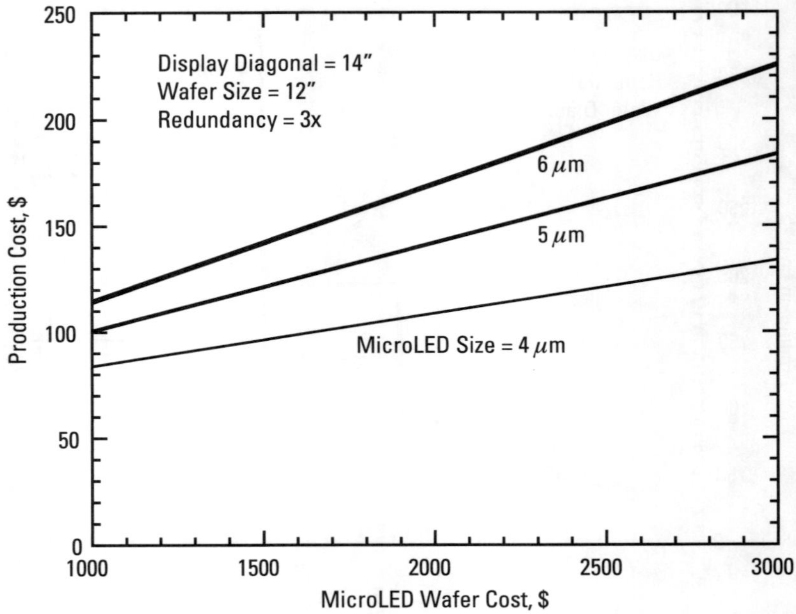


**Figure 7.25** Calculated production cost of a 14" diagonal display versus microLED wafer cost for three microLED sizes.

# References


[1] Vose, M., *The Simple Genetic Algorithm: Foundations and Theory,* Cambridge, MA: MIT Press, 1999.

[2] Farineau, T., B. Rabenasolo, J. Castelain, Y. Meyer, and P. Duverlie, "Use of Parametric Models in an Economic Evaluation Step During the Design Phase," *International Journal of Advanced Manufacturing Technology,* Vol. 17, 2001, pp. 79–86.

[3] Corbett, J., M. Dooner, J. Meleka, and C. Pym, *Design for Manufacture: Strategies, Principles, and Techniques,* Addison Wesley Publishing Company, 1991.

[4] Boothroyd, G., P. Dewhurst, and W. Knight, *Product Design for Manufacture and Assembly,* Third Edition, Boca Raton, FL: CRC Press, 2010.

[5] White, K., R. Athay, and W. Trybula, "Applying DFM in the Semiconductor Industry," in *Seventeenth IEEE/CPMT International Electronics Manufacturing Technology Symposium,* 1995.

[6] Freddi, A., M. Salmon, A. Freddi, and M. Salmon, "Introduction to the Taguchi Method," in *Design Principles and Methodologies: From Conceptualization to First Prototyping with Examples and Case Studies* (A. Freddi and M. Salmon, eds.), Cham, Switzerland: Springer, 2019, pp. 159–180.

[7] Gygi, C., and B. Williams, *Six Sigma for Dummies,* Hoboken, NJ: John Wiley & Sons, 2012.

[8] Wilson, L., *How to Implement Lean Manufacturing*, New York: McGraw-Hill Education, 2015.

[9] Asiedu, Y., and P. Gu, "Product Life Cycle Cost Analysis: State of the Art Review," *International Journal of Production Research*, Vol. 36, No. 4, 1998, pp. 883–908.

[10] Saravi, M., L. Newnes, A. Mileham, and Y. Goh, "Estimating Cost at the Conceptual Design Stage to Optimize Design in Terms of Performance and Cost," in *Proceedings of the 15th ISPE International Conference on Concurrent Engineering (CE2008)*, London, 2008.

[11] Datta, P., and R. Roy, "Cost Modelling Techniques for Availability Type Service Support Contracts: A Literature Review and Empirical Study," *CIRP Journal of Manufacturing Science and Technology*, Vol. 3, No. 2, 2010, pp. 142–157.

[12] Matthews, J., and A. Blakeslee, "Defects in Epitaxial Multilayers: I. Misfit Dislocations," *Journal of Crystal Growth*, Vol. 27, pp. 118–125, 1974.

[13] P. Capper, S. Irvine, and T. Joyce, "Epitaxial Crystal Growth: Methods and Materials," in *Springer Handbook of Electronic and Photonic Materials*, 2nd Edition (S. Kasap and P. Capper, eds.), Cham, Switzerland: Springer, 2017, p. 319.

[14] Nakamura, S., "In Situ Monitoring of GaN Growth using Interference Effects," *Japanese Journal of Applied Physics*, Vol. 30, No. 8R, 1991, p. 1620.

[15] Chang, T., C. Lin, and S. Chang, "LTPO TFT Technology for AMOLEDs," *SID Symposium Digest of Technical Papers*, Vol. 50, No. 1, 2019, pp. 545–548.

[16] Moon, K., H. Im, S. Hong, and Y. Kim, "Advanced LTPO Technology for CMOS Driving," *SID Symposium Digest of Technical Papers*, Vol. 53, No. 1, 2022, pp. 612–615.

[17] Rahaman, A., H. Jeong, and J. Jang, "A High-Gain CMOS Operational Amplifier Using Low-Temperature Poly-Si Oxide TFTs," *IEEE Transactions on Electron Devices*, Vol. 67, No. 2, 2020, pp. 524–528.

[18] Kim, H., D. Jeong, S. Lee, and J. Jang, "A High-Gain Inverter with Low-Temperature Poly-Si Oxide Thin-Film Transistors," *IEEE Electron Device Letters*, Vol. 40, No. 3, 2019, pp. 411–414.

[19] H. Luo, S. Wang, J. Kang, et al., "Complementary LTPO Technology, Pixel Circuits and Integrated Gate Drivers for AMOLED Displays Supporting Variable Refresh Rates," *SID Symposium Digest of Technical Papers*, Vol. 51, No. 1, 2020, pp. 351–354.

[20] Liu, Y., S. Que, C. Liao, et al., "LTPO TFTs Based PWM Pixel Circuit for AM-Micro-LED Display with Falling-time< 10 $\mu$s," *SID Symposium Digest of Technical Papers*, Vol. 54, No. 1, 2023, pp. 1810–1813.

[21] Zhao, J., M. Zhao, Y. Guo, et al., "High PPI MicroLED Display Driver Circuit and Device Structure," *SID Symposium Digest of Technical Papers*, Vol. 54, No. 1, 2023, pp. 29–31.

[22] Ko, Y., D. Jeon, W. Jeong, M. Lim, and S. Lee, "Bit Depth of Drivers for Micro-LED Displays Adopting Low-Temperature Polysilicon Oxide Thin-Film Transistors," *IEEE Journal of the Electron Devices Society*, Vol. 11, 2023, pp. 161–166.

[23] Ahmed, K., Methods and Apparatus for In-Pixel Driving of Micro-LEDs, US Patent 11,676,529, 2023.

[24] Kang, K., J. Park, C. Park, and S. Lee, "A New Line-by-Line SWEEP Signal Generation Method for PWM Driving MicroLED TFT Pixel Circuit," *SID Symposium Digest of Technical Papers*, Vol. 54, No. 1, 2023, pp. 70–73.

[25] Ahmed, K., and A. Pancholi, Micro Light-Emitting Diode Display Fabrication and Assembly, US Patent 1,177,243, 2021.

[26] Ahmed, K., and A. Khakifirooz, Light Emitting Display, US Patent 11,275,245, 2022.

[27] Ahmed, K., A. Prakash, R. Woodbeck and S. Pabba, Structures for Micro LED Laser Release, US Patent Application 17/402,313, 2023.

[28] West, P., and K. Ahmed, Micro LED Laser Release from Silicon Wafer, US Patent Application 17/485,398, 2022.

[29] Sounart, T., K. Ahmed, A. Pancholi, and S. Liff, Micro-LED Displays Including Solder Structures and Methods, US Patent Application 16/946,166, 2020.

[30] Chang, P., MicroLED Display and Assembly, US Patent 10,128,307, 2018.

[31] Chang, P., C. Pawashe, M. Mayberry, and J. Tseng, Micro Pick and Bond Assembly, US Patent 10,242,892, 2019.

[32] Ahmed, K., K. Parikh, and P. Chang, Apparatus for Micro Pick and Bond, US Patent 10,217,729, 2019.

[33] Ahmed, K., "Micro LED Display: Technology and Manufacturing Challenges," in *Novel Patterning Technologies 2021,* Vol. 11610, SPIE, 2021.

[34] Li, J., B. Luo, and Z. Liu, "Micro-LED Mass Transfer Technologies," *in 21st International Conference on Electronic Packaging Technology (ICEPT)*, 2020.

[35] Ding, K., V. Avrutin, N. Izyumskaya, Ü. Özgür, and H. Morkoç, "Micro-LEDs, a Manufacturability Perspective," *Applied Sciences*, Vol. 9, No. 6, 2019, p. 1206.

[36] Linghu, C., S. Zhang, C. Wang, H. Luo, and J. Song, "Mass Transfer for Micro-LED Display: Transfer Printing Techniques," *in Semiconductors and Semimetals,* Vol. 106, Elsevier, 2021, pp. 253–280.

[37] Bower, C., S. Bonafede, A. Pearson, et al., "Mass Transfer Throughput and Yield Using Elastomer Stamps," *SID Symposium Digest of Technical Papers*, Vol. 52, No. 1, 2021, pp. 849–852.

[38] Chaji, R., E. Fathi, and A. Zamani, "Essentials of MicroLED Display Production," *SID Symposium Digest of Technical Papers*, Vol. 51, No. 1, 2020, pp. 323–327.

[39] Chen, F., J. Bian, J. Hu, et al., "Mass Transfer Techniques for Large-Scale and High-Density MicroLED Arrays International," *Journal of Extreme Manufacturing*, Vol. 4, No. 4, 2022, p. 042005.

[40] Chaji, R., and E. Fathi, "MicroLED Displays for Smartwatch and Smartphone," *SID Symposium Digest of Technical Papers*, Vol. 54, No. 1, 2023, pp. 658–660.

[41] Ahmed, K., A. Pancholi, and A. Khakifirooz, Micro Light-Emitting Diode (LED) Display and Fluidic Self-Assembly of Same, US Patent 10,361,337, 2019.

[42] Lee, D., S. Cho, C. Park, et al., "Fluidic Self-Assembly for MicroLED Displays by Controlled Viscosity," *Nature*, Vol. 619, No. 7971, 2023, pp. 755–760.

[43] Hu, H., A. Bibl, J. Higginson, and H. Law, Method of Forming a Micro LED Structure and Array of Micro LED Structures with an Electrically Insulating Layer, US Patent 8,573,469, 2013.

[44] Bibl, A., J. Higginson, H. Law, and H. Hu, Micro Device Transfer Head Heater Assembly and Method of Transferring a Micro Device, US Patent 8,349,116, 2013.

[45] Bibl, A., J. Higginson, H. Law, and H. Hu, Method of Transferring a Micro Device, US Patent 8,333,860, 2012.

[46] Nuzzo, R., J. Rogers, E. Menard, et al., Pattern Transfer Printing by Kinetic Control of Adhesion to an Elastomeric Stamp, US Patent 7,943,491, 2011.

[47] Ahmed, K., Micro Light-Emitting Diode Display Fabrication and Assembly Apparatus, US Patent 16/235,831, 2020.

[48] Ahmed, K., and A. Pancholi, Laser Transfer Printing for Making Micro LED Display Devices and Method, US Patent 16/053,559, 2020.

[49] Ahmed, K., A. Pancholi, S. Dasgupta, and C. Mair, Micro Light-Emitting Diode Display Fabrication and Assembly, US Patent 11,637,093, 2023.

[50] Ahmed, K., Yield Statistics for Fault Tolerant Micro LED Displays, *SID Symposium Digest of Technical Papers*, Vol. 51, No. 1, 2020, pp. 520–523.

# 8

# Advanced MicroLED Concepts

In 1965, Gordon Moore observed that the number of transistors on a chip could be expected to double annually for at least 10 years. At different time points in the ensuing decades, overall the chip transistor count has continued to increase, and conversely, the size of each transistor has decreased, at an amazing rate, and Gordon Moore's postulate became known as Moore's law. The projected scalability by Moore's law attracted huge investments in semiconductor technologies over approximately 50 years that resulted in amazing innovation. In this chapter, we propose and discuss a number of potential advanced research and development concepts that can be used to optimize future microLED devices and systems. These concepts may seed a number of research topics that can potentially culminate into a scalability law that attracts further investments in microLED technologies. This may be useful for researchers in academia and industry. The discussion is limited to the concept stage with the aim to facilitate brainsteering toward future device and system improvements. Brainsteering has been explained by Coyne and Coyne as an alternative to brainstorming to find breakthrough ideas [1]. The advantage of brainsteering is that it applies the design thinking process to creative idea generation. Energy is invested upfront to ensure that the actual problem to be solved is crystal clear.

## 8.1 Meta MicroLED

Short-reach optical interconnects (OIO) with microLEDs as light emitters promise $< 1$ pJ/bit energy consumption, 2 cents/Gbps system cost, and 2 Gb/s/channel bandwidth. Realizing these promises requires microLEDs with $\geq$ 1-GHz modulation frequency operating $< 1{,}000$ A/cm$^2$ bias current, total divergence angle < 30°, and emission linewidth < 10 nm at a peak emission wavelength of < 450 nm. MicroLEDs developed for display applications do not meet these requirements.

The present-day microLEDs suffer from numerous deficiencies. First, light emission in the microLED is spontaneous, and, thus, is limited in time on the order of 1 to 10 ns. Therefore, the modulation speed of the microLED is also limited by the spontaneous lifetime of the microLED. This limits the maximum modulation frequency to ~400 MHz. Second, light emission in the active region is isotropic such that only a fraction of the emission may leave the body through the opening in the top electrode. Third, spectral linewidth of the microLED is broad, of the order of 1.8 $kT$ where $kT$ is the thermal energy. This results in chromatic dispersion in optical multimode fibers (i.e., pulse broadening), which limits the maximum distance of transmission of light emitted by a microLED to ~1m. These deficiencies may be addressed by introducing a microcavity in the microLED stack. In the past, LEDs with optical resonant microcavities typically used DBRs for the front and rear reflectors [2–5]. DBRs typically consist of a stack of alternating semiconductor materials with different refractive indices and quarter-wavelength thickness. A larger number of layers are required to achieve high reflectivity if the difference in refractive indices is small like in the case of III-N materials. A larger number of layers could increase electrical resistance losses due to the large number of interfaces or if some of the layers are difficult to dope. Also, it might be difficult to maintain material quality with a larger number of layers—particularly if the layers do not have the same lattice constant. DBRs are particularly difficult to fabricate for alloys of AlInGaN, because the Al alloys are difficult to dope (p-type is more difficult than n-type), and because there is a large lattice mismatch between AlGaN and GaN compounds. If one finds an alternative to using DBRs for III-N materials, the placement of the active electroluminescent region within a Fabry-Perot resonant cavity can result in several clear advantages over conventional microLEDs. First, enhanced spontaneous emission in micro RCLEDs results from the placement of the optical cavity into the resonant Fabry-Perot cavity. The probability for spontaneous emission is proportional to the optical matrix element of the initial and final electron state and proportional to the optical mode density. The carrier lifetime change is due to the strongly varying optical mode density in a Fabry-Perot cavity. The optical mode density in a Fabry-Perot resonator is strongly enhanced for on-resonance wavelengths. While off-resonance optical transitions have a longer lifetime, on-resonance transitions have a shorter lifetime. Spontaneous emission of the RCLED is therefore channeled into the optical resonance modes of the cavity. As a consequence, on-resonance transitions of the RCLEDs are enhanced. Second, emission of light through the top contact side of the RCLED device is enhanced due to the highly reflective mirror adjacent to the bottom confinement layer. Light emission in conventional

LEDs is typically close to isotropic and typically takes place through the substrate. In the RCLED structure, however, emission through the substrate is blocked by a bottom mirror that has a much higher reflectivity than the top reflector mirror. As a consequence, light propagating along the optical axis of the cavity exits the cavity predominantly through the top mirror. The anisotropic emission spectrum of the RCLED can enhance the emission through the top side by a factor of two. Third, the improved spectral purity of the RCLED makes the device well suited for optical fiber communication purposes. Conventional LEDs have spectral linewidths determined by the density of states in the conduction and valence band and the thermal energy of carriers or typical linewidths on the order of 1.8 $kT$, where $kT$ is the thermal energy. A far better spectral purity can be achieved with the RCLED. The emission linewidth is a function of the finesse of the cavity. Thus, the linewidth is not a fixed parameter but can be designed by means of the cavity characteristics.

Here, a meta microLED structure that is amenable to high-volume manufacturing is proposed. The device has an active layer composed of a quantum well that is sandwiched between a p-GaN and an n-GaN layer. The active layer is sandwiched between a top mirror and a bottom mirror. The top and bottom mirrors are made of dielectric metasurface mirrors, thus the name meta microLEDs. The structure is shown in Figure 8.1. The device resembles a VCSEL structure, but it does not have an emission threshold. Since the linewidth of the meta microLEDs is typically less than 5 nm at peak wavelength < 450 nm, then a WDM data communication system can be fabricated with these meta microLEDs.

Now, we explain how the linewidth and peak emission may be optimized by designing the optical cavity. The spontaneous emission spectrum from a cavity, $SE(\lambda)$, is modified from the as-grown spontaneous emission as represented by the photoluminescence $PL(\lambda)$. In addition to Fabry-Perot effects, the emission is also dependent on the position of the well within the cavity. This is due to the interference between coherent spontaneous wavepackets emitted in opposite directions from the individual emission events. The emission for a single well in a cavity may be described by the following expression:

$$SE(\lambda) = \left(1 - R_f\right) \left| \frac{1 + R_b \exp\left(-i4\pi n_{eff} t_b / \lambda\right)}{1 - R_f R_b \exp\left(-i4\pi n_{eff}\left(t_f + t_b\right) / \lambda\right)} \right|^2 \bullet PL(\lambda) / \int_0^\infty PL(\lambda) \bullet d\lambda \quad (8.1)$$

where $R_f$ and $R_b$ are the reflection coefficients of front and back mirrors, respectively, $\varphi_f$ and $\varphi_b$ are the phase shift due to front and back mirrors, respectively, $t_f$ is the distance between the quantum well and the front mirror, $t_b$ is the distance between the quantum well and the back mirror, $\lambda$ is the free-space

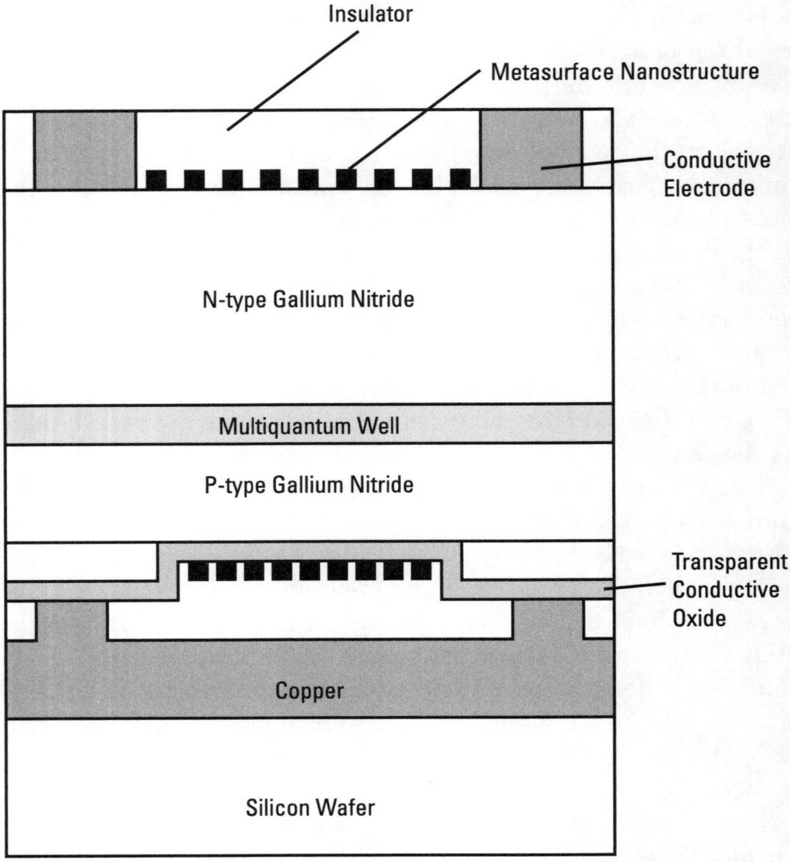


**Figure 8.1** Schematic cross section of a meta microLED. The meta microLED has a top mirror (metasurface nanostructure) and a bottom mirror (metasurface nanostructure). An active cavity is sandwiched between the top and bottom mirrors. The bottom mirror has a reflectivity near 100% and the top mirror has reflectivity near 90%. Unlike VCSELs, the device does not have a threshold. The absence of a threshold makes the device much less sensitive to junction temperature.

wavelength, and $n_{eff}$ is the effective refractive index of the cavity. For simplicity, $R_b$ and $R_f$ are assumed to have no dependence on $\lambda$, which can be realized by properly designing the metasurface mirrors. The calculated spectral emission is shown in Figure 8.2 along with the native stack spectrum, $PL(\lambda)$. Indeed, $SE(\lambda)$ has a narrower emission than $PL(\lambda)$, which has been realized experimentally [6]. The dominant wavelength is obtained from the condition

$$4\pi n_{eff}\left(t_f + t_b\right)/\lambda_p + \phi_f + \phi_b = 2\pi n \tag{8.2}$$

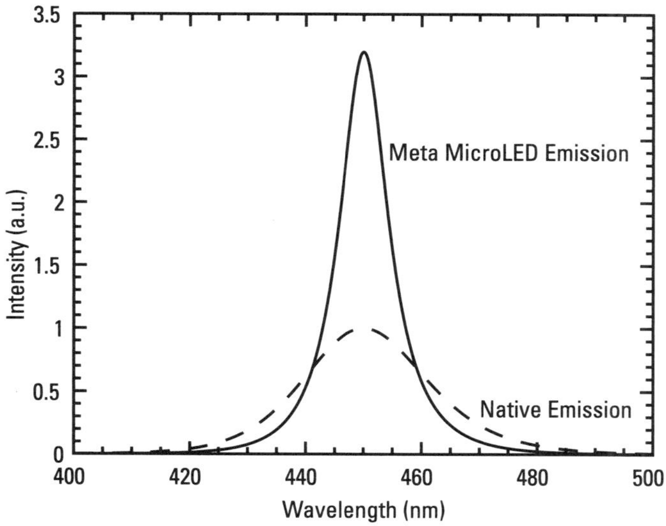


**Figure 8.2** Calculated *PL* and *SE* for a cavity with $R_b = 1$ and $R_f = 0.8$, $n_{eff} = 2.4$, $t_f = tb = 1.5\lambda_p/n_{eff}$, $\phi_f = \phi_b = 0$. Narrower FWHM (6.5 nm) spectra are obtained compared to the case without a cavity (25 nm).

where $n$ is an integer. It can be seen that if the phase shift at the front and back mirrors are tuned by properly designing the metasurface, one can possible tune the dominant wavelength $\lambda_p$.

## 8.2 Meta Photodetector

A meta microLED may be used as a photodetector, where a reverse biased electrical potential is applied through the electrodes between the p-side and the n-side of the layered structure [7]. A photodetector will absorb light in the active layer of the resonant cavity, thereby driving electron/hole pairs from the active layer to be collected to form a photocurrent. The standing wave effect (SWE) indicates the enhancement in absorption coefficient due to the cavity. For symmetric cavity, one can write [8]

$$\alpha_c = \alpha_0 \bullet \left[ 1 + \frac{2\rho_b}{2\pi \bullet (t_q / \lambda) \bullet (1 + \rho_b^2)} \sin\left(2\pi \frac{t_q}{\lambda}\right) \right] \tag{8.3}$$

where $t_q$ is the thickness of the quantum well absorbing layer, $\lambda$ is the peak emission wavelength, $\alpha_0$ is the absorption coefficient of the active layer without a cavity, and $\alpha_c$ is the effective absorption coefficient in the active layer with the cavity. Since $t_q/\lambda << 1$, we can write

$$\alpha_c \approx \alpha_0 \bullet \left[1 + \frac{2\rho_b}{1+\rho_b^2}\right] \tag{8.4}$$

If $\rho_b^2 = 0.81$, for example, we find $\alpha_c \approx 2\alpha_0$.

In other words, the absorption coefficient can be doubled due to the standing wave effect. This has positive effects on the responsivity of the meta microLED when used as a photodetector in an optical data communication system.

## 8.3 Technologies for Efficient Scaled MicroLEDs

Currently, to commercialize microLEDs, there are still many technical and cost difficulties to overcome. In manufacturing microLEDs, MOCVD is mainly employed to grow epitaxial material on a sapphire substrate to form an LED epitaxial wafer. Then, the LED epitaxial wafer is etched to form a plurality of etched grooves and mesas thereon. Thereafter, the LED epitaxial wafer is sliced along the etched grooves to complete the making of the LED epitaxies. During the process of etching LED epitaxial wafer, defects and dangling bonds occurs on sidewalls of the mesas formed with the etched grooves, which causes nonradiative recombination in the etched sidewalls of the LEDs, and further affects luminous brightness of the LEDs [9]. Traditional LEDs have the mesas far larger than the etched sidewalls, and therefore an effect of the nonradiative recombination on the overall luminous brightness is rather small, usually ignorable. However, the mesas are extremely small for microLEDs, and therefore the effect of nonradiative recombination on the etched sidewalls are also extremely large. Hence, how to reduce the nonradiative recombination occurring on the etched sidewalls becomes the main problem for commercializing microLEDs.

To solve the problem of the conventional technology, multiple ideas have been proposed for manufacturing methods for reducing nonradiative recombination of microLED, which can effectively repair the defects and dangling bonds on the etched sidewalls of the mesas that later become the microLEDs.

### 8.3.1 Passivation of Sidewalls

One solution provides manufacturing methods for reducing nonradiative recombination of microLED. This solution mainly repairs the defects and dangling bonds for the etched LED epitaxial wafer and then performs ALD on the repaired LED epitaxial wafer to form a passivation layer on the etched sidewalls of the mesas. This prevents the nonradiative recombination occurring on the etched sidewalls of the mesas that later become the microLEDs. The result is to effectively improve the luminous brightness and conversion efficiency of the microLEDs.

One method includes placing of the etched LED epitaxial wafer into a reaction chamber and transferring a repair gas into the reaction chamber. The repair gas reacts with dangling bonds and/or defects of the etched sidewalls and repairs the dangling bonds and/or defects of the LED epitaxial wafer. Thereafter, an ALD is performed to the repaired LED epitaxial wafer, and then to form a passivation layer on the etched sidewalls of the mesas.

Another method for reducing nonradiative recombination of a microLED includes providing an AC voltage to an AC coil adjacent to the reaction chamber to transform the repair gas (e.g., nitrogen, oxygen, or ozone) within a reaction chamber into a plasma, wherein, the repair gas in the plasma state reacts with the etched LED epitaxial wafer and repairs at least dangling bond or at least one defect on the etched LED epitaxial wafer. A second ALD is performed to dispose the passivation layer on a top surface of the mesa.

Figure 8.3 illustrates a process flow for performing passivation of sidewall damage and preparing the microLED for transfer from the growth substrate to a display backplane.

### 8.3.2 MicroLED with Current Confinement Structures

As explained above, the microLED sidewalls may be characterized by unsatisfied bonds, chemical contamination, and structural damage (particularly if dry-etched). Injected carriers recombine nonradiatively at states associated with these defects. Thus, the perimeter of an LED may be optically dead, and the overall efficiency of the microLED is reduced. The characteristic distance over which the sidewall surface effect occurs is related to the carrier diffusion length, which may typically be 1–10 $\mu$m in a III-N material system. Thus, the efficiency degradation is particularly severe in microLEDs in where the lateral dimensions approach the carrier diffusion length. Such nonradiative recombination may have a significant effect on microLED device efficiency, particularly when the microLED is driven at low current densities (e.g., below ~1 A/cm$^2$). By moving the microLED sidewalls and/or lateral edges of the active layer (e.g., including one or more quantum wells) to an interior of the p-n diode layer, nonradiative recombination at the sidewalls may be avoided. Thus, by forming a barrier layer within the p-n diode layer and laterally around the internally confined active layer, carrier diffusion from the active layer to the sidewalls is minimized. In this manner, the current injection path is directed internally through the LED and away from the sidewalls.

Alternatively, since either of the p-doped or n-doped layers in a p-n configuration may be considered as current spreading layers, either of the current spreading layers may be patterned such that it is narrower than the active layer

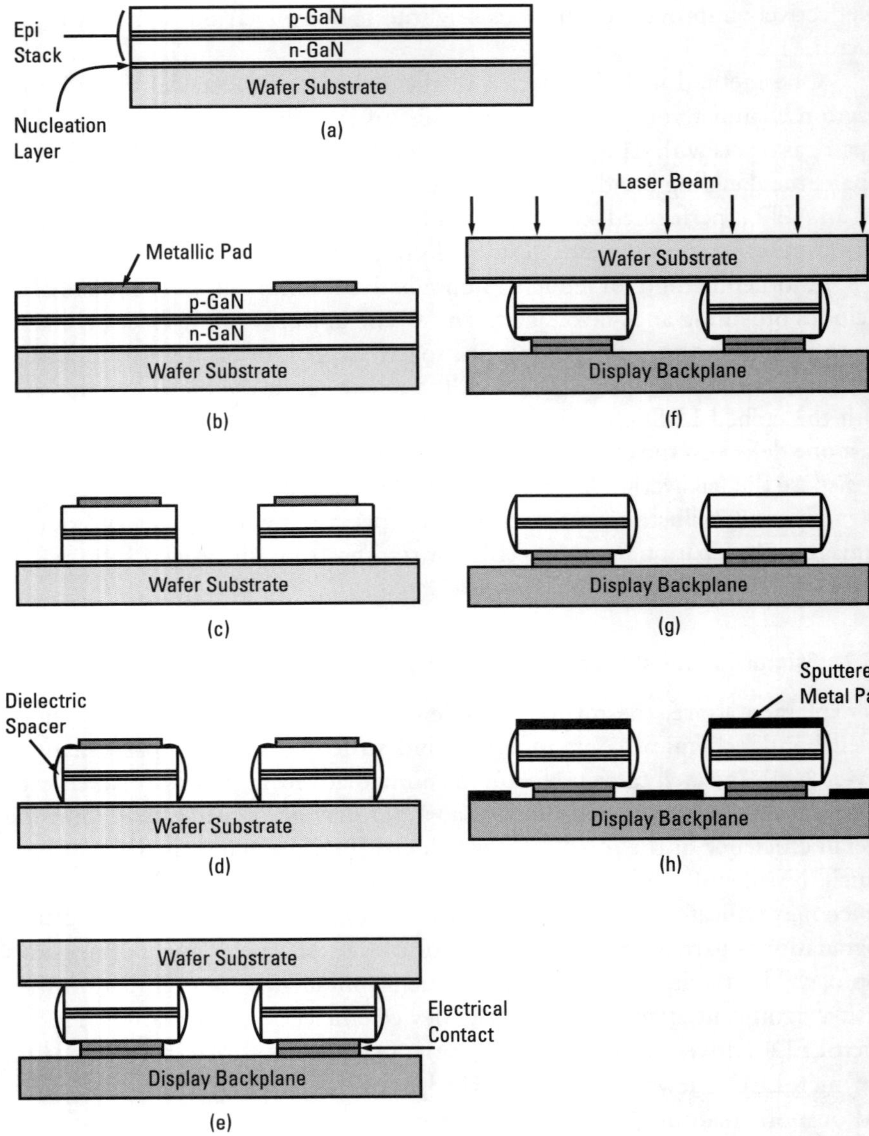


**Figure 8.3** Schematic illustration of process steps to produce passivated microLEDs that are transferrable from growth substrate to a display backplane: (a) start with wafer, grow epi stack on a nucleation layer that is also ablatable using laser irradiation; (b) deposit and pattern metal contacts for the anode; (c) singulate microLEDs using dry etch; (d) proper passivation treatment such as annealing in a reactive gas that passivates the defects on the sidewalls, followed by CVD process to deposit a dielectric on the sidewalls; (e) flip chip bonding of microLEDs to the display backplane; (f) laser release of the microLEDs by irradiation of a laser beam through the backside of the growth substrate; (g) clean of surface; and (h) sputtering of cathode metal electrode.

including the p-n diode. For example, the bottom current spreading layer (e.g., p-doped layer) is patterned to form a pillar structure with reduced width. In this manner, when a potential is applied across the LED, the current injection area within the active layer is modified by the relationship of the areas of the bottom current spreading layer pillar and top current spreading layer. In operation, the current injection area is reduced as the area of the bottom current spreading layer pillar configuration is reduced. In this manner, the current injection area can be confined internally within the active layer away from external or side surfaces of the active layer. In Figure 8.4, exemplary processing sequences are described for forming an array of microLEDs with confined current injection. The microLEDs manufactured using this sequence will be ready for transfer

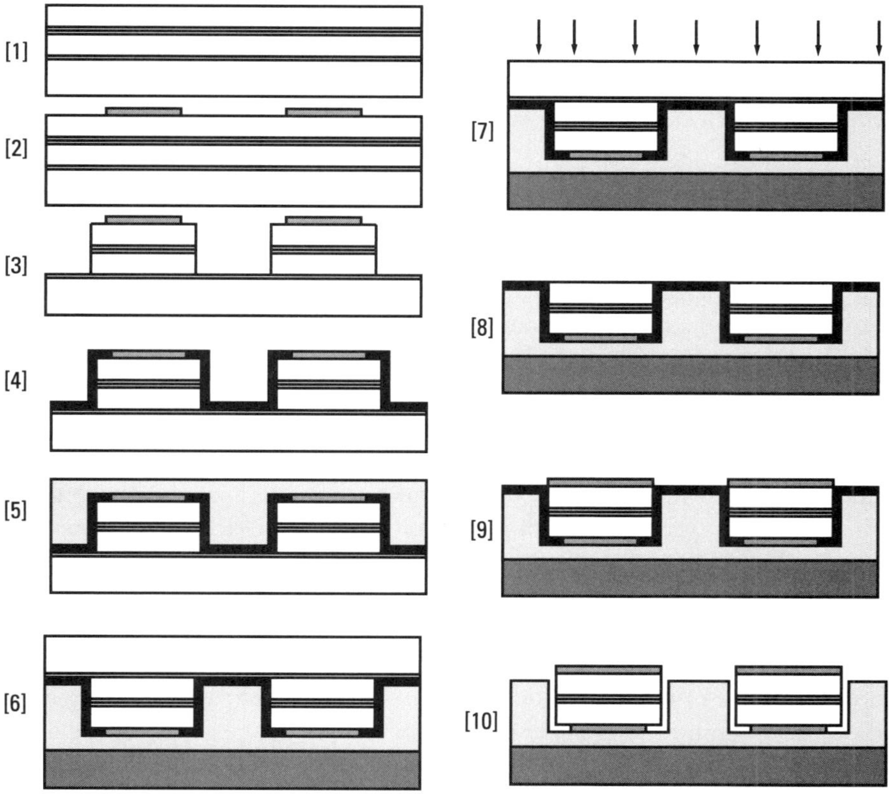


**Figure 8.4** Schematic illustration of process steps to manufacture transferrable microLEDs that have restricted injection away from the sidewalls aiming at avoiding nonradiative recombination at the sidewalls of a microLED mesa. The process sequence is: (1) epi stack growth; (2) deposition and patterning of contacts; (3) etching microLED mesas; (4) ALD of sacrificial dielectric; (5) deposition of bonding dielectric; (6) flip chip bonding to a carrier substrate; (7) laser-induced separation of growth substrate; (8) surface clean; (9) deposition and patterning of contacts; (10) wet etching of sacrificial dielectric.

later using any appropriate transfer technique to a different substrate (e.g., a display backplane).

### 8.3.3 MicroLED with Sidewall Spacer Stack

Baek et al. mitigated the edge effect of microLEDs by applying the sidewall gate voltage [10]. Cho et al. also demonstrate highly efficient nanorod LEDs passivated by the triple dielectric layers [11]. The use of a triple dielectric layer results in the formation of an internal dipole [12] that results in reduction of current crowding near the sidewalls, thus substantially reducing nonradiative recombination via sidewall defects. The physical origins of such interfacial dipoles are not clear. Several possible mechanisms have been proposed for high-k/$SiO_2$ interfaces, including oxygen vacancies model [13], an electronegativity and group electronegativity model [14, 15], and an oxygen density model [16]. An example structure and the corresponding energy band diagram are shown in Figure 8.5.

## 8.4 Tunnel Junction MicroLED

Current commercially available III-nitride LEDs use an active region in a biased p-n junction to allow for electron and hole injection. However, p-type gallium nitride (p-GaN) is difficult to contact electrically and has relatively low hole concentration and mobility. This means that p-GaN cannot be used as a current spreading layer and that traditional p-contacts will add significant voltage to devices. Current spreading layers, such as metals and transparent and conductive oxides (TCOs), are usually employed to enhance the current spreading performance. However, these current spreading materials are light absorbing in the visible light spectrum, which can harm the optical efficiency of Ill-nitride devices such as LEDs.

One approach is to anneal the p-type GaN layer using RTA as a production technique to realize p-type magnesium activation. In this process, the wafer is removed from the MOCVD growth system and loaded into a special infrared furnace capable of reaching 1000°C in less than 10 seconds and cooling back below the decomposition temperature just as fast. The anneal may also be done in situ [17].

Modified MOCVD deposition techniques, such as plasma-assisted MOCVD, may produce relatively more reactive species at low growth temperatures as compared with conventional MOCVD processes [18].

One alternative approach is to utilize n-type Ill-nitride materials as the current spreading layer to reduce light absorption while maintaining excellent electrical conductivity feature, as shown in Figure 8.6. The use of n-type

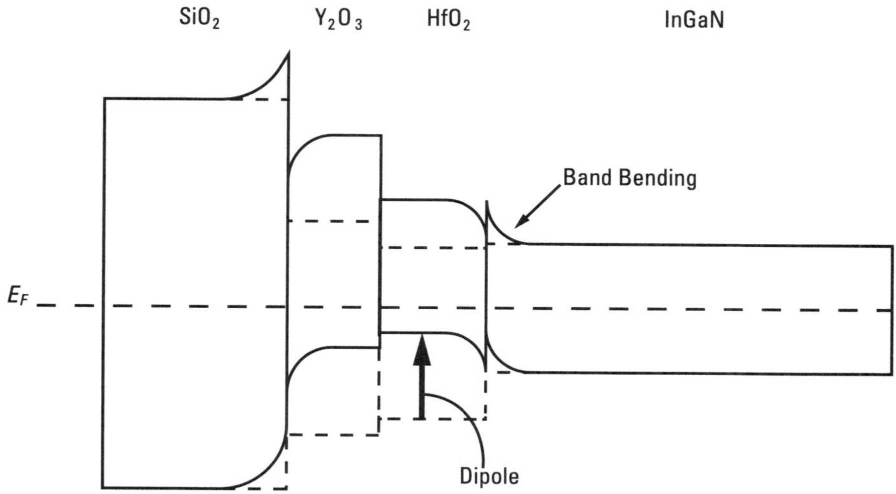


**Figure 8.5** Simplified band diagram for hafnium oxide/ytterbium oxide/silicon dioxide ($HfO_2$/$Y_2O_3$/$SiO_2$/Si) stacks. The dashed lines are for the case assuming no dipole at the high-k/$SiO_2$ interface. A dipole forms as shown due to the oxygen vacancies model [13], an electronegativity and group electronegativity model [14, 15], and an oxygen density model [16]. The dipole results in band bending in the quantum well, forming a barrier for electrons to exist there, substantially reducing nonradiative recombination via the sidewall defects.

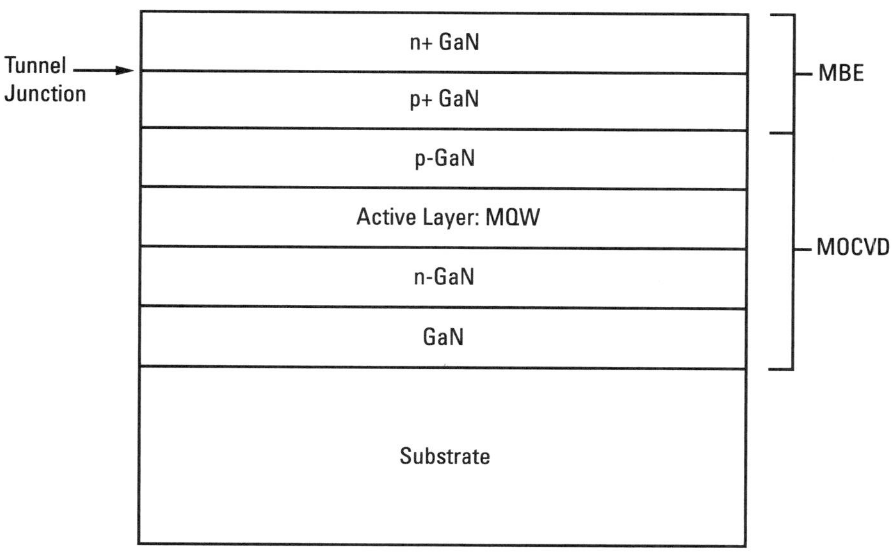


**Figure 8.6** Schematic cross section illustration of the concept of using tunnel junctions for microLEDs.

Ill-nitride materials for current spreading is commonly referred as tunnel junction (TJ). A low-resistance tunnel junction on top of p-GaN would allow for current spreading in n-type GaN (n-GaN) on both sides of the device, as well as the use of low-resistance n-type contacts on both sides of the device. A tunnel junction is a diode comprised of a very highly doped (n+/p+) interface that allows for electrons to tunnel between the valence band and conduction band. This was first demonstrated by Esaki [19] in highly doped Ge homojunctions with very thin depletion regions.

In principle, a highly doped Esaki-type homojunction diode should provide the lowest-loss tunnel junction. However, there have been a number of difficulties in achieving high-quality tunnel junctions in the GaN material system. For example, GaN is a wide bandgap semiconductor, so the barrier for tunneling is high. Several approaches to reducing the tunneling barrier have been attempted, including bandgap engineering via polarization (AlN interlayers) [20], and reducing the bandgap with an InGaN interlayer [21]. However, all of these approaches are associated with losses, either in terms of voltage or series resistance increases, or optical losses in the final device performance. In another example, Mg-doped p-GaN grown by MOCVD is compensated by hydrogen as grown, and it must be annealed after growth to remove the hydrogen. This anneal can only work if the p-GaN is not covered by n-GaN, as hydrogen cannot easily diffuse through n-GaN. This limits the effectiveness of tunnel junctions and prevents their widespread use.

One way to remove hydrogen from the p-type layer after TJ growth, also known as activation, is to use sidewall activation, where hydrogen is diffused out from the sidewall of p-type layer. The p-type layer is activated through a sidewall of the p-type layer after the removal of defects from the sidewall, thereby increasing a hole concentration in the p-type layer.

In yet another example, a hybrid epitaxial growth of III-nitride layers may be used [22, 23]. A hybrid growth method for III-nitride tunnel junction devices uses MOCVD to grow one or more light-emitting or light-absorbing structures and ammonia-assisted or plasma-assisted MBE to grow one or more tunnel junctions. Unlike p-GaN grown by MOCVD, p-GaN grown by MBE is conductive as grown, which allows for its use in a tunnel junction. Moreover, the doping limits of MBE materials are higher than MOCVD materials. MBE growth can occur in a hydrogen-free ambient, so that p-GaN is activated as-grown. MBE growth can occur far from thermodynamic equilibrium, thus enabling high doping levels without the formation of compensating defects found in MOCVD. However, MBE machines are expensive, difficult to scale to large wafer diameters and throughputs, and not always robust, and thus may not be well suited for industrial implementation [24].

Another example includes using sputter deposition to grow one or more tunnel junctions. Sputter deposition is a type of physical vapor deposition (PVD) method used to form thin films of various materials and microstructures. This is achieved by bombarding a target material with ionized atoms of an inert gas, such as argon, or a reactive gas, such as oxygen or nitrogen. As a result of this bombardment, atoms of the target material are ejected and transported in the gas phase onto a substrate where they condense and form a thin film. The source of these ions is typically from a plasma that is formed by applying a large negative potential to a cathode (i.e., the target material) under high vacuum conditions. The plasma is sustained in part due to the formation of secondary electrons produced during interactions between ions and the target surface. The ionization process can be enhanced through the use of magnetic fields in magnetron sputtering systems. The plasma is typically generated using either a radio frequency (RF), DC, or pulsed DC power supply. Although several demonstrations of sputter deposited GaN thin films exist, they have yet to be shown to behave as tunnel junction contacts to p-GaN. This is in part due to the fact that p-GaN is quite sensitive to plasma damage, since most sputtering techniques expose the surface of the substrate (i.e., p-GaN layer) to the same plasma that is used to bombard the target. The solution to this issue is either to protect the p-GaN from this type of damage, or minimize its exposure to the plasma. An alternative sputtering approach is to generate the plasma remotely in order to minimize its negative effects on the p-GaN surface. One technique to achieve this is to use electron cyclotron resonance (ECR) plasma sources. In this case microwave power is coupled to the plasma at the ECR frequency in order to produce high-energy electrons that ionize the neutral input gas to produce and maintain a dense, low-pressure plasma with a high degree of ionization. This process produces low-energy ions that mitigate plasma damage. ECR plasmas are typically used with gaseous precursors in chemical vapor deposition (CVD) systems. By using ECR plasma deposition to grow the n-GaN layer on top, the p-GaN remains activated while being buried beneath the n-GaN. This could allow for the regrowth of additional LED epitaxial layers by MOCVD on top of the first LED, because the hydrogen cannot diffuse through the top n-GaN layer [25].

Tunnel junctions have been used to realize high-efficiency GaN-based red microLEDs [26] and stacked blue and green microLEDs [27, 28]. The blue/green microLED stack is shown in Figure 8.7. A cascaded blue/green microLED structure will allow for use of relatively larger microLEDs (with improved low-current efficiency) since there is an area saving by stacking the blue and green microLEDs. However, the challenge will be in interconnecting these devices with a display backplane, for example.

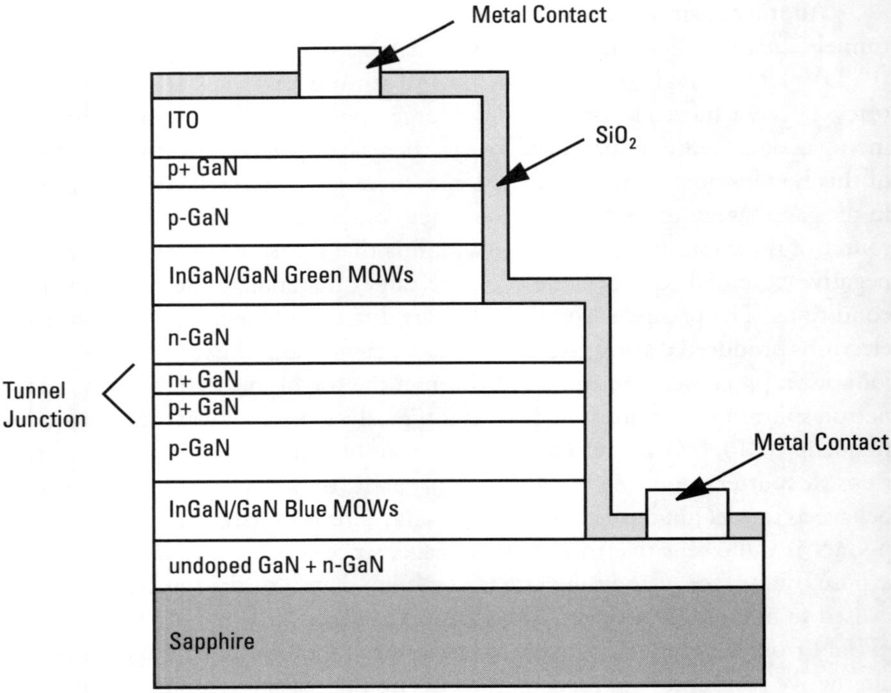


**Figure 8.7** Schematic structure of the cascaded blue/green microLED structure. (Adapted after [27].)

## 8.5 Structures to Enable Laser Release of MicroLEDs

If the nucleation layer shown in Figure 8.4 were made of a material that can be ablated by shining a pulsed laser on it through the growth wafer, one can void grinding and etching the growth wafer during the process of transferring microLEDs to a new substrate, as shown in part 7 of Figure 8.4. The concept of laser ablation of a transition metal nitride nucleation/buffer layer is schematically illustrated in Figure 8.8.

Currently, nonconductive sapphires are being extensively used as substrates for GaN layers grown by a MOCVD technique. A lattice mismatch of about 15% between the GaN and sapphire layers means a buffer layer is needed for growth of GaN on the sapphire substrate. The best buffer/nucleation layer discovered was an AlN layer deposited at a relatively low temperature, and the use of this layer made it possible for epitaxial growth of an GaN layer with a mirrorlike surface. Although a lattice mismatch of about 2.5% exists between GaN and AlN, the AlN buffer layer was believed to enhance GaN nucleation and growth due to a relatively low AlN/GaN interface energy.

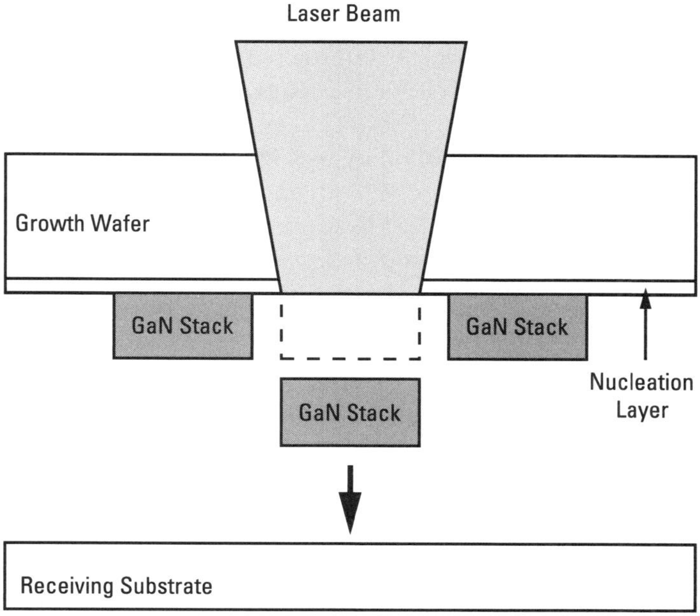


**Figure 8.8** Schematic illustration of epi stack on transition metal nitride nucleation/buffer layer to enable laser release of microLEDs.

MOCVD-grown, continuous, flat GaN layers may also be grown on metallic TiN buffer layers deposited on Sapphire substrates [29–32]. Three important conditions were found: (a) the Sapphire substrate surface plane should be $(11\bar{2}0)$, (b) the titanium nitride (TiN) layer surface plane should be (111), and (c) the TiN buffer layer nitrogen content should be higher than that of stoichiometric TiN. Reduction of TiN layer thickness reduces TiN buffer layer surface roughness. Threading dislocation density in GaN layers grown on TiN buffer layers was much lower than that in GaN layers grown on AlN. It is possible to ablate/vaporize thin (10–20 nm) TiN layers using a laser with appropriate pulse width and energy [33–38].

Moreover, hafnium nitride has the sodium chloride (NaCl)-type structure, a lattice constant of 0.452 nm, and a mismatch of only +0.35% for GaN(0001)/HfN(111). It is a refractory metal and has been studied as a diffusion barrier in Si technology. Due to the small (0.02%) mismatch for the coincident-site lattice involving six hafnium nitride (HfN) unit cells and five Si unit cells, HfN can be grown epitaxially on Si [39]. Like AlN, HfN is stable with regard to formation of $Si_3N_4$, but should offer better diffusion resistance. Epitaxial hafnium nitride films of ~200 nm thickness may be deposited by reactive dc magnetron sputtering on Si (111) and (001) substrates using the process of Shinkai and Sasaki [39].

Although most GaN growth efforts on Si focused on the (111) surface due to its hexagonal symmetry, Si (001) is more commonly used in microelectronics. GaN grown on Si(001) often results in a mixture of wurtzite- and zincblende-structure grains [40]. HfN (111) provides a hexagonal template for GaN nucleation while HfN (001) does not [41, 42]. Other researchers demonstrated growth of GaN on ScN [43, 44] and zirconium nitride (ZrN) [45]. All of these metals may be vaporized by exposure to a pulsed laser with the appropriate wavelength, pulse duration, and pulse energy.

## 8.6 Superpixel Concept

Demand is increasing for higher-resolution displays, as well as for thinner, lighter-weight, and lower-cost electronic devices with larger screens. OLED or liquid crystal display (LCD) technologies feature a TFT substrate. More recently, it has been proposed to replace the TFT substrate with a matrix of microcontrollers bonded to the display substrate and build a microLED display by integrating a matrix of microLEDs on the microcontroller substrate, in which each microcontroller is to switch and drive a plurality of microLEDs [46–48]. This concept is illustrated in Figure 8.9. This integration scheme may allow for significant freedom in designing the pixel driver chips. In such a configuration, the size of the pixel driver chips is not limited by the pitch between microLEDs. In this aspect, larger pixel driver chips with more functionality (e.g., with embedded memory) can potentially be integrated into the display panel. For an exemplary RGB display panel (pixels including a red-emitting, green-emitting, and blue-emitting LED) with 40 pixels per inch (PPI) may have an approximately 211–$\mu$m subpixel pitch, whereas an exemplary RGB display panel with 440 PPI may have an approximately 19–$\mu$m subpixel pitch. Rather than locating the pixel driver chips between the microLEDs on the display panel, the pixel driver chips are embedded within the display substrate allowing scalability of the display panel to high-resolution display with high PPI. The pixel driver chips may be located directly beneath the microLEDs and directly beneath the display area of the display panel. Pixel driver chips for driving and switching the microLEDs are embedded within the display substrate and electrically connected with the microLEDs through a front side redistribution layer (RDL). MOSFET processing techniques may be used for fabrication of the pixel driver chips on single crystalline silicon as opposed to TFT processing techniques on amorphous silicon (a-Si) or LTPS.

## 8.7 MicroLEDs with Color Conversion Layers

One of the challenges of microLED displays is the creation of efficient GaN-based red and green subpixels. Currently, the efficiency of red GaN-based mi-

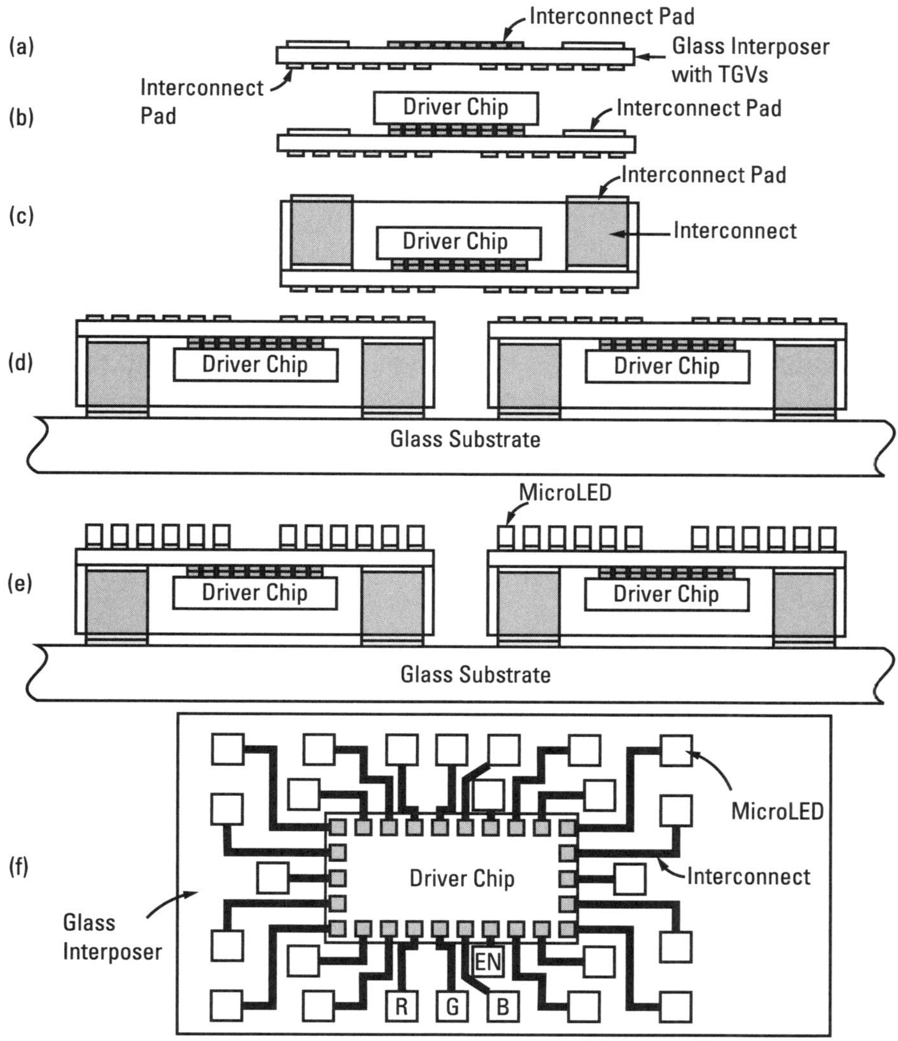


**Figure 8.9** Schematic illustration of process sequence for making a superpixel: (a) deposition of interconnects on glass interposer, (b) bonding the driver chip to one side of the interconnects on the glass interposer, (c) making superpixel interconnect and pads, (d) transferring superpixel modules to another glass substrate, (e) transferring microLEDs on the interconnect pads, and (f) schematic top view of the layout of the superpixel.

croLEDs is approximately 5 to 10 times lower than desired to realize energy-efficient microLED displays compared to OLED displays. In the absence of efficient GaN-based red and green subpixels, an efficient blue pixel converted to red and green by use of QDs has been proposed. This configuration is illustrated in Figure 8.10.

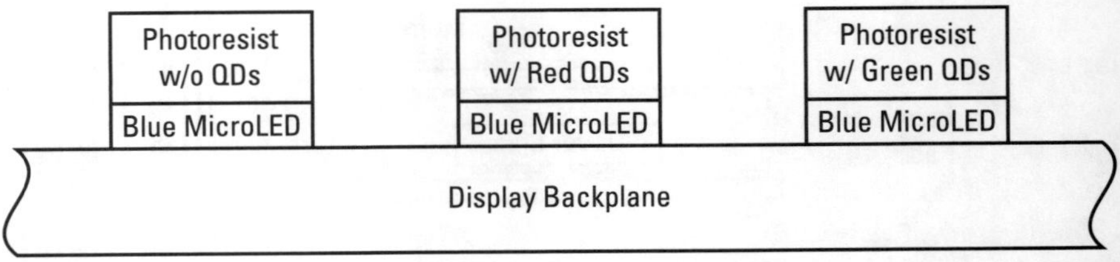


**Figure 8.10** Simplified schematic illustration of a microLED display RGB pixel based on using blue microLED emitters and red and green quantum dots.

As used herein, a QD can refer to a crystalline inorganic particle that is spherically or nearly spherically shaped and has diameters between 2 and 10 nm. Optical properties of QDs (e.g., emission wavelength) are exquisitely sensitive to the precise size of the particle, and thus allow one to tune them simply by controlling their size. For a given QD, the emission band is dependent on the size of the quantum dot. QDs may be based on cadmium sulfide (CdS). With respect to Cd-free QDs, however, an indium phosphide (InP)-based QD material system has been claimed to be able to match the color performance of the industry's best cadmium-based materials without requiring an exemption to the European Union's RoHS Directive. InP is a direct gap material with a band gap of 1.27 eV, which is suitable for achieving visible emission in the quantum confinement regime. As-prepared InP QDs generally show weak luminescence because of the existence of nonradiative carrier recombination originating from surface states. However, after over coating with a ZnS shell, InP QDs become highly luminescent. InP QDs are also attractive due to the stronger covalent bond as compared with the ionic bond in CdS QDs, increasing their photostability.

## 8.8 Patterning QD Films

Methods to deposit QDs on a display have been wasteful of the depositing material, which may also be too expensive. Spin-coating a photoresist containing QDs has been described by researchers for applying QDs on display surfaces. Although this may be a reliable process, most of the expensive QD material is etched away and wasted. Methods are needed to enable the application of only as much QD material as is necessary, with little to no waste.

### 8.8.1 Inkjet Printing

In an effort to minimize such problems, inkjet printing systems have been developed for forming the color conversion patterns on the substrates by depositing such patterns on the substrates in the form of special inks, as shown in

Figure 8.11. The inkjet systems deposit the ink on the substrate through an inkjet head. However, the inkjet head includes a plurality of nozzles, and if even only one of such nozzles becomes dysfunctional, the number of passes that the inkjet printing head must make increases. For example, if the inkjet head has 100 nozzles, and the sixtieth nozzle is damaged, only the first to fifty-ninth nozzles and the sixty-first to hundredth nozzles are available, and thus, in order to deposit ink over the entire target region of the substrate, the inkjet head must be moved, or offset, by a selected interval so as to deposit ink on the region corresponding to the sixtieth nozzle. As a result, processing time and costs are substantially increased. Additionally, since all of the nozzles of the inkjet head must be kept in good operating condition, downtime increases and process stability margins deteriorate. The flat-panel display industry has been attempting to employ inkjet printing to manufacture display devices and, in particular, color filters. However, one problem with effective employment of inkjet print-

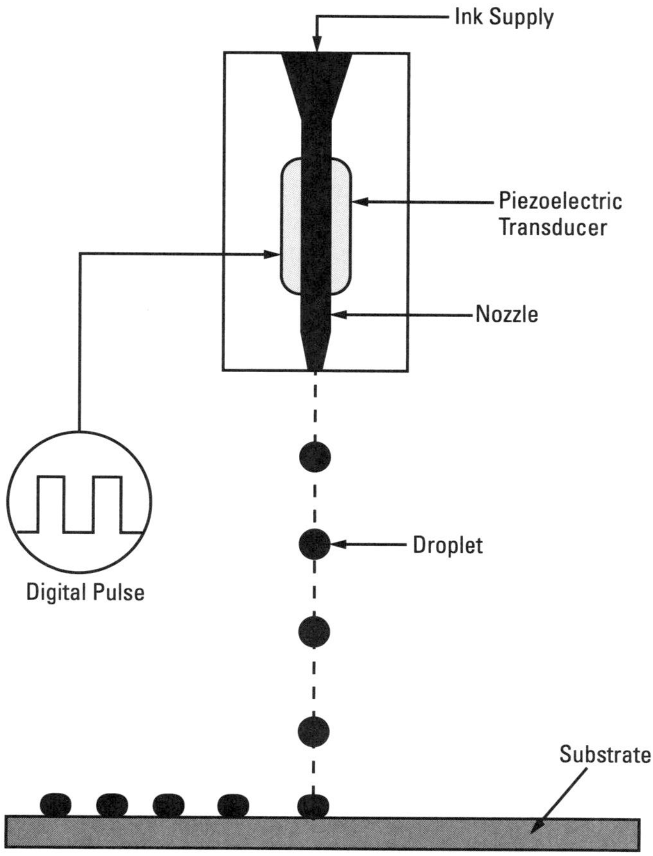


**Figure 8.11** Inkjet printing of QDs.

ing is that it is difficult to inkjet ink or other material accurately and precisely on a substrate while having high throughput. Examples techniques described herein address such issues. In some techniques, redundant nozzles are used in printing heads. In some techniques, stripes (not patches) of QD material are fabricated on red subpixels to address throughput issues.

### 8.8.2 Selective Deposition

Selective deposition of colloidal QDs on specific areas of display backplane that takes advantage of photocatalytic and photoinduced superhydrophilic properties of titanium dioxide ($TiO_2$) may be considered [49]. In this method, a conductive oxide layer, such as an ITO layer, of a display backplane is first coated with a thin film of titanium oxide or dioxide ($TiO_2$) using a sol-gel method, for example. The surface of the titanium oxide or dioxide film is then modified with fluoroalkylsilane by using a self-assembly method. The surface of the titanium oxide or dioxide becomes hydrophobic after the treatment with fluoroalkylsilane (i.e., the contact angle of water may be greater than 100°). The receiving substrate is then irradiated with ultraviolet light through a photomask to create a pattern with different degrees of wettability on different areas. The irradiation changes the contact angle of water on the irradiated surface to 0°, while no change occurs for the nonirradiated surface. Not to be bound by theory, but as best understood, the change in the contact angle of the irradiated portion derives from the photocatalytic and photoinduced superhydrophilic properties of titanium oxide or dioxide, where $TiO_2$ is a unique photocatalyst that does not exhibit irreversible photocorrosion, but which does display photoinduced superhydrophilic properties. As an example, in order to selectively deposit colloidal QD films on a display backplane, the display backplane is inserted or dipped into an aqueous suspension containing the QDs to fabricate a pattern consisting of a colloidal crystal film. The liquid surface is concave above the hydrophilic surface, while it is convex over the hydrophobic area. Colloidal crystals form over the hydrophilic areas during the lifting process, while no film or essentially no film is formed on the hydrophobic regions. Advantages to implementing the method described herein may include low manufacturing cost as achieved by using a lesser amount of color conversion film(s) material (which can be very expensive).

Figure 8.12 is a schematic cross-section illustration of the process sequence for selective deposition of QDs on microLED displays. There are five alternatives for creating domelike color-conversion films:

1. If the surface is hydrophilic, the chemical composition of the surface can be modified by applying a hydrophobic coating on top. Subse-

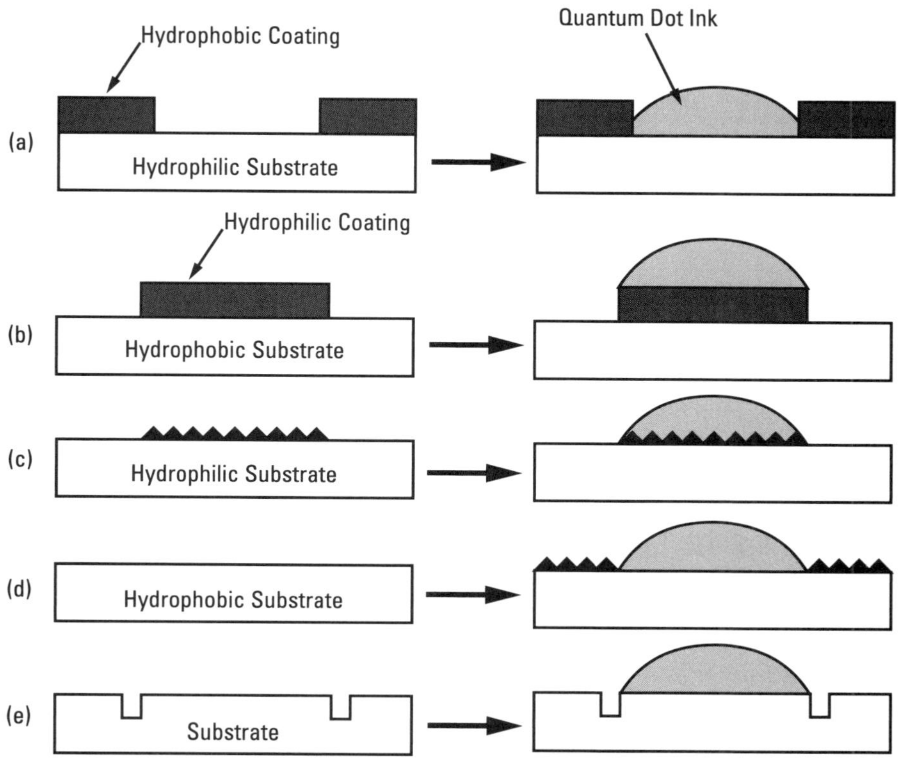


**Figure 8.12** Schematic cross-section illustration of process sequence for selective deposition of QDs on microLED displays.

quently, this coating can be selectively removed by laser machining to create a receptor site that is hydrophilic.

2. Hydrophilic sites on a hydrophobic substrate can be created by applying a hydrophilic coating at the desired positions.
3. If the substrate is hydrophilic, increasing the roughness of the hydrophilic receptor site by use of the laser.
4. If the substrate is hydrophobic, the increased roughness yields higher apparent contact angles, and therefore limits the liquid spreading.
5. Creating edges/obstacles by material removal from a laser track.

An edge (or trench) around the receptor site can be created by removing material from the tracks of a laser path that follows the perimeter of the receptor site. The edges of the tracks will provide a location for the pining of the liquid-solid-vapor interface, and sharp edges can be accurately machined by a proper selection of the laser processing parameters. This approach will work for hydrophobic as well as hydrophilic substrates.

## 8.9 Structures Enabling Thin QD Films

Conventionally, the QD active layer has a minimum thickness to be able to absorb most of the light to which the QD color conversion material is responsive. For example, an active layer made with crystalline InP QDs typically has a minimum thickness between 5 and 10 $\mu$m. This size is very thick compared to microLEDs (e.g., $4 \times 4\ \mu$m in area and approximately 1 $\mu$m in thickness or height), so the QD film can appear as a tube on top of the microLED, which can have negative consequences such as unexpected optical effects related to a shape of the radiation pattern, viewing angle, and so on. For example, a blue microLED can be used with an InP-based QD film (e.g., in a photoresist) to generate red light. Conversion of blue light to red via QD film produces an effective EQE of less than 4%. This efficiency is less than half of a target efficiency (e.g., 10%) to achieve power reduction in microLEDs compared to OLEDs.

One way to improve the effective EQE for red emitters is to use a light trapping structure that includes two mirrors that sandwich a microLED (e.g., a blue microLED) and a color conversion film (e.g., a QD film) [50, 51]. This is shown in Figure 8.13. A first mirror (e.g., a top mirror) is a wavelength-selective mirror (or reflect array) positioned on top of the color conversion film over a microLED device. The first mirror is implemented as a grating or lattice, for example, designed to selectively reflect blue light (e.g., wavelength ~467 nm ±10 nm) into the QD film and be transparent to red light (e.g., wavelength ~630 nm ±10 nm), green light (e.g., wavelength ~532 nm ±10 nm), and so on. The second mirror is a broadband mirror positioned at the bottom of the microLED device. The broadband mirror is used to pump (e.g., emit) blue light into the color conversion film. To improve external quantum efficiency, reflectivity of the bottom mirror is to be high (e.g., greater than 99% reflectivity for blue light).

The example light trapping structure improves conversion efficiency (e.g., from blue light to red light, green light) and also reduces leakage, such as blue leakage out of red, green, and/or other color emitters used in a microLED display system. The wavelength-selective mirror (e.g., a blue-selective mirror) also prevents excitation of the QD films from exposure to ambient light, for example.

A selective mirror (also referred to as a metamirror) is implemented using a 2D high-contrast grating (HCG) structure, a 2D array of spherical dielectric nanoparticles, and so on. The example 2D high-contrast grating structure is a structure having two different dielectric materials. The dielectric materials have

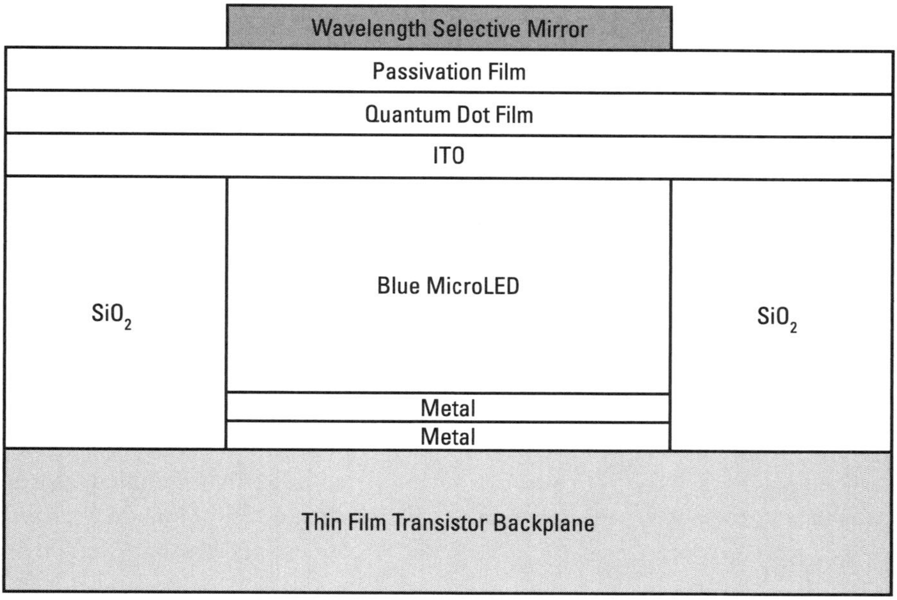


**Figure 8.13** Schematic cross-section illustration of the light trapping structure. The top mirror is a metasurface mirror that selectively reflects blue light and selectively transmits red (or green) light.

refractive indices that form a ratio of at least 1.5. The HCG structure exhibits a high reflectivity over a broad wavelength range (e.g., $\Delta\lambda/\lambda$ of approximately 10%–35%). A high-contrast grating can be defined lithographically using one or more techniques including deep ultraviolet (DUV) lithography, e-beam, focused ion beam, or nano-imprinting techniques. A desired wavelength control is achieved by varying a duty cycle and/or a period of the HCG structure.

## 8.10 Method to Extend QD Film Lifetime

One of the challenges facing QD-based microLED displays is that their brightness may be limited by their lifetime, which gets shorter at higher brightness. For instance, the QD color conversion films in red emitters are exposed to very high brightness during pulse width modulation driving of the underlying blue microLEDs, which is necessary to reduce power consumption. This compromises the lifetime and high brightness of microLED displays that use QD color conversion for a red (or green) emitter. Accordingly, microLED displays that utilize QD color conversion may be particularly susceptible to burn-in and other display degradation problems, among other example issues. Indeed, for device applications requiring high-brightness microLED displays, enhanced solutions may be applied to extend the lifetime of the display (e.g., by 2×) before a consumer can see burn-in issues and has to replace the device. An improved microLED display system may utilize multiple redundant subpixels controlled by graphics circuitry to rotate use of these redundant subpixels and address at least some of the issues identified above [52]. For instance, redundant subpixels and associated driving circuitry (example shown in Figure 8.14) may be provided in the improved display to drive different subpixels at different times (or rotating the use of these different redundant subpixels) and thereby extend the average lifetime of a microLED display with QD color conversion. For instance, pixel driver circuits may be provided to independently address different redundant subpixels at specific time periods during the use of the display. Such a rotation scheme is used by using different redundant subpixels at different times (e.g., according to a frequency of rotation of 8 hours, 24 hours, or another time period). Such displays may realize in the lifetime of a corresponding microLED displays with QD color conversion being more than doubled, as well as realizing low power consumption. Similarly, such a technology may enable

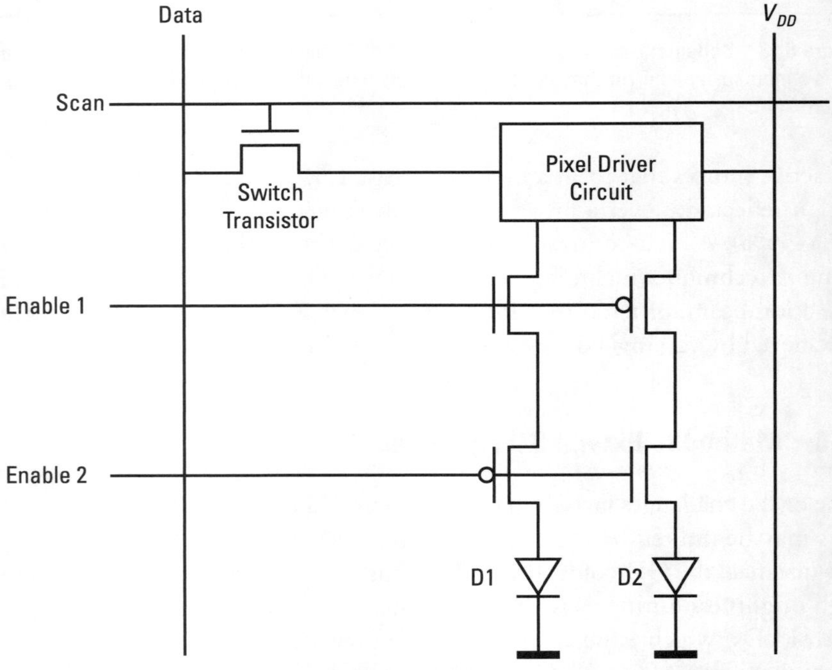


**Figure 8.14** Diagram of an example pixel driver architecture. Enable 1 and Enable 2 inputs may be provided to be signaled by controller circuitry to select which of the redundant emitters to enable within a given rotation window. For instance, Enable 1 and Enable 2 will be HIGH sequentially in time, and complementary to each other such that one is HIGH and the other is LOW and vice versa, resulting in either emitter D1 or emitter D2 being enabled for driving using the pixel driver circuit.

devices with more than double the brightness of a traditional device, but with a comparable lifetime, among other example advantages.

## 8.11 Remote Epitaxy for Fabrication of MicroLEDs on 300-mm Silicon Wafers

It is economically desirable to grow microLEDs on the largest silicon wafers (i.e., 300 mm diameter) as shown in Chapter 7. However, microLEDs are usually fabricated from functional semiconductors such as III-N semiconductors or III-V semiconductors. The lattice constants of these functional semiconductors typically do not match the lattice constants of silicon substrates. Lattice constant mismatch between a substrate and an epitaxial layer on the substrate can introduce strain into the epitaxial layer, thereby preventing epitaxial growth of thicker layers without defects. Therefore, non-silicon substrates are usually employed as seeds for epitaxial growth of most functional semiconductors. However, non-silicon substrates with lattice constants matching those of functional materials can be costly and therefore limit the development of non-silicon electronic/photonic devices.

One method of addressing the high cost of non-silicon substrates is the layer-transfer technique, in which functional device layers are grown on lattice-matched substrates and then removed and transferred to silicon substrates. The remaining lattice-matched substrates can then be reused to fabricate another device layer, thereby reducing the cost. However, existing layer-transfer techniques, such as chemical liftoff, optical liftoff, and controlled spalling, usually suffer from one or more drawbacks. For example, chemical liftoff is usually slow and tends to contaminate the surface of the growth substrate, thereby rendering it challenging to reuse the growth substrate. Optical liftoff also reduces the reusability of the growth substrate (e.g., to less than five times of reuse) because the optical beams employed to remove the device layer are also likely to damage the surface of the growth substrate. Controlled spalling usually has a higher throughput compared to chemical/optical liftoff, but it can be challenging to precisely remove the entire device layer from the growth substrate.

To address the drawbacks in conventional layer-transfer methods, remote epitaxy technique to fabricate semiconductor devices has been recently explored [53–58]. In this technique, shown in Figures 8.15 and 8.16, a device layer (also referred to as a functional layer) is epitaxially grown on a release layer, which in turn is disposed on a growth substrate that is lattice-matched to the device layer. As used herein, lattice-matching refers to situations in which two lattice constants are different by less than 10%. The release layer is made of a 2D material to support van der Waals epitaxy (VDWE), in which the device layer has only van der Waals interactions with the underneath release layer. A van der Waals interaction is not a chemical bond between two materials. Instead, it originates from the dipole interactions between atoms. Compared to ionic or covalent bonding, the van der Waals force is much weaker. As a result, when the device layer is deposited on the release layer, the device layer grows unstrained and forms a lattice having the lattice constant that is identical to its bulk lattice constant.

In remote epitaxy, as shown in Figure 8.15, the epitaxial registry of adatoms can be remotely assigned by the underlying growth substrate via modulating the distance between the growth substrate and the device layer (also referred to as the interaction gap). Theoretical simulation suggests that such remote epitaxy is feasible if the gap between the substrate and the epitaxial layer is smaller than ~0.9 nm. In other words, the growth substrate, although physically separated from the device layer by the release layer, still has a significant orienting effect on the device layer during epitaxial growth because the release layer is so thin. The grown device layer can then be readily released from the release layer, thereby allowing multiple reuses of the growth substrate.

The atomically thin release layer in remote epitaxy can be constructed from various materials. For example, the release layer can include a graphene monolayer. Any other appropriate 2D material can also be used.

The fabrication of the epitaxial layer can be carried out using any suitable semiconductor fabrication technique known in the art. For example,

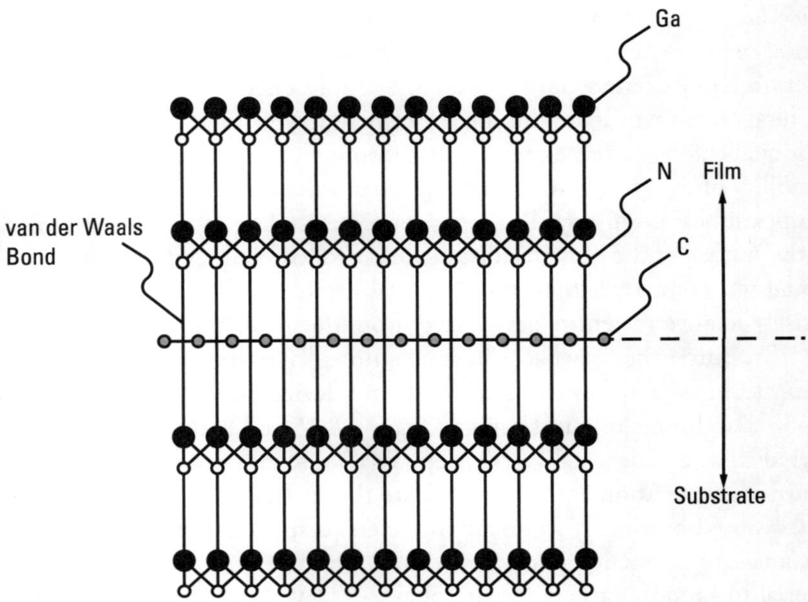


**Figure 8.15** Schematic illustration of the concept of remote epitaxy of GaN film on a substrate (e.g., GaN/sapphire) through a graphene film.

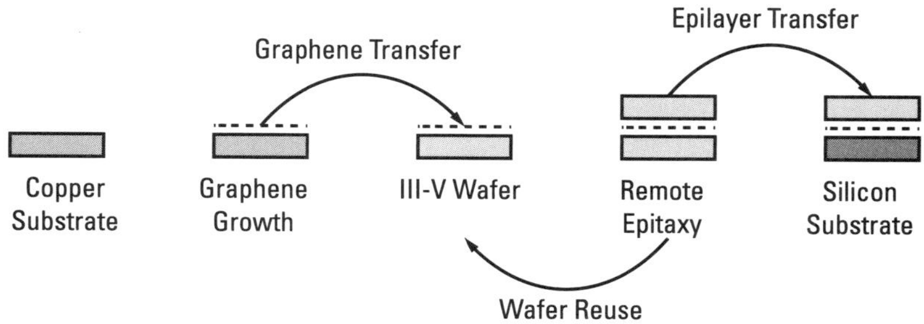


**Figure 8.16** Schematic illustration of the concept of remote epitaxy of GaN film on a substrate (e.g., GaN/sapphire) through a graphene film, then transfer of the GaN film onto a silicon wafer.

low-pressure MOCVD can be used to grow the epitaxial layer (e.g., a GaN film) on the release layer. Vertical GaN growth rate in this case can be around 20 nm per min.

A flexible (001) AlGaInP LED manifested device performance similar to that grown on a rigid substrate without the graphene monolayer [53].

## References


[1] Coyne, K., and S. Coyne, *Brainsteering: The Better Approach to Breakthrough Ideas,* Harper Collins, 2011.

[2] Cho, A. Y., E. F. Schubert, L.- W. Tu, and G. J. Zydzik, Light Emitting Diode, US Patent 5226053A, 1993.

[3] Benisty, H., H. D. Neve, and C. Weisbuch, "Impact of Planar Microcavity Effects on Light Extraction—Part I: Basic Concepts and Analytical Trends," *IEEE Journal of Quantum Electronics,* Vol. 34, No. 9, 1998, pp. 1612–1631.

[4] Baets, R., "Micro-Cavity Light Emitting Diodes," in *Semiconductor Quantum Optoelectronics,* Boca Raton, FL: CRC Press, 2020, pp. 213–264.

[5] Song, Y.- K., M. Diagne, H. Zhou, A. V. Nurmikko, R. P. S. Jr., and T. Takeuchi, "Resonant-Cavity InGaN Quantum-Well Blue Light-Emitting Diodes," *Applied Physics Letters,* Vol. 77, No. 12, 2000, pp. 1744–1746.

[6] Schubert, E., Y. Wang, A. Cho, L. Tu, and G. Zydzik, "Resonant Cavity Light-Emitting Diode," *Applied Physics Letters,* Vol. 60, No. 8, 1992, pp. 921–923.

[7] Hunt, N., E. Schubert, and G. Zydzik, Photodetector with a Resonant Cavity, US Patent 5,315,128, 1994.

[8] Ünlü, M., K. Kishino, H. Liaw, and H. Morkoç, "A Theoretical Study of Resonant Cavity-Enhanced Photodetectors with Ge and Si Active Regions," *Journal of Applied Physics,* Vol. 71, No. 8, 1992, pp. 4049–4058.

[9] Ahmed, K., Passivated Micro LED Structures Suitable for Energy Efficient Displays, US Patent 10,153,401, 2018.

[10] Baek, W., D. Geum, J. Park, and S. Kim, "Enhanced External Quantum Efficiency in the Low-Current Region Using Three Terminal GaN-Based Blue Micro-Light-Emitting Diodes," *SID Symposium Digest of Technical Papers*, Vol. 53, No. 1, 2022, pp. 545–548.

[11] Cho, H., D. Kim, S. Lee, C. Yoo, and Y. Sim, "Efficiency Enhancement of Submicron-Size Light-Emitting Diodes by Triple Dielectric Layers," *Journal of the Society for Information Display*, Vol. 31, 2023, p. 289–297.

[12] Zhu, L., K. Kita, T. Nishimura, K. Nagashio, S. Wang, and A. Toriumi, "Interfacial Dipole at High-k Dielectric/SiO2 Interface: X-Ray Photoelectron Spectroscopy Characteristics," *Japanese Journal of Applied Physics*, Vol. 50, No. 3R, 2011, p. 031502.

[13] Shiraishi, K., K. Yamada, K. Torii, et al., "Oxygen-Vacancy-Induced Threshold Voltage Shifts in Hf-Related High-k Gate Stacks," *Thin Solid Films*, Vol. 508, No. 12, 2006, pp. 305–310.

[14] Jagannathan, H., V. Narayanan, and S. Brown, "Engineering High Dielectric Constant Materials for Band-Edge CMOS Applications," *ECS Transactions*, Vol. 16, No. 5, 2008, p. 19.

[15] Kirsch, P., P. Sivasubramani, J. Huang, et al., "Dipole Model Explaining High-k/Metal Gate Field Effect Transistor Threshold Voltage Tuning," *Applied Physics Letters*, Vol. 92, No. 9, 2008, p. 092901.

[16] Kita, K., and A. Toriumi, "Origin of Electric Dipoles Formed at High-k/SiO2 Interface," *Applied Physics Letters*, Vol. 94, No. 13, 2009, p. 132902.

[17] Razeghi, M., In-Situ P-Type Activation of III-Nitride Films Grown via Metal Organic Chemical Vapor Deposition, US Patent 11,600,496, 2023.

[18] Brown, K., K. Griffin, D. Bour, and O. Kryliouk, Plasma-Assisted MOCVD Fabrication of P-Type Group III-Nitride Materials, US Patent Application 13/413,009, 2012.

[19] Esaki, L., "New Phenomenon in Narrow Germanium p-n Junctions," *Physical Review*, Vol. 109, No. 2, 1958, pp. 603–604.

[20] Simon, J., V. Protasenko, C. Lian, H. Xing, and D. Jena, "Polarization-Induced Hole Doping in Wide-Band-Gap Uniaxial Semiconductor Heterostructures," *Science*, Vol. 327, No. 5961, 2010, p. 60.

[21] Krishnamoorthy, S., F. Akyol, and S. Rajan, "InGaN/GaN Tunnel Junctions for Hole Injection in GaN Light Emitting Diodes," *Applied Physics Letters*, Vol. 105, No. 14, 2014, p. 141104.

[22] E. Young, B. Yonkee, J. Leonard, et al., Hybrid Growth Method for III-Nitride Tunnel Junction Devices, US Patent 11,217,722, 2022.

[23] Yonkee, B., E. Young, J. Leonard, T. Margalith, J. Speck, S. DenBaars, and S. Nakamura, III-Nitride Tunnel Junction with Modified PN Interface, US Patent 10,685,835, 2020.

[24] David, A., M. D'evelyn, C. Hurni, N. Young, and M. Cich, III-Nitride LED with Tunnel Junction, US Patent 10,490,696, 2019.

[25] Yonkee, B., A. Mughal, D. Hwang, et al., Methods for Fabricating III-Nitride Tunnel Junction Devices, US Patent 10,985,285, 2021.

[26] Li, P., H. Li, H. Zhang, Y. Yang, et al., "Red InGaN Micro-Light-Emitting Diodes (> 620 nm) with a Peak External Quantum Efficiency of 4.5% using an Epitaxial Tunnel Junction Contact," *Applied Physics Letters*, Vol. 120, No. 12, 2022.

[27] Li, P., H. Li, Y. Yao, et al., "Hybrid Tunnel Junction Enabled Independent Junction Control of Cascaded InGaN Blue/Green Micro-Light-Emitting Diodes," *Optics Express*, Vol. 31, No. 5, 2023, pp. 7572–7578.

[28] Li, P., H. Li, Y. Yao, et al., "Demonstration of High Efficiency Cascaded Blue and Green Micro-Light-Emitting Diodes with Independent Junction Control," *Applied Physics Letters*, Vol. 118, No. 26, 2021.

[29] Uchida, Y., K. Ito, S. Tsukimoto, et al., "Epitaxial Growth of GaN Layers on Metallic TiN Buffer Layers," *Journal of Electronic Materials*, Vol. 35, 2006, pp. 1806–1811.

[30] Ito, K., Y. Uchida, S. Lee, et al., "Effects of TiN Buffer Layer Thickness on GaN Growth," *Journal of Electronic Materials*, Vol. 38, 2009, pp. 511–517.

[31] Watanabe, T., K. Ito, S. Tsukimoto, et al., "Growth of GaN on Nitriding TiN Buffer Layers," *Materials Transactions*, Vol. 46, No. 9, 2005, pp. 1975–1978.

[32] Chen, N., W. Lien, C. Shih, P. Chang, T. Wang, and M. Wu, "Nitride Light-Emitting Diodes Grown on Si (111) using a TiN Template," *Applied Physics Letters*, Vol. 88, No. 19, 2006.

[33] Ahmed, K., A. Prakash, R. Woodbeck, and S. Pabba, Structures for Micro LED Laser Release, US Patent Application 17/402,313, 2023.

[34] Ahmed, K., A. Pancholi, and A. Khakifirooz, Micro Light-Emitting Diode Displays Having Color Conversion Devices and Assembly Approaches, US Patent 11,610,936, 2023.

[35] Kumar, B., K. Ahmed, A. Keates and J. Gupta, Micro-LED Display Architecture for High Volume Manufacturing, US Patent Application 17/710,662, 2023.

[36] Ahmed, K., A. Pancholi, J. Heck, T. Sounart, H. Frish, and S. Dasgupta, III-N Multichip Modules and Methods of Fabrication, US Patent 11,211,245, 2021.

[37] West, P., and K. Ahmed, Micro LED Laser Release from Silicon Wafer, US Patent Application 17/485,398, 2022.

[38] Sounart, T., K. Ahmed, A. Pancholi, and S. Liff, Micro-LED Displays Including Solder Structures and Methods, US Patent Application 16/946,166, 2020.

[39] Shinkai, S., and K. Sasaki, "Influence of Sputtering Parameters on the Formation Process of High-Quality and Low-Resistivity HfN Thin Film," *Japanese Journal Applied Physics*, Vol. 38, 1999, p. 2097.

[40] Yang, B., A. Trampert, O. Brandt, B. Jenichen, and K. Ploog, "Structural Properties of GaN Layers on Si (001) Grown by Plasma-Assisted Molecular Beam Epitaxy," *Journal of Applied Physics*, Vol. 83, No. 7, 1998, pp. 3800–3806.

[41] Xu, X., R. Armitage, S. Shinkai, K. Sasaki, C. Kisielowski, and E. Weber, "Epitaxial Condition and Polarity in GaN Grown on a HfN-Buffered Si (111) Wafer," *Applied Physics Letters*, Vol. 86, No. 18, 2005.

[42] Armitage, R., Q. Yang, H. Feick, et al., "Lattice-Matched HfN Buffer Layers for Epitaxy of GaN on Si," *Applied Physics Letters*, Vol. 81, No. 8, 2002, pp. 1450–1452.

[43] Moram, M., M. Kappers, T. Joyce, P. Chalker, Z. Barber, and C. Humphreys, "Growth of Dislocation-Free GaN Islands on Si(111) using a Scandium Nitride Buffer Layer," *Journal of Crystal Growth*, Vol. 308, No. 2, 2007, pp. 302–308.

[44] Moram, M., M. Kappers, Z. Barber, and C. Humphreys, "Growth of Low Dislocation Density GaN using Transition Metal Nitride Masking Layers," *Journal of Crystal Growth*, Vol. 298, 2007, pp. 268–271.

[45] Oliver, M., J. Schroeder, D. Ewoldt, et al., "Organometallic Vapor Phase Epitaxial Growth of GaN on ZrN/AlN/Si Substrates," *Applied Physics Letters*, Vol. 93, No. 2, 2008.

[46] Huitema, E., V. Patel, T. Nauta, X. Li, and H. Hu, Display with Embedded Pixel Driver Chips, US Patent 10,665,578, 2020.

[47] Song, S., S. Han, H. Ahn, et al., Display Apparatus and Method of Manufacturing the Same, US Patent 11741886B2, 2022.

[48] Hin, T., and H. Wong, Flipchip Interconnected Light-Emitting Diode Package Assembly, US Patent Application 17/132,359, 2021.

[49] Ahmed, K., and A. Keates, Micro Light-Emitting Diode Displays Having Colloidal or Graded Index Quantum Dot Films, US Patent 11,515,297, 2022.

[50] Ahmed, K., Micro LED Apparatus Including Color Conversion Structures and Methods of Manufacturing the Same, US Patent 11,430,921, 2022.

[51] Ahmed, K., "Design of a Transparent Dielectric Metamirror for Micro LED Displays," *SID Symposium Digest of Technical Papers*, Vol. 52, No. 1, 2021, pp. 788–791.

[52] Ahmed, K., V. Sinha, and M. Bartscherer, Redundant Sub-Pixels in a Light-Emitting Diode Display, US Patent Application 16/914,309, 2020.

[53] Kim, Y., S. Cruz, K. Lee, et al., "Remote Epitaxy through Graphene Enables Two-Dimensional Material-Based Layer Transfer," *Nature*, Vol. 544, No. 7650, 2017, pp. 340–343.

[54] Singh, A., K. Ahn, D. Yoo, S. Lee, A. Ali, G. Yi, and K. Chung, "van der Waals Integration of GaN Light-Emitting Diode Arrays on Foreign Graphene Films using Semiconductor/Graphene Heterostructures," *NPG Asia Materials*, Vol. 14, No. 1, 2022, p. 57.

[55] Badokas, K., A. Kadys, J. Mickevičius, et al., "Remote Epitaxy of GaN via Graphene on GaN/Sapphire Templates," *Journal of Physics D: Applied Physics*, Vol. 54, No. 20, 2021, p. 205103.

[56] Han, X., J. Yu, Z. Li, et al., "Remote Epitaxy and Exfoliation of GaN via Graphene," *ACS Applied Electronic Materials*, Vol. 4, No. 11, 2022, pp. 5326–5332.

[57] Lee, S., M. Abbas, D. Yoo, et al., "Pulsed-Mode Metalorganic Vapor-Phase Epitaxy of GaN on Graphene-Coated c-Sapphire for Freestanding GaN Thin Films," *Nano Letters*, Vol. 3, 2023, p. 11578–11585.

[58] Choi, J., J. Jeong, X. Zhu, et al., "Exceptional Thermochemical Stability of Graphene on N-Polar GaN for Remote Epitaxy," *ACS Nano*, Vol. 17, No. 21, 2023, pp. 21678–21689.

[59] Shinkai, S., and K. Sasaki, "TBD," *Japanese Journal of Applied Physics Part 1*, Vol. 38, 1999, p. 2097.

# 9

# Potential Applications for MicroLEDs

MicroLEDs offer extraordinarily high luminance, high energy efficiency, low cost, and long lifetime. These characteristics are highly desirable in various applications, but their usage has, to date, been primarily focused on next-generation display technologies. In this chapter, a number of potential nondisplay application areas of the microLEDs are discussed. The discussion is limited to the concept stage with the aim to facilitate brainsteering toward new applications. Brainsteering has been explained by Coyne and Coyne as an alternative to brainstorming to find breakthrough ideas [1]. The advantage of brainsteering is that it applies the design thinking process to creative idea generation. Energy is invested upfront to ensure that the actual problem to be solved is crystal clear.

## 9.1 Thermal Processing

In semiconductor and display manufacturing, a substrate may be subjected to thermal processing to change the atomic structure of the substrate, to facilitate deposition of a material on the substrate, and/or to remove, or facilitate removal of, a material from the substrate. To the extent the thermal process is sensitive to the temperature of the thermal process, temperature nonuniformity on the substrate during processing can lead to nonuniformity in process results. For example, if a material is deposited on a substrate during thermal processing, the rate of deposition may depend on the local temperature of the substrate or at a location near the substrate surface. Differences in the deposition rate may lead to differences in a thickness of the material deposited across the substrate, which can lead to unacceptable nonuniformity in the functionality of devices formed on the substrate.

Temperature nonuniformities on the substrate during processing can arise from thermal and optical properties of various structures in the processing chamber, such as different objects and surfaces with different thermal and optical properties and different orientations within the processing environment of the chamber. Other sources of processing nonuniformity may also impact the result of the process. In processing systems with circular or cylindrical geometry, nonuniformities can have radial patterns and/or azimuthal patterns. Radial patterns of nonuniformity are typically addressed by heating adjustments in radial zones. Addressing azimuthal patterns arising from discrete chamber structures, such as substrate support and transportation structures, is more challenging.

As device (e.g., transistor) geometries continue to scale down, the uniformity of semiconductor processes become more demanding. Nanoscale nonuniformities are increasingly problematic at advanced dimension CMOS nodes. There are continuing needs for processing apparatus and methods that reduce processing nonuniformity in thermal processing chambers.

Figure 9.1 describes a heating system and a corresponding method of heating a surface of an object to a processing temperature of at least 100°C, wherein the heating system comprises microLEDs and is adapted to heat an area element of the heating surface with a plurality of microLEDs (e.g., 49, 100, 400) at the same time. The heating system may be part of a reactor for processing semiconductor structures. The light emitted by means of the microLEDs overlaps at the heating surface. Differences of the characteristic of one single microLED may be blurred at the heating surface such that a homogeneous

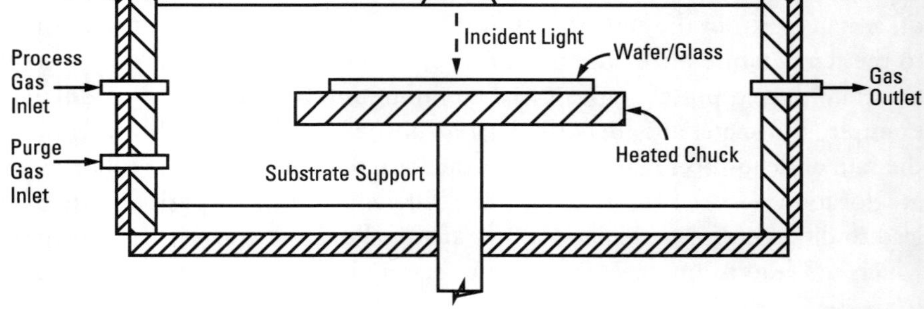


**Figure 9.1** A schematic illustration of a thermal processing apparatus/chamber utilizing an array of microLEDs as a heat source. A processing gas may be flowed through the chamber to produce a specific desired change in material properties, or to activate dopants, for example.

temperature distribution across a processing surface of a, for example, wafer may be enabled.

The object may be an OLED substrate (glass, plastic wafer, foils, etc.), a semiconductor wafer (Si, GaAs, etc.) or a carrier like a susceptor on which one or more of such wafers may be placed for processing semiconductor layers. The processing temperature strongly depends on the material to be processed like a plastic or Si wafer. In OLED processing temperatures of 100°C, 150°C, or 200°C may be preferred. Processing of GaAs may require a processing temperature above 500°C, wherein the processing of InGaN layers used for LED fabrication may require even processing temperatures above 600°C.

MicroLEDs are used to illuminate the heating surface of the object. The optical energy provided by the microLEDs heats a processing surface to the desired temperature. The processing surface may be at least partly identical with the heating surface. The processing surface of a wafer may in this case be directly illuminated by means of the microLEDs. Alternatively, the heating surface and the processing surface may be separate surfaces. The backside of a wafer may, for example, be illuminated by means of the microLEDs and the front side of the wafer may comprise the processing surface. Furthermore, one or more wafers may be placed on a carrier-like a graphite susceptor. At least a part of one side of the carrier may be illuminated by means of the microLEDs such that the wafer provided on the opposite side of the carrier is indirectly heated to the desired temperature. The heating system may provide a homogenous temperature distribution of the processing surface by illuminating an area element of the heating surface with at least 49 microLEDs at the same time. Furthermore, reliability of the heating system may be improved because failure of one microLED may cause only a minor change of the optical power provided by the microLED array to the area element. It may thus be advantageous to provide 100, 200, 500, 1,000, or more microLEDs to heat an area element of the heating surface at one moment in time. An increased number of microLEDs may reduce the power requirements regarding the single microLED emitter. It may in this case be possible to use medium-power microLEDs even in high-temperature applications with processing temperatures of 800°C, 900°C, or even more than 1000°C.

Nonuniform heating can be produced intentionally by controlling of the pattern of microLEDs that are lit in an array, as shown in Figure 9.2.

As shown in Figure 9.3, the microLED array pitch (P) and the divergence angle ($\alpha$) of a microLED can be used to control the uniformity of a heating pattern on a substrate. Simulations can be used to adjust the pitch of microLEDs in an array to produce intentionally nonuniform heating to compensate for a pattern on the heated substrate that otherwise causes nonuniform heating with respect to other parts of the wafer where the pattern on the heated sub-

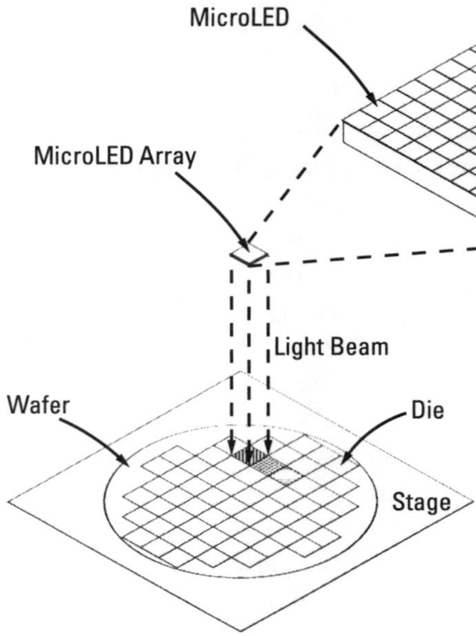


**Figure 9.2** Schematic illustrating how an array of microLEDs illuminates a particular die on the wafer. By controlling the number and pattern of microLEDs in the arrays that are lit, different thermal processing temperatures may be provided for each die as desired.

strate is significantly different. This can also be used to produce combinatorial experimentation with annealing temperature on various parts of the substrate.

Figure 9.4 illustrates the use of a microLED array to heat a susceptor through a window in the reactor. The susceptor heats a wafer. The uniformity of the temperature can be controlled without using raster anneal and a laser beam. The smaller size of microLEDs (down to 30 $\mu$m) may be useful in enhancing the light extraction efficiency due to sidewall reflections. The thermal processing chambers described herein have directed energy sources configured to heat specific locations of a substrate disposed in the chambers for processing thereof.

Figure 9.5 illustrates a concept for using microLEDs to perform selective annealing on specific dies on the wafer/glass substrate.

## 9.2 Wafer/Glass Substrate Inspection System

Inspection processes are used at various steps during a semiconductor (display) manufacturing process to detect defects on wafers (glass backplane) to promote higher yield in the manufacturing process and thus lower cost of ownership. Inspection has always been an important part of fabricating semiconductor devices, for example. As the dimensions of semiconductor devices decrease,

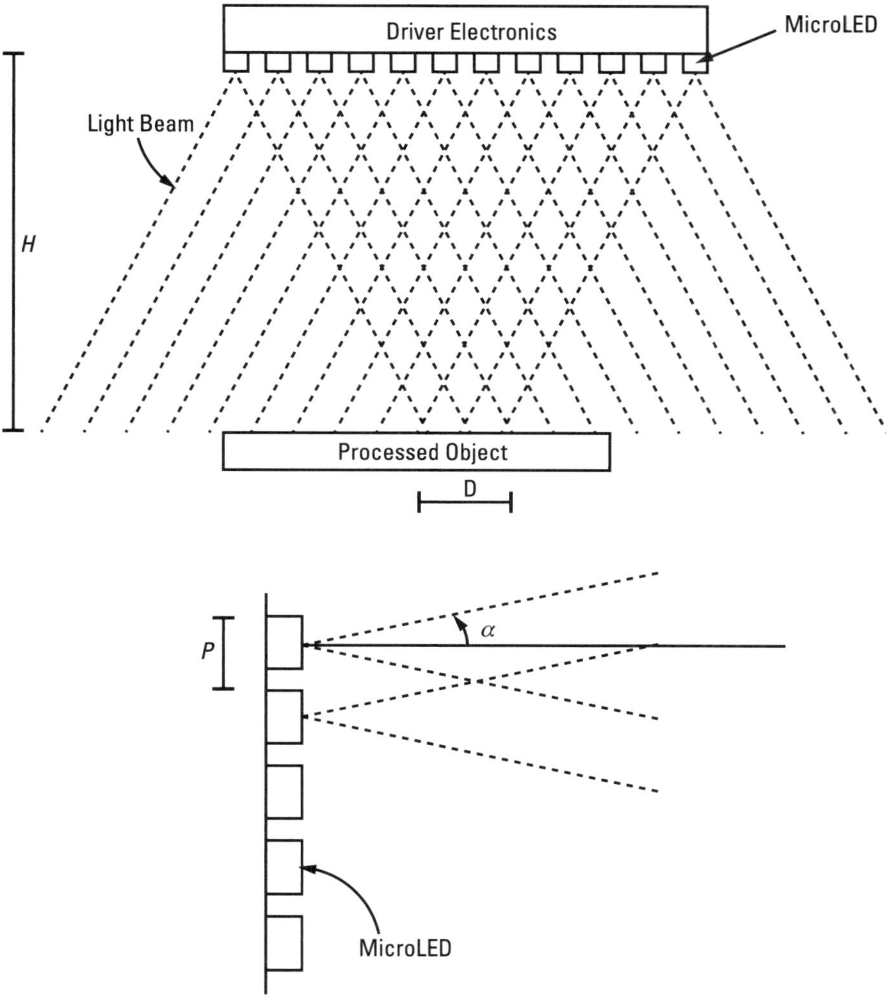


**Figure 9.3** Schematic illustration of how control of the microLED array pitch (P) and the divergence angle of a microLED ($\alpha$) can be used to control the uniformity of a heating pattern on a substrate over area D using a plurality of microLEDs (UV laser or IR laser depending on the receiving substrate) to uniformly illuminate a relatively large area of a substrate for heating purposes. The front side of the substrate is heated in this example.

inspection becomes even more important to the successful manufacture of acceptable semiconductor devices because smaller defects can cause the devices to fail. Improved sensitivity to particles, anomalies, and other defect types, while maintaining overall inspection speed (in wafers per hour), is desired in wafer inspection systems. Dark field optical inspection systems typically use laser light to illuminate the wafer in a specific pattern—individual spots, lines, or areas—and collection optics to direct the scattered light on a corresponding set of sen-

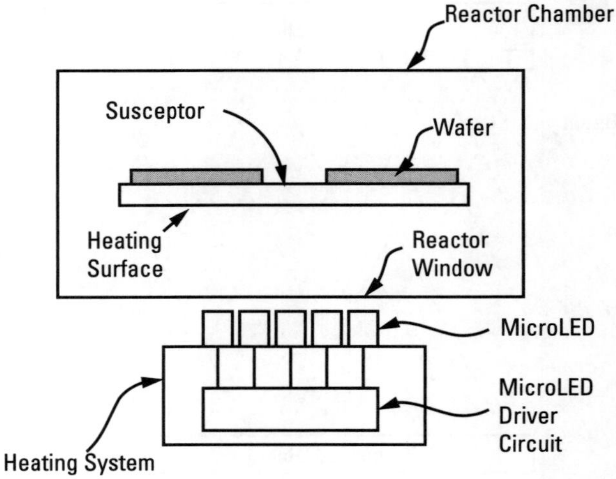


**Figure 9.4** Illustrates the use of a microLED array to heat a susceptor through a window in the reactor where the susceptor heats a wafer.

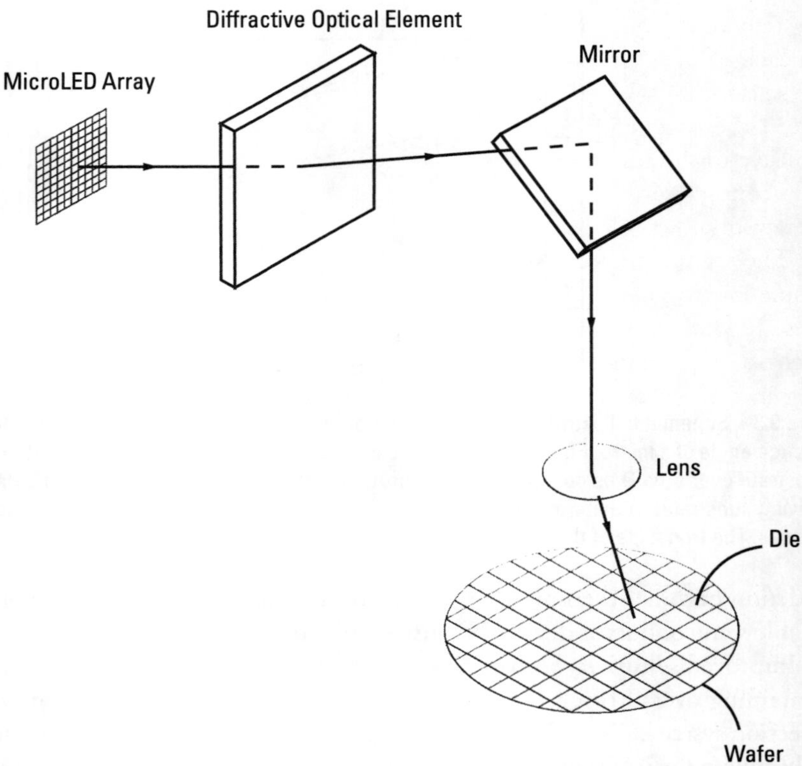


**Figure 9.5** Schematic illustration of a selective annealing system using microLED arrays.

sors. One advantage of an inspection system where a large area (on the order of 1 mm × 1 mm) of the wafer is illuminated at once, as opposed to a spot (on the order of microns) or a line (on the order of microns wide by mm long), is that many varieties of two-dimensional sensors exist that can capture information on thousands to millions of individual detectors in parallel. Furthermore, spot-illuminated inspection systems are practically limited to dozens of spots due to the complexities of illumination optics and of integrating individual sensors thereby limiting achievable throughput. One further disadvantage of spot and line scanning systems is the illumination energy is concentrated in relatively small areas, increasing the power density on the inspected surface, which can undesirably alter the sample properties. Accordingly, it would be advantageous to identify inspection systems and/or methods that do not have one or more of these disadvantages.

Here a system that includes a microLED-based illumination subsystem configured to simultaneously form multiple illumination areas on the wafer with substantially no illumination flux between each of the areas is described. The system also includes a scanning subsystem configured to scan the multiple illumination areas across the wafer. In addition, the system includes a collection subsystem configured to simultaneously and separately image light scattered from each of the areas onto two or more sensors. Characteristics of the two or more sensors are selected such that the scattered light is not imaged into gaps between the two or more sensors. The two or more sensors generate output responsive to the scattered light. The system further includes a computer subsystem configured to detect defects on the wafer using the output of the two or more sensors.

The scanning and/or imaging inspection time may be reduced by using multiple inspection beams, each beam having generally similar properties. The beams are focused onto the wafer surface and are scanned across the surface in tandem. Using a multiplicity of inspection beams produces a corresponding saving in time to scan and/or image the wafer surface compared to the time taken if only a single beam is used.

Different configurations of the inspection system based on microLEDs are shown in Figures 9.6, 9.7, and 9.8.

## 9.3 MicroLED Pattern Printer—Maskless Lithography

The high and rising cost of photomasks (largely driven by writing times exceeding 24 hours) is driving the exploration of maskless lithography for applications requiring throughput about 1 $cm^2/s$. To try and avoid the high and rising costs of photomasks, optical maskless lithography (OML) promises no fundamental limit to throughput [2]. Active matrix-addressable UV microemitters are highly

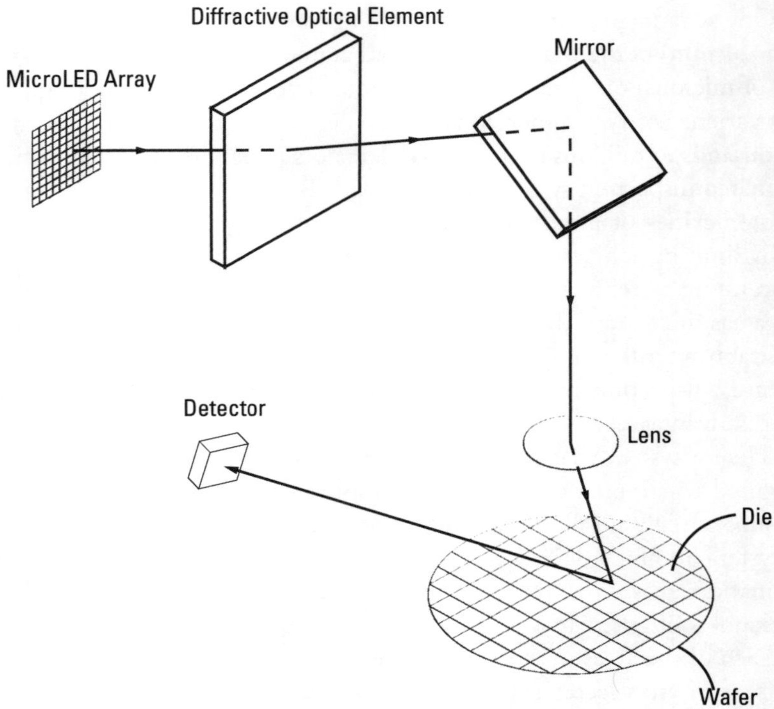


**Figure 9.6** Schematic illustration of a wafer inspection system based on an illumination subsystem that is in turn based on an array of microLEDs.

attractive as specialized photolithographic and photochemistry exposure tools as arbitrary image patterns can be generated and transferred to a UV-sensitive material such as a photoresist without the need to manufacture expensive photomasks [3–8]. As a result, it offers more flexibility in the photolithography process and a compact system. The concepts of maskless lithography and mask lithography are illustrated in Figure 9.9.

A maskless exposure system that has multiple maskless optical engines arranged in an (N × M) matrix that form and project a pattern onto a large glass substrate is shown in Figure 9.10. A first-stage system is capable of driving the maskless optical engines in a first direction, while a second stage-system is capable of holding and moving the substrate in a second direction perpendicular to the first direction. The system includes a control system that processes data and synchronizing movement of the first- and second-stage systems and a vision system that detects the positions of the second-stage system to synchronize movements with the multiple optical engines.

A schematic illustration of the concept of parallel processing using maskless lithography with the aid of multiple arrays of microLEDs is shown in Figure 9.11.

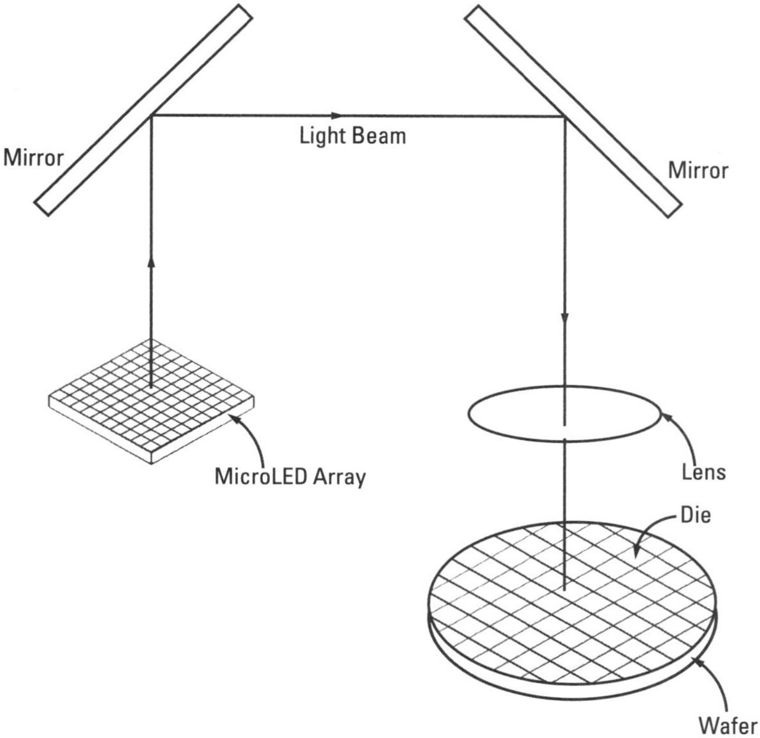


**Figure 9.7** Schematic illustration of a wafer illumination system based on the use of an array of microLEDs.

## 9.4 Dynamic Structured Light Projector

This application is in the field of projectors and relates specifically to structured light illumination that can be used in three-dimensional (3D) scanning for sensing, imaging, 3D printing, and computer-integrated manufacturing (CIM) [9–13].

Computed reconstruction of a 3D object can be achieved by projecting a known pattern, such as vertical or horizontal bars or spots, either random or deterministic, on the object, as shown in Figure 9.12. As the bars deform or spots deviate when striking surfaces, vision systems can calculate the depth and surface information of the object. The high-resolution structured light system includes one or more image capture devices, such as a camera and/or an image sensor and a projector. The projector is configured to project a binary pattern so that the projector can operate at high throughput. Each microLED emitter produces a light beam and is electronically controlled/tuned, being switchable on and off. The array of light sources provides dynamic pattern projection by turning on and off selected microLED(s). The diffractive optical element (DOE) is

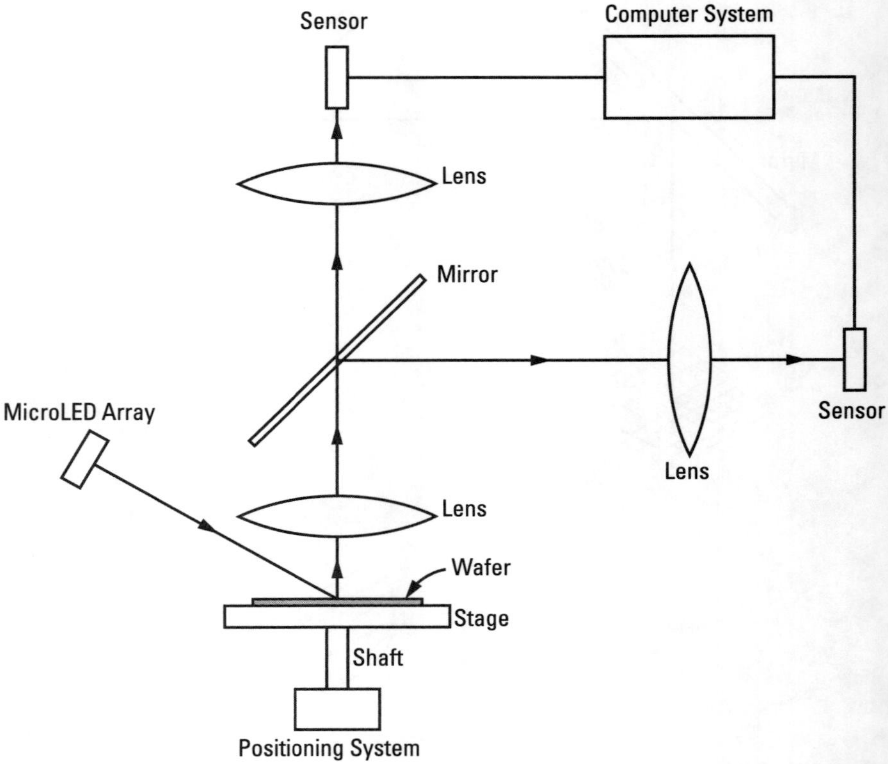


**Figure 9.8** Schematic illustration of a possible implementation of the wafer inspection system concept shown in Figure 9.6.

two-dimensional, having a two-dimensional structure of the grating, varying over its length and height dimensions. Being nonperiodic, the DOE does not require collimation of the beam light before passing through the DOE or focusing of the light beam after the DOE, enabling it to work directly with the light sources toward the object on which the SL pattern is generated.

State-of-the-art light projectors used in such reconstruction applications include spatial light modulators (SLM) such as DLP, LCD, and liquid-crystal-on-silicon (LCoS) with incoherent LED or lamp light sources. These projectors usually have a limited number of spatial pixels, have limited, high, etendue of the power flux and have low light efficiency due to multiple layers structure. The raster structure of the projectors imposes limitations on the state-of-the-art light projectors to be used as a source for structured light for three-dimensional scanning. Accordingly, power losses, acquisition time, frame rate, object size, contrast of projected structured light (SL) intensity patterns in any background light are compromised and consequently the resolution and working distance range of the entire 3D scanning system is reduced.

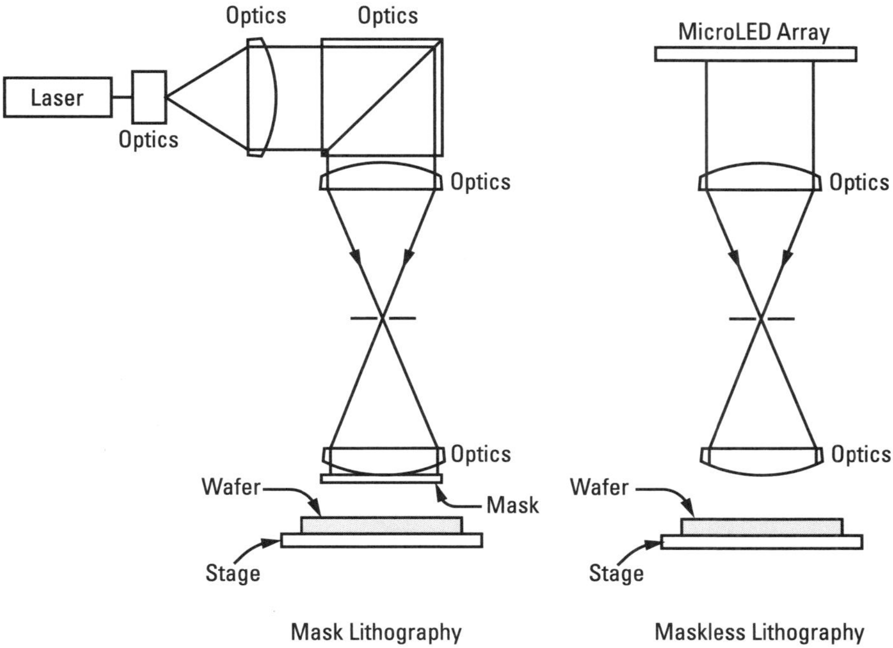


**Figure 9.9** Schematic illustration of the concept of maskless lithograph and comparison to the mask lithography concept.

A microLED-based structured light projector is highly efficient, for example, in its use of light power and in that it is cost effective and provides high-resolution structured light patterns. The projector can be used in 3D imaging of objects within 1m with high resolution. A key advantage of using microLEDs as opposed to lasers for a light source is the avoidance of speckle noise.

## 9.5 Structured Light Probe

Polyp size assessment during gastrointestinal endoscopy is crucial for therapeutic decision making. Indeed, polyp size affects several factors during the diagnosis and treatment cycle: (a) it is correlated with the likelihood of malignancy within the polyp, (b) it affects the choice of treatment for polypectomy, and (c) it is the main determinant in postpolypectomy surveillance risk stratification. In daily clinical practice, endoscopists estimate the diameter of polyps only by visual inspection, relying on their own experience. Expertise may increase precision, but discrepancies between endoscopic and pathologic measurements have been a challenge. Usually, endoscopists overestimate the real size of the polyp and this is particularly true for the left colon. Open biopsy forceps of known

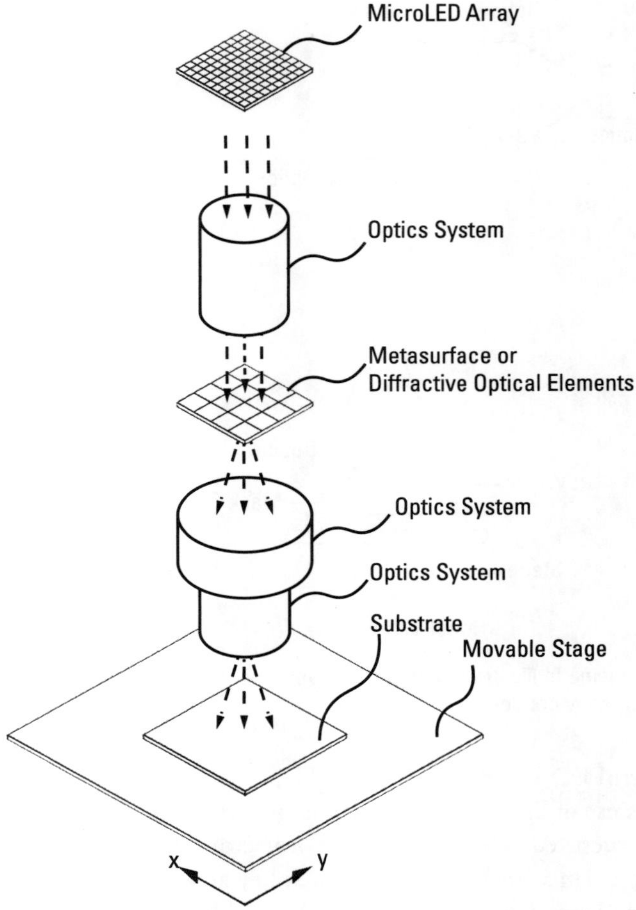


**Figure 9.10** Schematic illustration of a microLED-based maskless lithography (pattern printer) system. An array of UV microLEDs emits light toward a substrate through an optics system to print a pattern on the substrate.

size and endoscopic rulers have been proposed to improve precision, as well as comparison with an open snare, but results are often inconsistent [14, 15].

The proposed system consists of a flexible structured light microLED pattern projector (Figure 9.13) and is adapted from the work done using laser as a light source [16]. An array of light beams from an array of microLEDs is transmitted through a plastic imaging optical fiber (diameter = 1–3 mm) up to its tip. The light pattern/grid is dialed by turning on/off various microLEDs in the microLED array so a known shape and size is projected onto the tissue. The image of the grid is captured by the scope camera. By knowing the relative position of camera and projector, it is possible to geometrically find the 3D position and distance of all grid points projected onto the polyp.

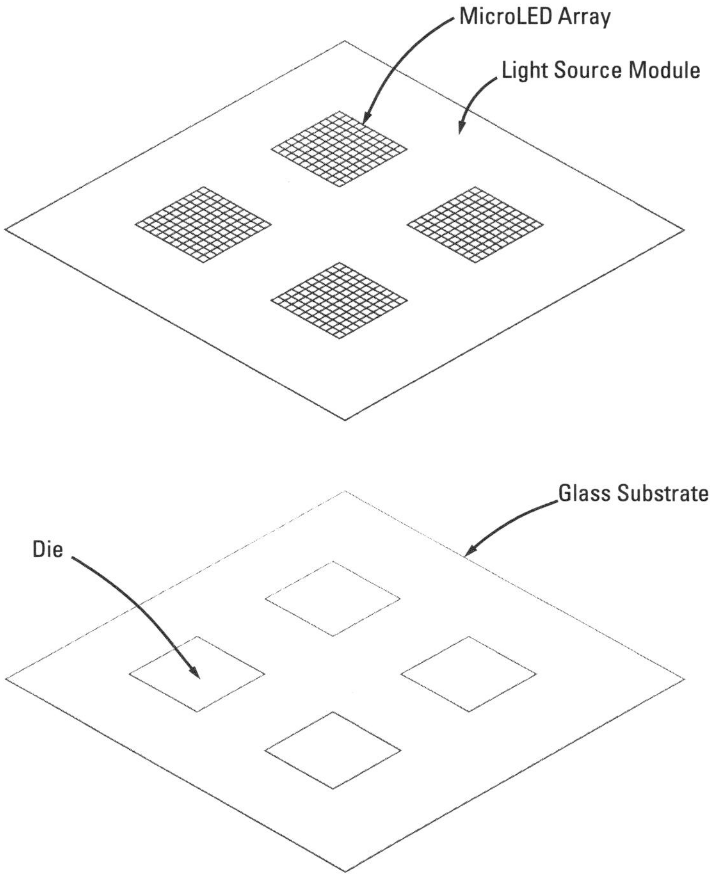


**Figure 9.11** Schematic illustration of the concept of parallel processing using maskless lithography with the aid of multiple arrays of microLEDs.

A cross section illustration of the plastic imaging fiber is shown in Figure 9.14.

## 9.6 Hyperspectral Imaging of Biological Tissues

Here we discuss apparatuses for generating, calibrating, sample focusing, and processing hyperspectral images of molecular samples at high speed. Two example classes of apparatuses include a line scanning apparatus and a staring apparatus. Both classes of apparatuses involve consideration of sufficient illumination, high data acquisition rates, efficient data processing, and calibration. Illumination may be provided by an array of blue microLEDs, possibly with

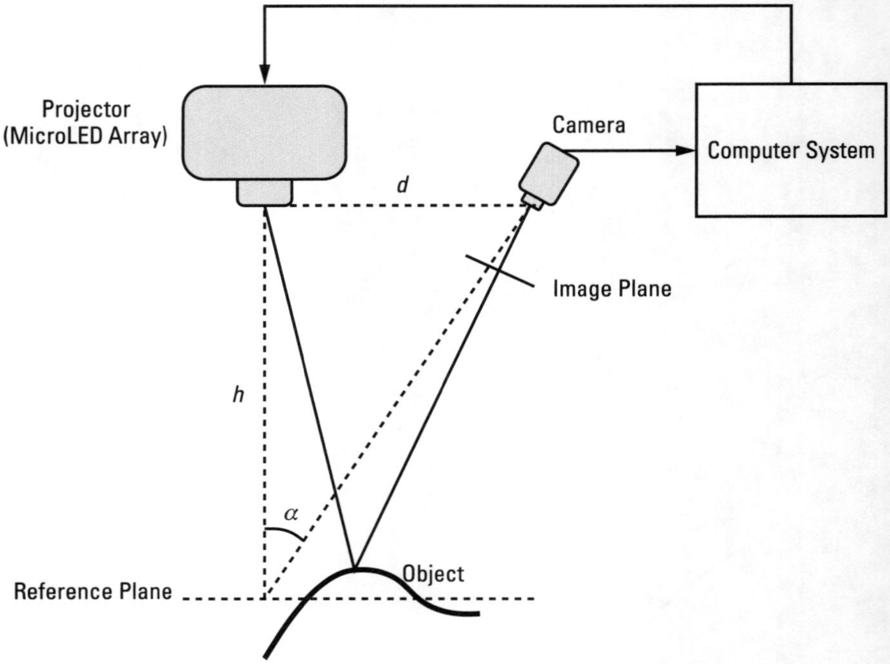


**Figure 9.12** Computed reconstruction of a 3D object can be achieved by projecting a known pattern, such as vertical or horizontal bars or spots, either random or deterministic.

different peak wavelengths. One or more microLEDs can illuminate one pixel on the biological sample.

### 9.6.1 Motivation

In biomedical research, there is increasing demand for quantitative multiplexed measurement methods (i.e., analyzing multiple proteins, nucleic acids, or other cellular structures (e.g., analytes) in tandem). In quantitative multiplexed measurement methods, numerous biologic molecules (e.g., circulating tumor cells (CTCs), labeled tissue sections, and exosomes) can be analyzed at the same time. Analyzing multiple proteins, nucleic acids, or other cellular structures (hereby referred to as analytes) in tandem, can be useful to understanding information, such as how individual components in complex biological systems interact with one another for drug discovery, diagnostics, basic research, and other applications. Multiplexed measurements can be used in the fields of genomics or proteomics and other emerging areas to analyze different biologic molecules in one or multiple samples. However, such techniques are difficult to carry out in real time due to time constraints and the amount of data to be

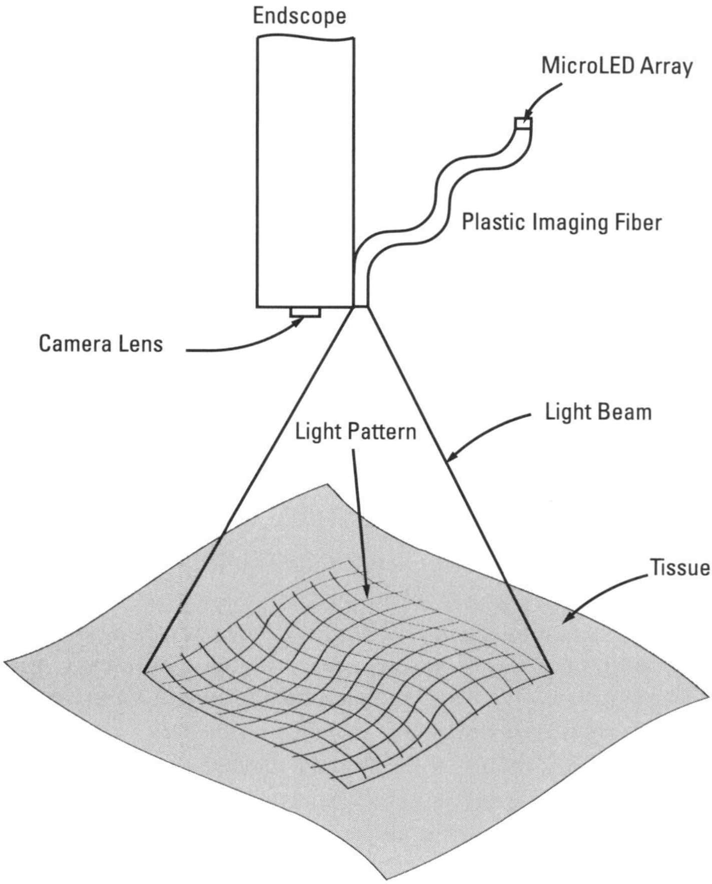


**Figure 9.13** Basic functioning of the structured light probe. A grid of known shape and size is projected from the probe onto the tissue, where it will appear deformed by the local morphology.

collected and analyzed. Real-time analysis can be beneficial for various applications, such as in the practice of medicine and/or diagnosis.

Imaging biological molecules may be performed either directly based on absorption (e.g., absorption by oxyhemoglobin, deoxyhemoglobin, or melanin), with endogenous fluorescence (inherent to the sample, e.g., NADH or flavins) or indirectly by use of a label that indicates the presence of the molecule as by fluorescence (fluorescent dyes, quantum dot, phosphors, or other nanoparticles), chemiluminescence, scattering (metal or other nanoparticle), or absorption (dyes). For ease of reference, these various fluorophores, chromophores, or scatterers can be referred to as labels, even though the label may be the molecule of interest itself. To generate quantitative, multiplexed images of the labels in

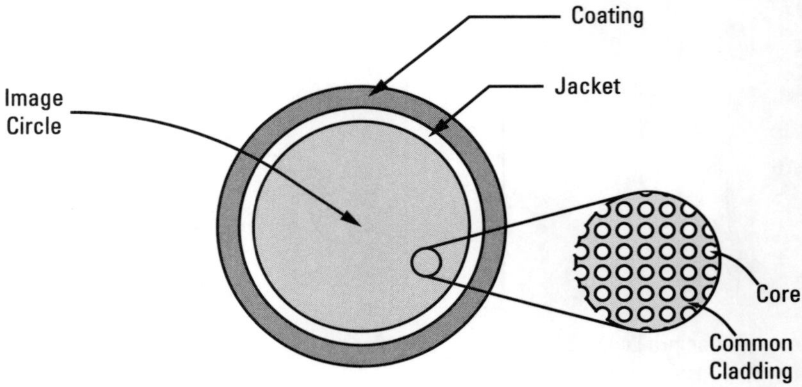


**Figure 9.14** Schematic illustration of the cross section of a plastic imaging fiber.

a high-throughput manner, the imaging apparatus, data acquisition, and data processing operate at a threshold speed.

The fluorescence resonance energy transfer (FRET) is a phenomenon that if two fluorescent dyes different from each other are positioned within a distance of 1 to 10 nm, a light emitted after a shorter wavelength dye is excited induces excitation of a longer wavelength excitation dye to emit fluorescence [17–22]. The concept of FRET is shown schematically in Figure 9.15. That is, after two different fluorescent dyes are attached to the back of two proteins with which an interaction is desired to be studied, by detecting fluorescence caused by fluorescence resonance energy transfer occurring by an interaction between the two proteins when the two fluorescent dyes are close to each other within 1 to 10 nm, a protein interaction can be analyzed. Miyawaki et al. [23] analyzed interaction between calmodulin and calmodulin-binding peptide by using the FRET principle and developed a novel protein interaction analysis system. The dyes absorb lights having intrinsic wavelengths different from each other and excite, and when the energy is emitted in the form of light or heat, the dyes are reinstated in a ground state and each dye emits a light having a unique wavelength range. By way of example, a fluorescent protein excited in the form of light having a wavelength of 488 nm emits fluorescence having a wavelength of 520 nm, which stimulates other fluorescent proteins in a pair, resulting in the emitting fluorescence having a wavelength of 630 nm. Therefore, by exciting proteins with light of 488 nm and detecting fluorescence having a wavelength of 630 nm, it is possible to analyze an interaction between the two proteins. This system is capable of analyzing a dynamic interaction between proteins in a live cell, but it is capable of detection only when two fluorescent proteins are positioned at a very short distance from each other (e.g., $<10$ nm).

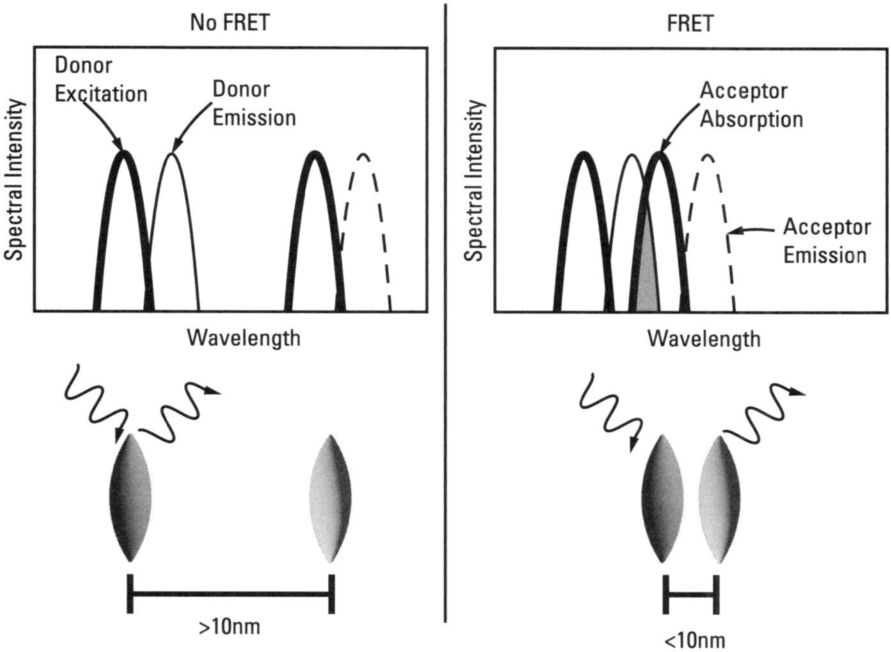


**Figure 9.15** Schematic illustration of the concept of FRET as a result of the interaction of two molecules. In this case the energy from the first molecule, the donor, can transfer into the second one, the acceptor. MicroLEDs emitting different wavelengths in the blue spectrum can excite donor proteins and a detector can be used to detect acceptor protein emission in the longer wavelength (e.g., red). Conditions for FRET include (a) a donor and acceptor pair where the emission spectra of the donor overlap with the excitation spectra of the acceptor (spectral overlap; gray shading), (b) the distance between the donor and acceptor must be less than approximately 10 nm; at larger distances there is no FRET, and (c) FRET efficiency is highest when the excitation and emission dipoles are oriented parallel and there is no FRET if they are perpendicular (not shown).

### 9.6.2 Theory

The rate of energy transfer $k_{ET}$ is according to Förster theory [24–26]

$$k_{ET} = \frac{9\ln 10}{128\pi^5} \bullet \frac{\kappa^2}{N_A n^4 \tau_0 r^6} \bullet \int_0^\infty F(\lambda) \bullet \varepsilon(\lambda) \bullet \lambda^4 \bullet d\lambda \tag{9.1}$$

where $N_A$ is the Avogadro constant, $n$ refractive index of solvent, $\tau_0$ is the radiative decay time of donor, $r$ is the distance between donor and acceptor molecule, $\varepsilon(\lambda)$ is the molar decadic extinction coefficient of acceptor, $\kappa^2$ is the orientation factor: $\kappa^2 = [\cos \varphi_{DA} - 3 \cos \varphi_D \cos \varphi_A]^2$, $\varphi_{DA}$ is the angle between transition dipoles of donor and acceptor, $\varphi_D$ is the angle between donor transition dipole and line connecting the dipoles, $\varphi_A$ is the angle between acceptor transition dipole and line connecting the dipoles, and $F(\lambda)$ is the normalized fluorescence spectrum of donor, normalized according to

$$1 = \int_0^{\infty} F(\lambda) \bullet d\lambda \tag{9.2}$$

The rate is proportional to the extinction coefficient of the acceptor dye in the wavelength range of the donor fluorescence (*overlap integral*, $J = \int_0^{\infty} F(\lambda) \bullet \varepsilon(\lambda) \bullet \lambda^4 \bullet d\lambda$).

As shown in (9.1), fluorescence resonance energy transfer is a phenomenon that is strongly dependent on the distance (proportional $r^{-6}$ ) between donor and acceptor. The transition from no to very effective energy transfer is very sharp (i.e., a high-fluorescence modulation can be achieved). Also from the above equation it is obvious that FRET can be considered like a spectroscopic microscope, providing us information about the distance and orientation on the molecular scale regardless of the size of the sample. Fluorophore involving FRET can be considered as analogous to roaming molecular spies with radio transmitters, radiating information to the experimenter about the state of affairs on the molecular scale, and informing us where the spies are located and how they are oriented.

The efficiency of energy transfer ($\eta$) is modulated by the distance between the two molecules ($r$):

$$\eta = \frac{1}{1 + \left(r / R_0\right)^6} \tag{9.3}$$

where $R_0$ is of the order of 5 nm and is called the Förster radius, which is the characteristic distance between molecules where the FRET efficiency is 50%. For most cell biology applications detecting interactions between two proteins, FRET is used as a binary readout, with high FRET indicating the presence of an interaction and no FRET indicating the absence of interaction. To assay protein-protein interactions in cells, fluorescent proteins are most commonly employed as the FRET donor and acceptor.

FRET may be used in biological applications for determining the binding between proteins or to study membrane structures or to study interactions between membranes. For those purposes, vesicles were developed that contain a fluorescence donor and/or acceptor for FRET.

If a microLED array illuminates specific pixels (area) on a biological sample, it might be possible to detect 2D maps where there is interaction between the donor protein and the acceptor protein based on the fluorescence signal level. It is also possible to use microLEDs emitting different excitation wavelengths to probe different types of proteins that get excited by different light wavelengths.

### 9.6.3 Requirements

To generate a hyperspectral image of a molecular sample, the total number of data points acquired is significantly larger than for conventional imaging, which acquires a few wavelengths for each point in the sample. For example, imaging of a standard biological tissue slide (e.g., 15 mm × 15 mm) results in 126 billion data points to generate a hyperspectral image of the sample using a 20× microscope objective and 96 wavelengths per sample point. Further, the plurality of analytes can be analyzed using fluorophores or other labels, which may have spectral overlap. Due to the spectral overlap, in order distinguish if an observed signal came from the desired fluorophore or a fluorophore whose emission spectra overlapped with the desired fluorophore, spectral imaging techniques can be used. Spectral imaging techniques can include acquiring many wavelength measurements for each spatial point in a molecular sample and using those data points to mitigate spectral overlap in a process called spectral unmixing or spectral decomposition. In this process, the wavelength measurements (e.g., the spectral data) is transformed into label quantifications. In order to make hyperspectral imaging practical for applications, such as those in biomedical research and medicine, it becomes imperative to increase the data acquisition rate of the hyperspectral imaging apparatus.

To perform imaging at high speeds involves various interrelated factors. For example, appropriate illumination power and illumination throughput efficiency as well as efficient capture of photons from multiple labels is beneficial because image integration or exposure times are shorter. Data processing speeds and efficiency are also beneficial because of the large data bandwidths and to avoid bottlenecks and minimize latency. Image correction methods are used to minimize or mitigate degradations of image quality due to illumination nonuniformity or to compensate for image distortions from hyperspectral imaging systems. Data compression is important to assist data processing and minimize file storage requirements.

### 9.6.4 Apparatus

The imaging apparatus (Figure 9.16) comprises a light source, an imaging spectrometer, an image sensor, control circuitry, and processing circuitry. An array of microLEDs may be used as the light source. The light source generates optical power for delivery at a molecular sample, which is of the order of 100 mW. The imaging spectrometer separates light emitted from the molecular sample into a plurality of different component wavelengths in the range 400 to 1,000

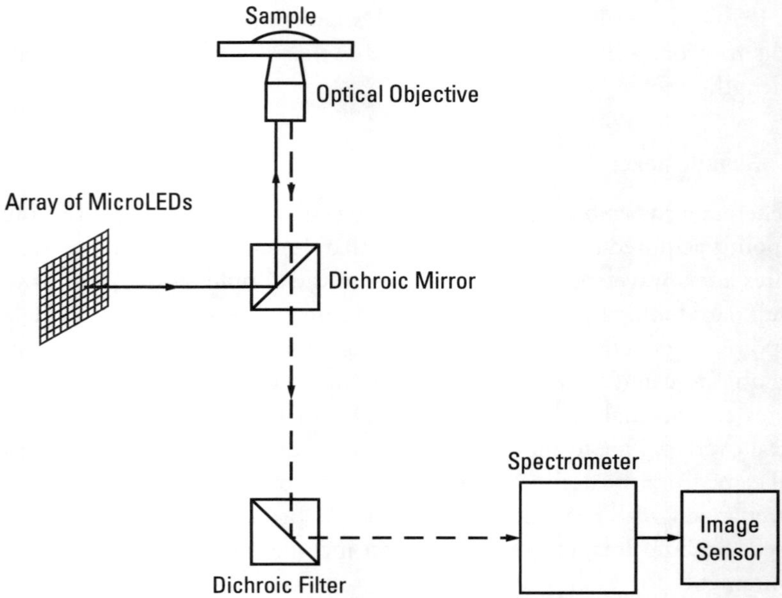


**Figure 9.16** Schematic of an imaging apparatus. The imaging apparatus comprises a light source (array of microLEDs), an imaging spectrometer, an image sensor, control circuitry, and processing circuitry.

nm. The control circuitry causes the image sensor to scan one or more regions of the molecular sample while the imaging spectrometer is aligned with the image sensor and collects hyperspectral image data of the molecular sample from the light emitted that corresponds to the plurality of different component wavelengths. The processing circuitry performs an image processing pipeline by transforming the hyperspectral image data into data that is representative of a quantification of emitters, absorbers, and/or scatterers present in the one or more regions of the molecular sample.

The hyperspectral imaging apparatuses described above can be used to extract a large amount of information from an observed molecular sample. The ability to perform the selection and analysis with the same apparatus can reduce or minimize the risk of cross contamination of the samples due to handling and transport. The detection and real-time analysis can be carried out at video rates. Applications of the method include microscopy, high-throughput in vitro assays, and in vivo imaging. For microscopy, this method can allow rapid-imaging cytometry or rapid identification of rare cell types. For in vitro diagnostics, it can allow accurate use of more labels in large-format assays such as gene or protein arrays, microfluidic droplet arrays, or large-format multiwall plates. For in vivo imaging, it can allow real-time monitoring of multiple-label concentrations.

A key advantage of using microLEDs as light sources for this application is the possibility of using different excitation wavelengths to accommodate the possibility of different responses from different labels in the sample under test. MicroLEDs are compact, low-cost, have a long lifetime, and are easily replaced. The spectral power distribution of a microLED is fairly narrow, with half-bandwidths of about 20 to 30 nm, and can be reduced to ~5 nm using a resonant cavity structure as discussed in Chapter 8. Indeed, microLEDs produce highly saturated, nearly monochromatic light and are ideal for constructing the compact and inexpensive FRET and cytometer devices.

## 9.7 Flow Cytometry

Flow cytometry is a technology that simultaneously measures and then analyzes multiple physical characteristics of single particles, usually cells, as they flow in a fluid stream through a beam of light. The properties measured include a particle's relative size, relative granularity or internal complexity, and relative fluorescence intensity. These characteristics are determined using an optical-to-electronic coupling system that records how the cell or particle scatters incident laser light and emits fluorescence. A flow cytometer is made up of three main systems: fluidics, optics, and electronics. The fluidics system transports particles in a stream to the laser beam for interrogation. The optics system consists of lasers to illuminate the particles in the sample stream and optical filters to direct the resulting light signals to the appropriate detectors. The electronics system converts the detected light signals into electronic signals that can be processed by the computer. For some instruments equipped with a sorting feature, the electronics system is also capable of initiating sorting decisions to charge and deflect particles. In the flow cytometer, particles are carried to the laser intercept in a fluid stream. Any suspended particle or cell from 0.2–150 $\mu$m in size is suitable for analysis. When particles pass through the laser intercept, they scatter laser light as shown in Figure 9.17. Any fluorescent molecules present on the particle fluoresce. The scattered and fluorescent light is collected by appropriately positioned lenses. A combination of beam splitters and filters steers the scattered and fluorescent light to the appropriate detectors. The detectors produce electronic signals proportional to the optical signals striking them. Data is collected on each particle or event. The characteristics or parameters of each event are based on its light scattering and fluorescent properties. The data is collected and stored in the computer. This data can be analyzed to provide information about subpopulations within the sample.

In conventional flow cytometry, a spatially incoherent single wavelength laser beam is incident on the sample. Due to the scattering of the tissue, the incident beam will form a scattered beam measured at an output as a speckle

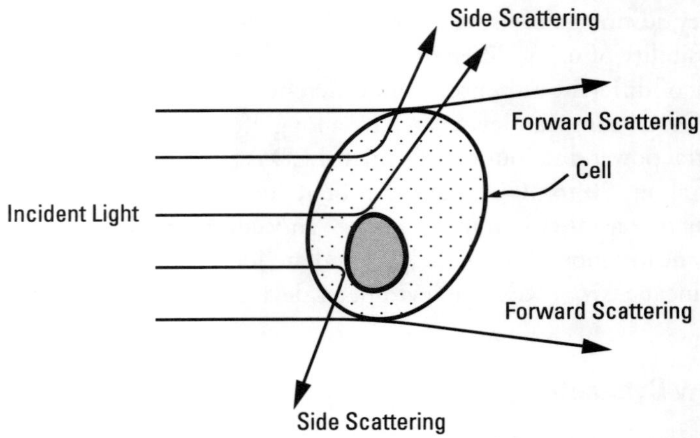


**Figure 9.17** Light scattering properties of a cell. Forward-scattered light is proportional to cell-surface area or size. Side-scattered light is proportional to cell granularity or internal complexity.

pattern. Alternatively, the laser light source may be replaced with a meta microLED (details were given in Chapter 8). A meta microLED has a small but finite linewidth (e.g., 5 nm). The intensity measurements can then be analyzed to derive information, such as cell type or cell count, of one or more cell types of interest. The flow cytometry system based on using meta microLEDs (incoherent light source) is shown in Figure 9.18.

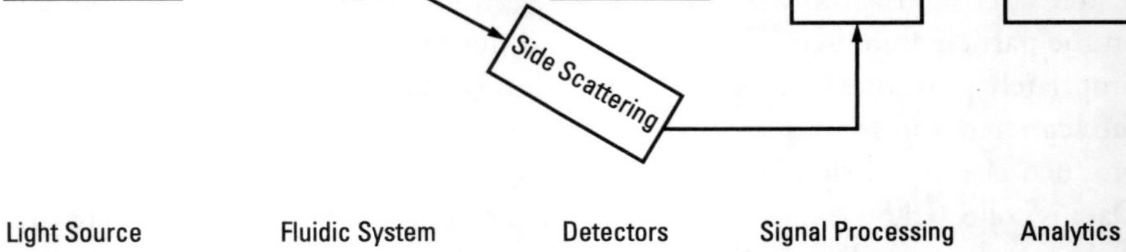


**Figure 9.18** Flow cytometry using meta microLEDs as a light source. Scattered and emitted light signals are converted to electronic pulses. Forward-scattered light (FSC) is proportional to cell-surface area or size. FSC is a measurement of mostly diffracted light and is detected just off the axis of the incident laser beam in the forward direction by a photodiode. Side-scattered light (SSC) is proportional to cell granularity or internal complexity. SSC is a measurement of mostly refracted and reflected light that occurs at any interface within the cell where there is a change in refractive index.

## References

[1] Coyne, K., and S. Coyne, *Brainsteering: The Better Approach to Breakthrough Ideas,* Harper Collins, 2011.

[2] Pease, R., "Maskless Lithography," *Microelectronic Engineering,* Vol. 78, pp. 381–392, 2005.

[3] Jeon, C., E. Gu, and M. Dawson, "Mask-Free Photolithographic Exposure Using a Matrix-Addressable Micropixellated AlInGaN Ultraviolet Light-Emitting Diode," *Applied Physics Letters,* Vol. 86, No. 22, 2005.

[4] Elfström, D., B. Guilhabert, J. McKendry, et al., "Mask-Less Ultraviolet Photolithography Based on CMOS-Driven Micro-Pixel Light Emitting Diodes," *Optics Express,* Vol. 17, No. 26, 2009, pp. 23522–23529.

[5] Suzuki, S., and Y. Matsumoto, "Lithography with UV-LED Array for Curved Surface Structure," *Microsystem Technologies,* Vol. 14, 2008, pp. 1291–1297.

[6] Guijt, R., and M. Breadmore, "Maskless Photolithography Using UV LEDs," *Lab on a Chip,* Vol. 8, No. 8, 2008, pp. 1402–1404.

[7] B. Guilhabert, D. Massoubre, E. Richardson, et al., "Sub-Micron Lithography Using InGaN Micro-LEDs: Mask-Free Fabrication of LED Arrays," *IEEE Photonics Technology Letters,* Vol. 24, No. 24, 2012, pp. 2221–2224.

[8] Kumar, V., and I. Kymissis, "MicroLED/LED Electro-Optical Integration Techniques for Non-Display Applications," *Applied Physics Reviews,* Vol. 10, No. 2, 2023.

[9] Geng, J., "Structured-Light 3D Surface Imaging: A Tutorial," *Advances in Optics and Photonics,* Vol. 3, No. 2, 2011, pp. 128–160.

[10] Zhang, S., "High-Speed 3D Shape Measurement with Structured Light Methods: A Review," *Optics and Lasers in Engineering,* Vol. 106, 2018, pp. 119–131.

[11] Salvi, J., S. Fernandez, T. Pribanic, and X. Llado, "A State of the Art in Structured Light Patterns for Surface Profilometry," *Pattern Recognition,* Vol. 43, No. 8, 2010, pp. 2666–2680.

[12] Ni, Y., S. Chen, Y. Wang, Q. Tan, S. Xiao, and Y. Yang, "Metasurface for Structured Light Projection Over 120* Field of View," *Nano Letters,* Vol. 20, No. 9, 2020, pp. 6719–6724.

[13] Dorrah, A., and F. Capasso, "Tunable Structured Light with Flat Optics," *Science,* Vol. 376, No. 6591, 2022, p. eabi6860.

[14] Izzy, M., M. Virk, A. Saund, J. Tejada, F. Kargoli, and S. Anand, "Accuracy of Endoscopists' Estimate of Polyp Size: A Continuous Dilemma," *World Journal of Gastrointestinal Endoscopy,* Vol. 7, No. 8, 2015, p. 824.

[15] Kaz, A., A. Anwar, D. O'Neill, and J. Dominitz, "Use of a Novel Polyp "Ruler Snare" Improves Estimation of Colon Polyp Size," *Gastrointestinal Endoscopy,* Vol. 83, No. 4, 2016, pp. 812–816.

[16] Visentini-Scarzanella, M., H. Kawasaki, R. Furukawa, et al., "A Structured Light Laser Probe for Gastrointestinal Polyp Size Measurement: A Preliminary Comparative Study," *Endoscopy International Open,* Vol. 6, No. 5, 2018, pp. E602–E609.

[17] Jones, G., and D. Bradshaw, "Resonance Energy Transfer: From Fundamental Theory to Recent Applications," *Frontiers in Physics*, Vol. 7, 2019, p. 100.

[18] Dos Santos, M., W. Algar, I. Medintz, and N. Hildebrandt, "Quantum Dots for Förster Resonance Energy Transfer (FRET)," *TrAC Trends in Analytical Chemistry*, Vol. 125, 2020, p. 115819.

[19] El Khamlichi, C., F. Reverchon-Assadi, N. Hervouet-Coste, L. Blot, E. Reiter, and S. Morisset-Lopez, "Bioluminescence Resonance Energy Transfer as a Method to Study Protein-Protein Interactions: Application to G protein Coupled Receptor," *Biology Molecules*, Vol. 24, No. 3, 2019, p. 537.

[20] Stanisavljevic, M., S. Krizkova, M. Vaculovicova, R. Kizek, and V. Adam, "Quantum Dots-Fluorescence Resonance Energy Transfer-Based Nanosensors and Their Application," *Biosensors and Bioelectronics*, Vol. 74, 2015, pp. 562–574.

[21] Sasmal, D., L. Pulido, S. Kasal, and J. Huang, "Single-Molecule Fluorescence Resonance Energy Transfer in Molecular Biology," *Nanoscale*, Vol. 8, No. 48, 2016, pp. 19928–19944.

[22] Bhuckory, S., J. Kays, and A. Dennis, "In Vivo Biosensing Using Resonance Energy Transfer," *Biosensors*, Vol. 9, No. 2, 2019, p. 76.

[23] Miyawaki, A., J. Llopis, R. Heim, J. McCaffery, J. Adams, M. Ikura, and R. Tsien, "Fluorescent Indicators for Ca2+ Based on Green Fluorescent Proteins and Calmodulin," *Nature*, Vol. 388, No. 6645, 1997, pp. 882–887.

[24] Jares-Erijman, E. A., and T. Jovin, "FRET Imaging," *Nature Biotechnology*, Vol. 21, 2003, p. 1387.

[25] Gust, A., A. Zander, A. Gietl, et al., "A Starting Point for Fluorescence-Based Single-Molecule Measurements in Biomolecular Research," *Molecules*, Vol. 19, 2014, p. 15824.

[26] Förster, T. H., *Action of Light and Organic Molecules*, New York: Academic Press, 1965.

# 10

# Epitaxial Growth of III-Nitride Light-Emitting Diodes

There are many great books on epitaxy of III-N materials (e.g., [1–4]). This chapter presents a systems engineer's perspective on epitaxial growth technologies for III-N that are important for making microLEDs.

For III-N epitaxial growth, both MOCVD and MBE have been standard methods. So far, MOCVD has been mostly used for GaN-based optoelectronic and electronic devices and utilizes metalorganic precursors for group-III elements (Ga, Al, and In) and nitrogen precursor, typically ammonia ($NH_3$), which are transported with $H_2$, $N_2$, or those mixed gas as carrier gas into a growth chamber. The metal-organic precursors are trimethylgallium (TMG), trimethylaluminium (TMA), and trimethylindium (TMI) for gallium, aluminum, and indium elements, where they react with $NH_3$ on the surface of a substrate for formations of GaN, AlN, and InN.

## 10.1 MBE Growth

MBE can be considered as a precise form of PVD. Solid source materials are placed in evaporation cells around a centrally placed, heated, substrate. Pressures less than $10^{-5}$ torr ensure that the mean free path of the vapor exceeds practical vacuum chamber dimensions (~1m), the molecular beam condition. UHV conditions are needed to ensure the absence of contamination from residual gases (from the chamber walls, etc.). A few seconds are typically required to grow one monolayer. The technique has been developed very successfully using a practical, empirical approach; thermodynamic analysis is difficult because the various parts of the system (sources, substrate, chamber wall) are at different temperatures.

In the molecular beam epitaxy technique, layers are grown by directing an atomic or molecular beam onto a heated substrate located in an ultrahigh-vacuum environment. The particles in the molecular beam adhere to the substrate, resulting in a lattice-matched layer. The strength or flow rate of the atomic/molecular beams can be adjusted to compensate for differences in the adhesion properties of the constituents making up the epitaxial layers.

Figure 10.1 shows a schematic of an MBE system for the growth of heterostructure devices. The substrate is heated by a molybdenum heating block inside a vacuum chamber held at a pressure of $10^{-7}-10^{-10}$ torr. Diagnostics, such as electron diffraction, mass spectrometer, and Auger analysis, can be

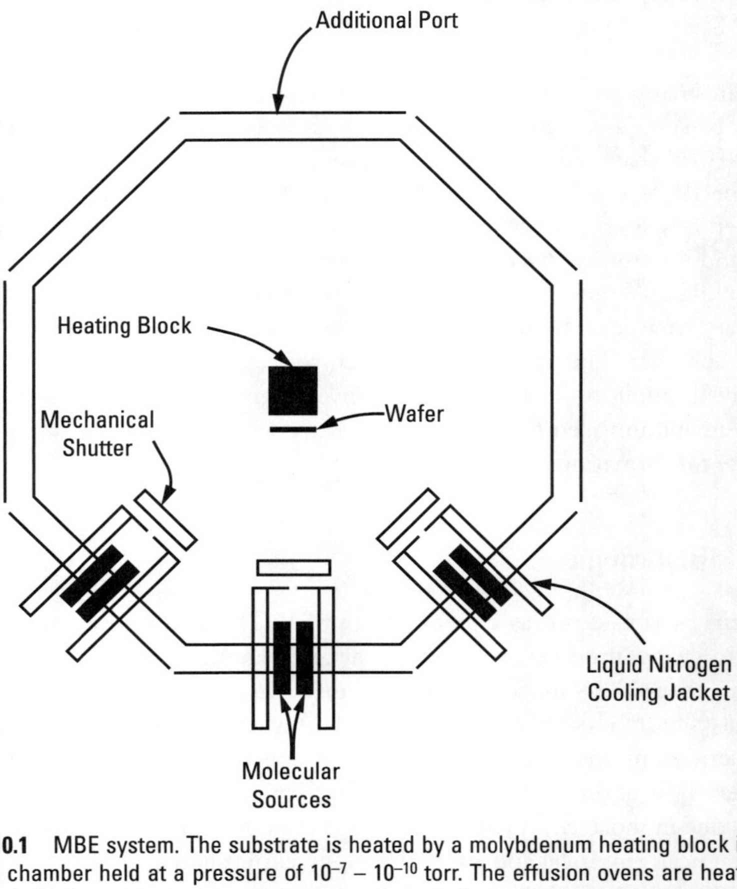


**Figure 10.1** MBE system. The substrate is heated by a molybdenum heating block inside a vacuum chamber held at a pressure of $10^{-7}-10^{-10}$ torr. The effusion ovens are heated to a sufficiently high temperature to generate an adequate beam flux on the substrate surface. The molecular beams can be started or stopped in less than the time it takes to grow a single atomic or molecular layer.

incorporated onto the MBE chamber to characterize the epitaxial layers during growth. The atomic and molecular sources (Ga, GaAs, In, arsine ($As_2$), phosphine ($P_2$), etc.) as well as the n- and p-type dopants are contained in independently heated effusion ovens surrounded by liquid nitrogen shrouds. The effusion ovens are heated to a sufficiently high temperature to generate an adequate beam flux on the substrate surface. The flux rate falls in the range of $10^{12} - 10^{14}$ atoms/(cm-sec) for the growth of heterostructures such as AlGaAs on GaAs. The required flux rate is dependent on the adhesion coefficient (i.e., the fraction of atoms in the beam adhering to the substrate surface). For many of the group III elements, specifically Al or Ga, the adhesion coefficient is nearly unity. On the other hand, the adhesion coefficient differs considerably for group V elements. As a result, the adhesion coefficient must be determined empirically for the range of operating substrate temperatures and beam intensities.

These molecular beams can be started or stopped in less than the time it takes to grow a single atomic or molecular layer. Stoichiometry of the film is controlled both by the substrate temperature and the rates at which the various component species are delivered to the growing film. In order to provide sources of species that cannot be evaporated, metal-organic (MO) sources are sometimes used, a technique called MOMBE.

Because films are grown under UHV conditions, physical and chemical properties of the film can be measured in situ using reflection high-energy electron diffraction (RHEED) and Auger electron spectroscopy (AES) studies, which improves experimental control over the structure of the resulting film. MBE-like technology has been used to grow crystalline films of a wide range of materials III–V semiconductors.

With MBE, the realization that structures of atomic dimensions could be fabricated opened up an entirely new area of condensed matter physics, the experimental investigation of structures exhibiting strong quantum size effects. During the growth of atomic overlayers it is desirable to incorporate dopant atoms in a controlled manner; using MBE, dopant profiles can be engineered on the atomic scale since dopant may be introduced at any time during the layer-by-layer growth. Although this is also true of other surface deposition techniques including CVD, the relatively low growth temperatures involved in MBE inhibit dopant diffusion and preserve atomically abrupt profiles.

In general, MBE is an excellent technique for research applications as well as for specialized devices for which abrupt junctions and thin layers are required but a high wafer volume is not necessarily needed.

### 10.1.1 MBE Growth of III-N Materials

For growth of the nitride semiconductor film by the MBE method, a solid of Ga, Al, In, or the like is preferably used as a group III source. A nitrogen ($N_2$)

gas, an $NH_3$ gas, a mixed gas prepared by adding hydrogen gas ($H_2$) to $N_2$, or the like may be used as a nitrogen source.

For III-nitrides growth with MBE, metal beam fluxes are provided by the conventional Knudsen cells while several different methods are used to provide nitrogen including ammonia, supersonic jet sources, ECR, RF sources, and ion sources. In the case of GSMBE, as was mentioned, ammonia is used as the nitrogen source in spite of its high thermal stability. Since nitrogen incorporation is difficult at low temperature when ammonia is used, plasma cells are widely used to provide the nitrogen species, which are often called plasma-assisted MBE. The generated nitrogen species is chemically so active that the growth temperature of nitrides is low. These kinds of cells include RF plasma cell and ECR. High quality nitride films have been obtained by both kinds of plasma-assisted MBE [5–10].

#### 10.1.1.1 AlN Growth with MBE

MBE growth of AlN films with both crystallographic polarities on nonpolar Si(111) substrates has been demonstrated [11]. The nucleation temperature was found to be responsible for AlN film formation with either Al- or N-face polarity.

#### 10.1.1.2 InN Growth with MBE

The growth of InN is the most problematic among III-nitrides due to its low dissociation temperature. InN epilayers start to decompose at temperatures above about 500°C and In-droplets easily appear on the surface. Once those In-droplets appear on the surface, they disturb the epitaxy itself and it is very difficult to continue the growth. The growth process is limited by the dissociation of InN itself and not by the reevaporation of excess In on the surface.

MBE shows an essential advantage over MOCVD for obtaining high-quality InN that has a low dissociation temperature. Using a very low growth temperature one can avoid the effect of the high equilibrium vapor pressure of N [11]. InN films grown by MBE generally show better crystalline quality than those grown by MOVPE [12–14]. Since most InN films are grown on GaN or AlN template/buffer layers, the polarity of InN is usually determined by the polarity of the GaN or AlN template. It is easy to understand that In polarity is obtained on Ga-polar GaN or Al-polar AlN while N-polarity is obtained on N-polar GaN or AlN. The nondoped InN shows high n-type conductivity. Since nondoped InN has been showing high n-type conductivity up until now, p-type doping is still very difficult.

#### 10.1.1.3 InGaN Growth with MBE

InGaN and InGaN quantum wells are key structures for the active region of LEDs. The energy bandgap of $In_{1-x}Ga_xN$ can be expressed by

$$E_g(x) = (1-x)E_g(\mathrm{InN}) + xE_g(\mathrm{GaN}) - bx(1-x)$$

where, $E_g$(InN) and $E_g$(GaN) are the bandgaps of InN and GaN, respectively, and *b* is the bowing parameter of $In_{1-x}Ga_xN$ . A bandgap bowing parameter of 1.43 eV is obtained by fitting the results of wurtzite In-rich $In_{1-x}Ga_xN$ (x = 0 – 0.5) grown by MBE.

The MBE process for growing InGaN quantum wells involves intricate control over the deposition of InGaN layers with specific indium compositions to create quantum-confined structures. Precise indium and gallium flux control—In, Ga, and N sources—are introduced into the MBE chamber. The growth temperature and flux rates of In and Ga are meticulously controlled to deposit ultrathin layers of InGaN with varying indium compositions. The indium content determines the bandgap energy of the quantum well structure. The growth process might involve the deposition of multiple layers of InGaN quantum wells separated by barrier layers. Each quantum well has a specific indium content, and the barrier layers typically consist of materials like GaN to confine the electrons and holes within the quantum well region. The growth temperature for InGaN quantum wells in MBE typically ranges from around 650°C to 750°C, although it can vary based on specific system configurations and desired material properties. The quality of InGaN on a Ga-polar GaN template was better than that of InGaN grown on an N-polar [15]. Both the hexagonal and cubic InGaN have been grown by MBE. A GaN or AlN buffer layer/template was usually used for the growth of InGaN. The growth of hexagonal InGaN was also influenced by the polarity.

#### 10.1.1.4 GaN Growth with MBE

Since the thermal stability of GaN is much higher than that of InN, the epitaxial temperature of GaN can be increased to higher temperatures up to 850°C. Therefore, the growth process of GaN is limited by the effective supply rate of Ga but not the dissociation of GaN itself. Excess Ga on the surface can be fairly easily reevaporated even after the appearance of Ga droplets. Epitaxy of GaN can be continued even after the appearance of Ga droplets by carefully adjusting the growth conditions to enhance the diffusion of N-species in the Ga droplets, resulting in the growth of GaN even beneath the Ga droplets.

For growth of the gallium nitride film by using $N_2$ and solid Ga, for example, excited plasma is generated by applying a high-frequency magnetic field (e.g., 800–900G) with a frequency of 13.56 MHz to molecular nitrogen ($N_2$). Film formation conditions include a temperature of the sapphire to be used as a substrate of 600°C to 800°C, a nitrogen gas flow rate of 2 to 10 standard cc/min (sccm), an RF power of 200 to 400W, and a treatment time of 30 to 120 min.

A typical growth procedure for a GaN film on c-sapphire using sapphire nitridation by MBE is shown in Figure 10.2. The growth temperatures are example. After thermal cleaning at 900°C and sapphire nitridation at 200°C, the LT-GaN buffer layer is grown at 650°C before the epitaxial growth of the GaN layer at 820°C.

#### 10.1.1.5 Doping of GaN

Doping is an important issue for any semiconductor including the nitrides. Undoped GaN is n-type with the lowest electron concentration at a level of $10^{16}$ $cm^{-3}$. Decreasing the electron concentration has been a very difficult problem in the history of nitride research. The greatest development for nitrides was the achievement of p-type doping by using Mg in the late 1980s.

##### *10.1.1.5.1 N-Type Doping*

Both Si- and Ge-doping are effective for getting high electron concentrations of n- type III-nitrides while Si-doping is more widely used due to its higher solubility in III-nitrides. They substitute for the Ga sites in the GaN and form shallow donors. The activation energy for Si determined by electrical methods was in the range of 12–22 meV. The electron concentration of Si-doped GaN grown by MBE was reported to be above $10^{20}$ $cm^{-3}$. Besides Si and Ge, Se is also used for n-type doping.

##### *10.1.1.5.2 P-Type Doping*

P-type doping of GaN has been difficult for a very long time and much research has been carried out on p-type doping of GaN and its alloys. P-type GaN was achieved first by MOCVD using Mg as a dopant in the late 1980s by Amano et

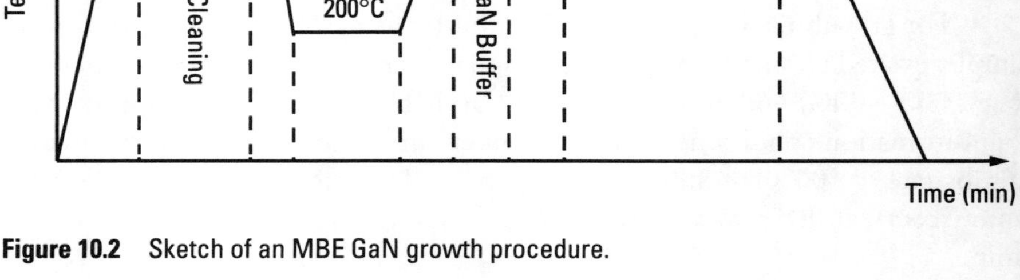


**Figure 10.2** Sketch of an MBE GaN growth procedure.

al. [16, 17]. They found that the Mg-doped GaN could be inverted into p-type GaN by low-energy electron beam irradiation (LEEBI) that might have the same effect as heating the GaN layer as reported by Nakamura et al. Nakamura found that the thermal annealing in vacuum or in nitrogen atmosphere was also effective for obtaining p-type material [18, 19]. It was found that this kind of thermal annealing was necessary for MOCVD-grown GaN in order to activate the Mg. During MOCVD growth, Mg-H complexes are formed, which improves the Mg incorporation. Thermal annealing is effective and necessary for removing the H and to activate the Mg. The activation of Mg impurity by thermal annealing results in a decrease of resistivity by more than 6 orders of magnitude.

The behavior of Mg-doping in MBE-grown GaN is different from that of MOCVD-grown GaN. As-grown Mg-doped GaN is p-type even in an H-containing environment. Thermal annealing is not necessary or does not even change the electrical characteristics of the doped GaN film [20]. The incorporation of Mg depends on the growth conditions of GaN. For example, Mg is easier to incorporate into GaN in N-rich growth conditions and at lower growth temperatures [21]. The larger the flow rate of $NH_3$ the better was the Mg-doping in the case of GSMBE growth. In the MBE growth of GaN the polarity had a large influence on the doping efficiency. Mg is easier to incorporate into Ga-polar GaN in comparison to an N-polar surface. It was reported that up to a factor of 30 times more Mg was incorporated into Ga-polar layers under certain conditions, as determined by secondary ion mass spectrometry [22]. This is different from MOCVD growth because MOCVD-grown GaN is usually Ga-polar. A high flux of Mg may invert the Ga-polarity to N-polarity, which will influence the Mg incorporation. Mg incorporation was reduced by factors of 10 for a lower growth temperature and a factor of 2 for a higher temperature [23]. The maximum Mg concentration they achieved was $3.5 \times 10^{20}$ $cm^{-3}$. Although the hydrogen does not play the same important role in MBE-grown GaN as in MOCVD-growth, the presence of hydrogen did enhance Mg incorporation rates for most growth conditions [22].

There are several reports about the thermal activation energy of Mg in GaN with a generally accepted value of 150–160 meV [24–26].

Other possible p-type dopants include carbon, beryllium, cadmium, and calcium. "Be" is expected theoretically to be a more promising candidate for p-type doping since its ionization energy is calculated to be ~60 meV when residing on Ga-lattice sites in wurtzite GaN [27, 28]. Carbon is generally thought to replace the position of the N atom in GaN and forms an acceptor. It is found that C can readily incorporate under both Ga-rich and N-rich growth conditions. No deterioration of structural quality was observed for the concentration of C between mid-$10^{17}$ and ~$10^{19}$ $cm^{-3}$ [29].

### 10.1.2 MicroLED Stack Growth with MBE

The MBE process for growing GaN-based microLEDs involves a sequence of steps to create epitaxial layers with precise thickness and composition. Here we present a generalized flow of the MBE process for growing GaN-based microLEDs.

The process begins with the selection of a suitable substrate, often sapphire or silicon carbide, which is cleaned thoroughly to remove any contaminants or impurities that could interfere with the epitaxial growth. The clean substrate is loaded into the MBE chamber under ultrahigh vacuum conditions to ensure a pristine environment for the growth process. The substrate is heated to a high temperature and annealed to further cleanse the surface and create a favorable starting point for epitaxial growth. A thin nucleation layer, usually made of materials like GaN or AlN, is deposited onto the substrate surface. This layer helps in achieving better crystalline quality and serves as a foundation for subsequent layers. The MBE system precisely deposits GaN-based semiconductor layers atop the nucleation layer. This involves introducing elemental Ga and N sources into the chamber, where they adsorb onto the substrate surface and form the desired crystal structure. During the growth process, intentional doping with impurities like Si or Mg is performed to modify the electrical properties of specific layers, such as creating p-type or n-type conductivity regions. This step is crucial for microLED functionality. The epitaxial growth process might involve multiple cycles of layer deposition, each with precise control over composition, thickness, and doping concentration to create the different semiconductor layers necessary for microLED operation (e.g., n-type, active, and p-type layers).

The growth temperature ranges in MBE for GaN-based microLEDs can vary based on the specific layer being deposited and the desired characteristics. The nucleation layer is typically grown at a lower temperature (500°C to 800°C) to facilitate the initial crystal formation and improve adhesion between the substrate and subsequent layers. The main GaN layers are deposited at higher temperatures (800°C) to achieve the required crystal quality and thickness for efficient LED operation. Varying growth conditions within this range can affect the defect density and crystal structure.

## 10.2 MOCVD Growth

One class of techniques for growth of group-III nitride structures is MOCVD. Such techniques achieve epitaxial growth by providing flows of precursors for both the group-III element(s) and nitrogen to a processing chamber where thermal processes act to achieve growth of a III-N film. The effectiveness of the growth may depend on a wide array of different factors, notably including the rate at which precursors are flowed into the processing chamber and the environmental conditions within the processing chamber.

In contrast to its main competitor—MBE—MOCVD is extremely hardware-dependent. Even in reactors that are similar but different in size, process development may be different. This poses a challenge for scaling MOCVD reactors from the currently dominant 6" wafer diameters to 12" wafer diameters as required by some applications. Currently most of the market is controlled by two companies: AIXTRON and Veeco. TNSC is a third power, popular in Japan. Figure 10.3 is a simplified diagram of an exemplary MOCVD system, illustrating the basic structure of a chamber in which individual growth steps can be performed. This system is suitable for performing thermal, subatmospheric CVD processes. In some instances, multiple-step processes can still be performed within an individual chamber before removal for transfer to another chamber. The major components of the system include, among others, a vacuum chamber that receives process and other gases from a gas or vapor delivery

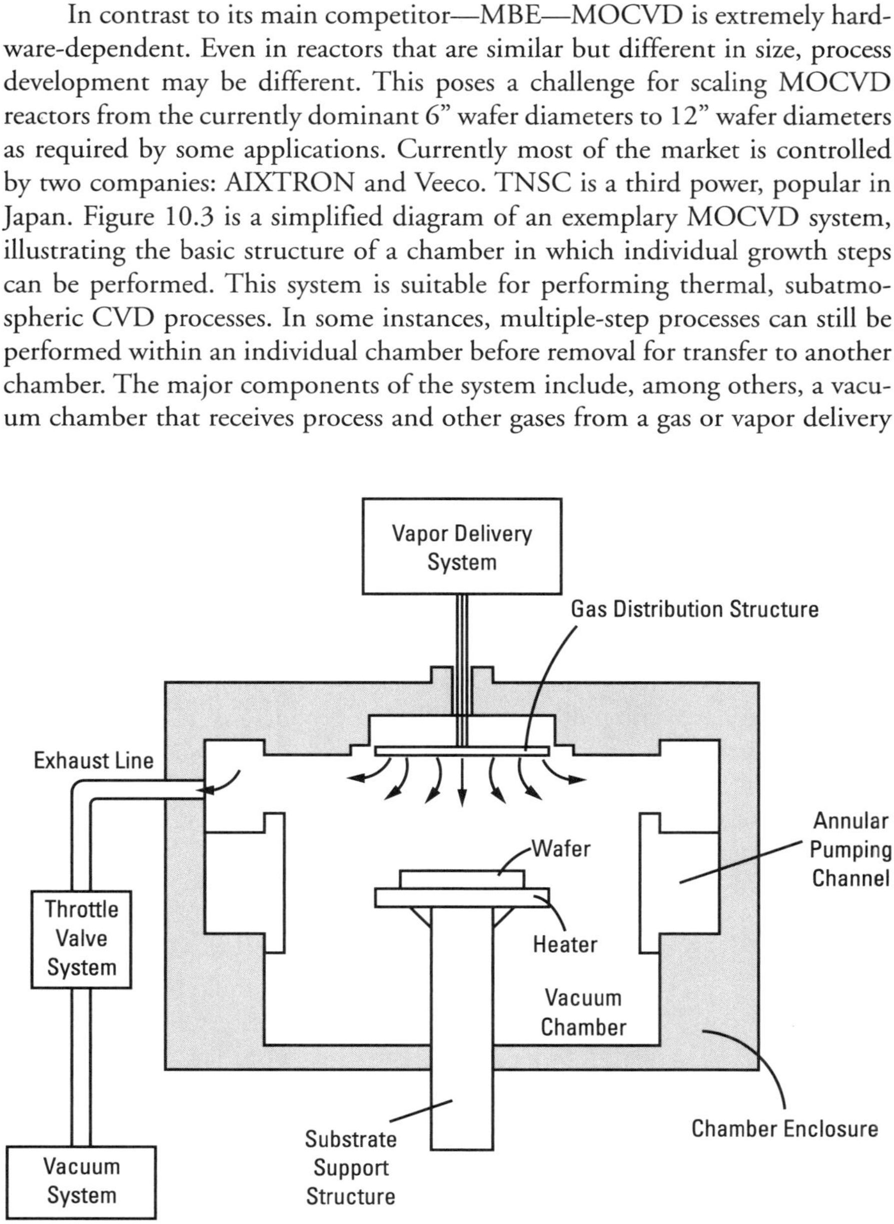


**Figure 10.3** A simplified schematic cross section of an MOCVD growth chamber. Gases are supplied into a vacuum chamber from a vapor delivery system and are distributed via a gas distribution structure (e.g., showerhead). The substrate is heated to a desired temperature and growth/deposition of epitaxial material proceeds.

system, a vacuum system, and a control system (not shown). These and other components are described in more detail below. While the drawing shows the structure of only a single chamber for purposes of illustration, multiple chambers with similar structures may be provided as part of a cluster tool, each tailored to perform different aspects of certain overall fabrication processes.

The MOCVD apparatus includes an enclosure assembly that forms a vacuum chamber with a gas reaction area above a substrate (e.g., wafer). A gas distribution structure disperses reactive gases and other gases, such as purge gases, toward one or more substrates held in position by a substrate support structure. Between the gas distribution structure and the substrate is a gas reaction area. A center board (not shown) includes sensors for providing information on the position of the substrate. Different structures may be used for heaters. For example, the heaters could include an electrically resistive heating element (not shown) enclosed in a ceramic. The ceramic protects the heating element from potentially corrosive chamber environments and allows the heater to attain temperatures up to about 1200°C. All surfaces of heaters exposed to the vacuum chamber are made of a ceramic material, such as aluminum oxide (alumina) or aluminum nitride. The heaters may also comprise lamp heaters. Such lamp heater arrangements are able to achieve temperatures greater than 1200°C, which may be useful for certain specific applications.

Reactive and carrier gases are supplied from the gas or vapor delivery system through supply lines to the gas distribution structure. For example, the supply lines may deliver gases into a gas mixing box to mix the gases before delivery to the gas distribution structure. The supply lines may also deliver gases to the gas distribution structure separately, such as in certain showerhead configurations. The gas or vapor delivery system includes a variety of sources and appropriate supply lines to deliver a selected amount of each source to chamber. Generally, supply lines for each of the sources include shutoff valves that can be used to automatically or manually shut off the flow of the gas into its associated line, and mass flow controllers or other types of controllers that measure the flow of gas or liquid through the supply lines. Depending on the process run by the system, some of the sources may actually be liquid or solid sources rather than gases. When liquid sources are used, gas delivery system includes a liquid injection system or other appropriate mechanism (e.g., a bubbler) to vaporize the liquid. Vapor from the liquids is then usually mixed with a carrier gas. During deposition processing, gas supplied to the gas distribution structure is vented toward the substrate surface, where it may be uniformly distributed radially across the substrate surface in a laminar flow. Purging gas may be delivered into the vacuum chamber from the gas distribution structure and/or from inlet ports or tubes (not shown) through the bottom wall of enclosure assembly. Purge gas introduced from the bottom of chamber flows upward from the inlet port past the heater and to an annular pumping channel. The vacuum system, which includes a vacuum pump (not shown), exhausts the gas through an exhaust line. The rate at which exhaust gases and entrained particles are drawn from the annular pumping channel through the exhaust line is controlled by a throttle valve system.

The temperature of the walls of deposition chamber and surrounding structures, such as the exhaust passageway, may be further controlled by circulating a heat-exchange liquid through channels (not shown) in the walls of the chamber. The heat-exchange liquid can be used to heat or cool the chamber walls depending on the desired effect. For example, hot liquid may help maintain an even thermal gradient during a thermal deposition process, whereas a cool liquid may be used to remove heat from the system during other processes or to limit formation of deposition products on the walls of the chamber. Typical heat-exchange fluids water-based ethylene glycol mixtures, oil-based thermal transfer fluids, or similar fluids. This heating, referred to as heating by the heat exchanger, beneficially reduces or eliminates condensation of undesirable reactant products and improves the elimination of volatile products of the process gases and other contaminants that might contaminate the process if they were to condense on the walls of cool vacuum passages and migrate back into the processing chamber during periods of no gas flow.

A system controller controls activities and operating parameters of the deposition system. The system controller may include a computer processor and a computer-readable memory coupled to the processor. The processor executes system control software, such as a computer program stored in memory. The processor operates according to system control software (program), which includes computer instructions that dictate the timing, mixture of gases, chamber pressure, chamber temperature, pedestal position, and other parameters of a particular process. Control of these and other parameters is affected over control lines that communicatively couple the system controller to the heater, throttle valve, and the various valves and mass flow controllers associated with the gas delivery system.

A class of III-V MOCVD reactors that avoids the need for bubbler temperature control makes use of direct liquid injection. An illustration of a direct-liquid-injection structure that may be used is provided in Figure 10.4 for a single group-III liquid metalorganic source. It will be understood that such a structure may be replicated one or more times for additional sources so that the gas or vapor delivery system shown in Figure 10.3 has access to sufficient sources to implement deposition processes for different materials. The group-III metalorganic liquid is driven into a vaporizer through a flow meter with a push gas provided with a push-gas source. Examples of suitable push gases include $H_2$ or $N_2$, although other push gases may be used. Metering by the flow meter permits the vaporization to be of a known mass of liquid. The vaporizer may also receive a carrier gas from a carrier-gas source, with the vaporized

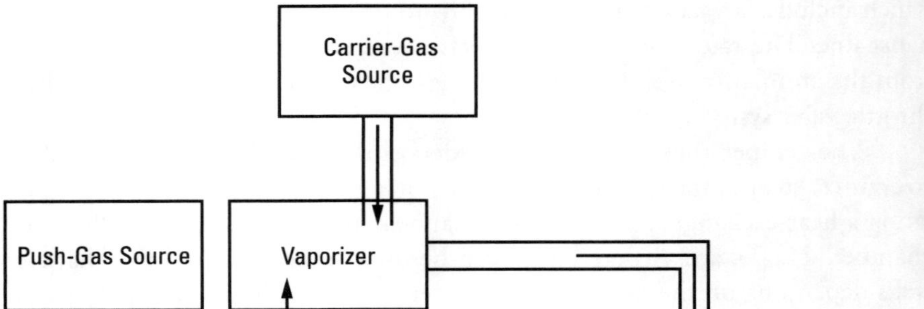


**Figure 10.4** Schematic illustration of the vapor gas delivery system from liquid metal organic precursors.

group-III precursor being delivered with the carrier gas to the processing chamber. Examples of suitable carrier gases also include $H_2$ and $N_2$, although alternative carrier gases may be used.

The use of direct liquid injection may also provide benefits to both the MOCVD growth process and to the quality of material that is grown. For instance, in the growth of III-N films, a more active nitrogen-rich growth ambient may be achieved with direct liquid injection of efficient nitrogen precursor liquids such as hydrazine $N_2H_4$ or its variants dimethylhydrazine ethylenediamine ($C_2H_8N_2$), phenylhydrazine 2,6-dimethylpyrazine ($C_6H_8N_2$), butylhydrazine, 1,4-diaminobutane ($C_4H_{12}N_2$), and so on. Injection of vapor from such precursors in combination with a flow of ammonia $NH_3$ to the processing chamber may reduce the formation of nitrogen vacancies. The formation of nitrogen vacancies is believed to have a generally detrimental effect on the optoelectronic properties of the III-N film that is deposited. Nitrogen vacancies in III-N films are believed to be nonradiative, a hypothesis that results from analogy with vacancies in other III-V semiconductor structures in which the group-V vacancies are known to be nonradiative. The use of direct liquid injection, particularly in combination with a gaseous nitrogen-precursor flow, results in fewer nitrogen vacancies being formed, which in turn causes the overall quantum efficiency of the deposited film to increase. It is also believed that by providing more activated nitrogen for reaction may double the quantum efficiency. This hypothesis is consistent with observations that improved optoelectronic properties are obtained in processes performed at higher $NH_3$ partial pressures.

In the case of deposition of aluminum nitride layers such as AlGaN or InAlGaN, direct liquid injection allows the otherwise strong parasitic gas-phase reaction between TMA and $NH_3$ to be overcome. This is avoided by use of an aluminum precursor in which the bond sites normally available for TMA-$NH_3$ adduct formation are already satisfied.

### 10.2.1 Reduced-Pressure MOCVD

Low-pressure MOCVD (reactor pressure ca. 1–100 torrs) has several desired features for fabricating sophisticated heterostructure devices such as microLEDs [30]. Briefly these are: (1) increased gas flow velocity leading to extremely sharp, high-quality interfaces, (2) reduced auto-doping due to rapid removal of out diffusing species, and (3) lower growth rate (~1 nm/s) permitting increased accuracy in controlling thin (e.g., <10 nm) layers such as the quantum well and quantum barriers.

### 10.2.2 Cluster Tool

The growth methods described below may be performed with a cluster tool (Figure 10.5) having a first housing that defines a first processing chamber and a second housing that defines a second processing chamber. The first processing chamber includes a first substrate holder and the second processing chamber includes a second substrate holder. A robotic transfer system is adapted to transfer substrates between the first and second substrate holders in a controlled environment. A gas delivery system is configured to introduce gases into the first and second processing chambers. A pressure-control system maintains selected pressures within the first and second processing chambers, and a temperature-control system maintains selected temperatures within the first and second processing chambers. A controller controls the robotic transfer system, the gas-delivery system, the pressure-control system, and the temperature-control system. A memory is coupled to the controller and comprises a computer-readable medium having a computer-readable program. The computer-readable program includes instructions for operating the cluster tool to fabricate a compound nitride semiconductor structure.

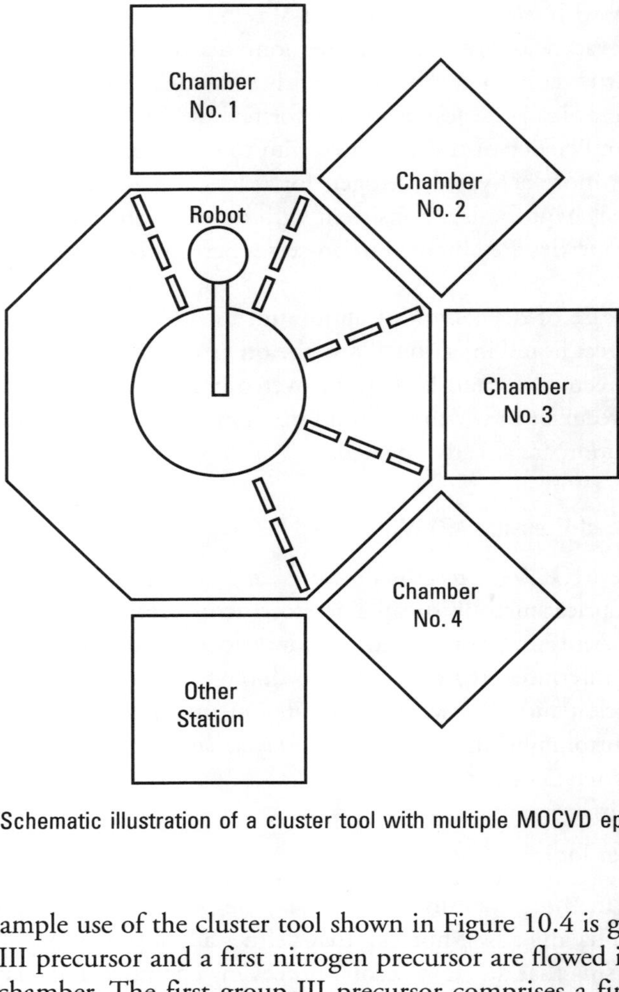


**Figure 10.5** Schematic illustration of a cluster tool with multiple MOCVD epitaxial growth chambers.

An example use of the cluster tool shown in Figure 10.4 is given here. A first group-III precursor and a first nitrogen precursor are flowed into the first processing chamber. The first group-III precursor comprises a first group-III element. A first layer is deposited over the substrate with a thermal chemical-vapor-deposition process within the first processing chamber using the first group-III precursor and the first nitrogen precursor so that the first layer comprises nitrogen and the first group-III element. The substrate is then transferred from the first processing chamber to a second processing chamber different from the first processing chamber after depositing the first layer. A second group-III precursor and a second nitrogen precursor are flowed into the second processing chamber. The second group-III precursor comprises a second group-III element not comprised by the first group-III precursor. The second layer is deposited over the first layer with a thermal chemical-vapor-deposition process within the second processing chamber using the second group-III precursor and the second nitrogen precursor.

The transfer of the substrate from the first processing to the second processing chamber may be done under different conditions. For instance, the transfer is made in an atmosphere having greater than 90% $N_2$; in another instance, it is made in an atmosphere having greater than 90% $NH_3$; and in still another instance, it is made in an atmosphere having greater than 90% $H_2$. The substrate may also be transferred in an atmosphere having a temperature greater than 200°C.

The precursor flows may be accompanied by carrier gas flows, examples of which include $N_2$ and $H_2$. In one embodiment, a third group-III precursor is flowed into the second processing chamber with the second group-III precursor and the second nitrogen precursor. The third group-III precursor comprises the first group-III element. Specific examples of group-III elements that may be used include the use of gallium as the first group-III element and the use of aluminum as the second group-III element, resulting in the first layer comprising a GaN layer and the second layer comprising an AlGaN layer. In another specific example, the first group-III element is gallium and the second group-III element is indium, resulting in the first layer comprising a GaN layer and the second layer comprising an InGaN layer. In still another specific example, the first group-III element is gallium and the second group-III element includes aluminum and indium, resulting in the first layer comprising a GaN layer and the second layer comprising an AlInGaN layer.

A transition layer may sometimes be deposited on the first layer in the second processing chamber before depositing the second layer. The first processing chamber may advantageously be adapted to provide rapid growth of material comprising nitrogen and a group-III element. The second processing chamber may advantageously be adapted to provide enhanced uniformity of deposited material comprising nitrogen and a group-III element.

A structure that may be grown using the cluster tool shown in Figure 10.5 is shown in Figure 10.6, although it is preferred that the entire layer stack is grown in a single run rather than assigning each layer to a single process in a separate growth chamber. This means frequent cycling of gas flows, pressure, and growth temperatures is required during a growth run with typical process temperatures for nitrides ranging from about 500°C to 1200°C and pressures from 50 mbar to nearly atmospheric pressure. To achieve acceptable quality of the films the growth is performed with high precursor flow such as $NH_3$ and TMG, and hence high partial pressures. A commonly used measure is the V/III-ratio, which relates the molar flow of the precursor elements, for example the molar ratio between the $NH_3$ and TMG. The V/III-ratio used for GaN film growth is in the range of 1,000–10,000. The significant disparity of thermal stability between group-III metalorganics and ammonia and the need for preserving the integrity of the solid film at high growth temperatures by sufficient

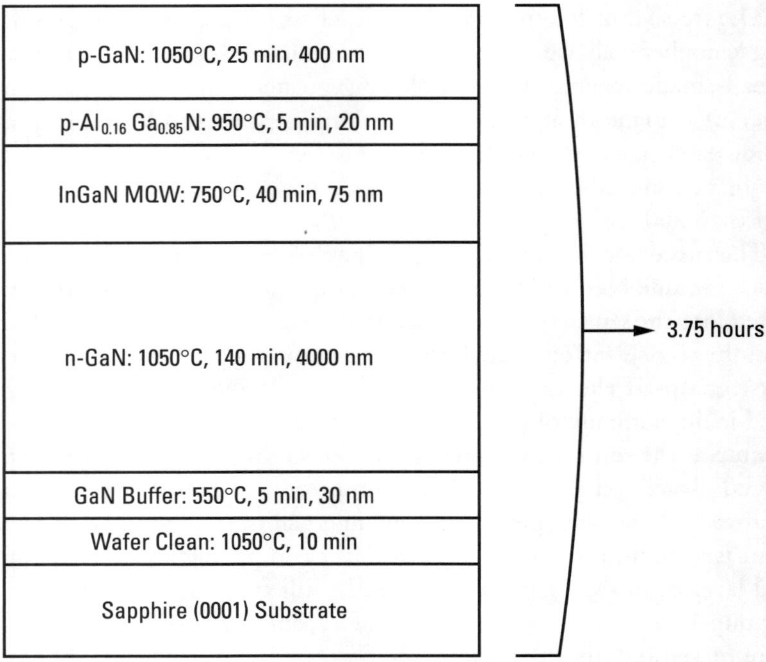


**Figure 10.6** Schematic cross section of a microLED stack, with typical layer thickness and growth time. A typical microLED epitaxial stack may take about 3–4 hours to grow.

partial pressures of $NH_3$ are among the causes for typically high V/III inlet ratios [31].

### 10.2.3 Substrate Effect on Growth

Nonconductive sapphires have been extensively used as substrates for GaN layers grown by a MOCVD technique. A lattice mismatch of about 15% between the GaN and sapphire layers means a buffer layer is needed for lateral growth of GaN on the sapphire substrate. The best buffer layer discovered was an AlN layer deposited at a relatively low temperature, and the use of this layer made it possible for epitaxial growth of an GaN layer with a mirrorlike surface. Although a lattice mismatch of about 2.5% exists between GaN and AlN, the AlN buffer layer was believed to enhance GaN nucleation and growth due to a relatively low AlN/GaN interface energy. Other nucleation layers have been demonstrated such as TiN and HfN. For example, MOCVD-grown GaN layers have been demonstrated on metallic TiN buffer layers deposited on sapphire substrates [32–35]. Three important conditions were found: (1) the sapphire substrate surface plane should be $(11\bar{2}0)$, (2) the TiN layer surface plane should be (111), and (3) the TiN buffer layer nitrogen content should be higher than that of stoichiometric TiN. Reduction of TiN layer thickness reduced TiN buffer layer surface roughness. Threading dislocation density in GaN layers grown on TiN buffer layers was much lower than that in GaN layers grown on AlN. Another example is the growth of MOCVD GaN on hafnium nitride (HfN(111)). HfN has the NaCl-type structure, a lattice constant of 0.452 nm, and a mismatch of only +0.35% for GaN(0001). It is a refractory metal and has been studied as a diffusion barrier in Si technology. Due to the small (0.02%) mismatch for the coincident-site lattice involving 6 HfN unit cells and 5 Si unit cells, HfN can be grown epitaxially on Si [36]. Like AlN, HfN is stable with regard to formation of $Si_3N_4$, but should offer better diffusion resistance. One unexpected benefit is the use of HfN or TiN as a laser release layer when transferring microLEDs from growth wafer to another substrate.

Finally, although most GaN growth efforts on Si focused on the (111) surface due to its hexagonal symmetry, Si(001) is more commonly used in microelectronics. However, GaN grown on Si(001) often results in a mixture of wurtzite- and zincblende-structure grains [37].

### 10.2.4 Selective Area Growth

Selective area growth (SAG), also referred to as selective area epitaxy (SAE) or selective epitaxy, is a technique for growing an epitaxial layer solely in some selected part of a substrate; these areas are defined by windows cut through a mask layer (see Figure 10.7). At appropriate conditions growth proceeds only in the mask windows where the crystalline substrate surface is uncovered. The growth material is supplied by various paths. In addition to direct impingement of species on the windows area diffusion provides additional material. A basic requirement for selective epitaxy is the suppression of growth on the mask. Such conditions are favored by a large diffusion length and a small sticking coefficient of adatoms on the mask. Growth conditions and mask material must then appropriately be chosen to obtain the essential selectivity. Precursor molecules used in MOCVD have much smaller sticking coefficients than elemental particles used in MBE; the selectivity in MOCVD is hence much larger than in MBE, and usually polycrystalline growth on the mask is observed in MBE in addition to epitaxial growth in the windows [1].

Selective area growth of GaN has been studied extensively since the 1990s to reduce the dislocations density in GaN films. From dot patterned GaN openings, Akasaka et al. showed GaN columns growth with the diameter of 5 $\mu$m [38]. Hersee et al. reported array fabrication of GaN wires sized by 221 nm using selective area growth. It was described that pulsed growth had to be used for growing GaN nanowires to confine the lateral growth [39]. Pulsed growth is also referred to as migration enhanced growth. The method may be described as a two-step method comprising an initial nanowire growth step

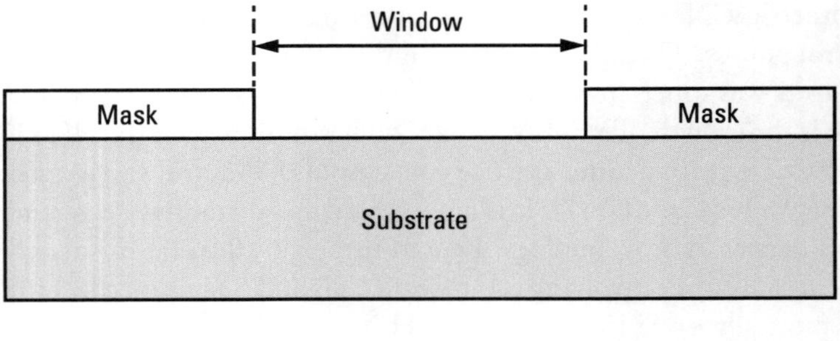


**Figure 10.7** Schematic showing the concept of selective epitaxial growth. Reactive species provided by the MOCVD or MBE systems reach the substrate via two paths: (1) direct impingement, and (2) diffusion along the mask. (Adapted from [1].)

referred to as a selective growth step wherein both precursor gases are provided. The initial growth step is followed by a secondary step of pulsed growth wherein precursor gases are provided one at the time. However, successful nanowire growth can be achieved without pulsed growth through decreasing $NH_3$ flow rate, thus controlling the supersaturation [40].

### 10.2.5 Low-Temperature MOCVD Epitaxy

Historically, III-N MOCVD films have used $NH_3$ for fabrication of optoelectronic devices such as microLEDs. However, lower thermal budgets needed to make InGaN films with high indium mole fractions for red emission have exposed limitations with ammonia usage in light-emitting diode processing. Specifically, growth rates for InGaN films deposited with ammonia at reduced temperatures are prohibitively slow (e.g., ~0.01 nm/s at 400°C) and grossly inefficient in ammonia usage. A more reactive nitrogen source can enable acceptable growth rates at temperature lower than ~650°C, where alloy stability is significantly increased and nitride source to precursor ratio can be reduced [41]. For example, gaseous hydrazine ($N_2H_4$), which is significantly more reactive than ammonia, has been considered theoretically and experimentally [42–48]. Replacement of ammonia had not occurred due to the lack of safety and purity of commercially available hydrazine. A safer solution for the delivery of hydrazine into MOCVD reactors could enable low-temperature epitaxy of III-N materials. Low-temperature (LT) MOCVD growth, however, has been associated with unintentional impurity incorporation. LT GaN grown with dimethylhydrazine exhibited lower-quality films with higher impurity incorporation compared to LT GaN grown with ammonia [45]. Pulsed growth methods using standard precursors have also been investigated as a more viable approach to LT GaN [49] and LT InGaN [50]. It remains to be seen if high-quality InGaN quantum-well-grade films can be grown with high indium mole fraction as needed for making efficient red GaN-based microLEDs.

## 10.3 Epitaxy Cost of Ownership

The cost of ownership of microLED epitaxial growth equipment such as MOCVD or MBE contributes substantially to the microLED system cost. This is due, in part, to the low throughput of the epitaxial growth technology for MBE (maximum growth rate ~4 $\mu$m/h), or the use of costly, highly refined chemical precursors for MOCVD.

For MBE, material consumption represents approximately 25% of the cost of ownership (CoO), while equipment depreciation represents ca. 45% of the CoO [4]. This has led to prohibitively high capital expense that has prevented its use in relatively low-cost LED manufacturing. Recently, a linear MBE (LMBE) design was proposed to alleviate some of these concerns by replacing a single, multipurpose MBE growth chamber with a continuous line of interconnected chambers, each whose purpose is to grow a separate layer needed in a III-V solar cell [51]. The in-line system is connected at opposite ends by rapid wafer loading and unloading chambers. Production cost for archetype single-junction GaAs solar cells was estimated to reduce from $25/Wp for conventional MBE to $14/Wp using LMBE. However, this is still much higher than MOCVD-based manufacturing cost of ~$5/Wp. It remains to be seen if LMBE can be used for III-nitride devices such as microLEDs.

The multiwafer planetary MOCVD reactors with ever-higher productivity results in significant dependence of the cost of ownership of MOCVD on the efficient utilization of the precursor materials, the depositable wafer area, the uniformity across the wafers, their reproducibility from wafer to wafer and run to run, and the number of runs per day [52]. For MOCVD, the precursor utilization efficiency is defined as the ratio of group III atoms incorporated into the grown layers to the number of group V atoms entering the reactor through the metal-organic sources. Optimizing the reactor's growth efficiency for novel geometries is a time-consuming process that has to take into account details relating to both reactor hardware and process parameters. High efficiencies are frequently achieved by adjusting the parameters that also affect film thickness uniformity, so the solution must balance optimizing the efficiency while ensuring high levels of uniformity for all relevant materials within the microLED structure. For example, GaN is deposited by MOCVD using trimethylgallium, $Ga(CH_3)_3$, and ammonia, $NH_3$, at 800°C to 1000°C. The kinetics of the decomposition chemistry between the two precursors is highly mismatched: $NH_3$ has a very slow decomposition compared to the decomposition of $Ga(CH_3)_3$ to $GaCH_3$. This forces the use of very high N/Ga precursor ratios (500–1,000) for MOCVD of high-quality GaN, leading to 99.9% of the $NH_3$ used in GaN MOCVD ending up as a waste gas, neutralized by bubbling through large amounts of acid to abate it. Given that $NH_3$ is manufactured by the energy-consuming Haber-Bosch process, the GaN MOCVD process—an essential process for low energy consumption—is far from sustainable [53]. The price of TMI is ~$12/g, the price of TMG is ~$1/g, the TMG, TMI material utilization rate is approximately 30%, and price of $NH_3$ is ~$2/kg. Prices can vary widely depending on the production location and company's leverage and supply chain. Such high dependence of CoO of MOCVD epitaxy on precursor cost might change with the migration to single-large-wafer epitaxial reactors to meet cost requirements of microLEDs driven by wafer size.

The other factor that strongly impacts the CoO is yield, which can be considered in terms of microLED chips. The epitaxy process influences the uniformity of microLED properties on each wafer and from wafer to wafer. MicroLED materials such as InGaN and AlGaInP are more growth temperature dependent. Functional yield requirements for making microLED displays is 99.9999% or higher without using redundancy. The use of redundancy can reduce this requirement to only 99.9%, alleviating the requirements on growth temperature uniformity, and would reduce the CoO [54].

An exact comparison of the cost of ownership of MBE and MOCVD is not straightforward [55, 56]. MBE has longer individual campaigns (e.g., 6–12 months [4]) with less setup time variability. MOCVD has shorter maintenance periods and more flexibility for source and reactor configuration changes. MBE has a lower material cost per wafer. MOCVD has a higher safety risk, increasing scrutiny of legislative bodies worldwide. MBE's overhead time does not scale with run rate and contribution per wafer increases with wafer volume. MOCVD's overhead scales with run rate.

More research is needed to determine whether microLED costs are primarily driven by capital expenses related to a particular growth technology (MBE versus MOCVD), or by other potentially less cost-elastic sources.

## 10.4 Nanowire Light-Emitting Diode Growth

Bottom-up InGaN-based nanostructures (e.g., nanowires) offer an alternative approach to overcome the efficiency cliff of microLEDs in the visible spectrum. The bottom-up approach has a major advantage over a top-down etching approach due to the reduced density of surface defects at the edge of the device mesa, commonly associated with plasma-based etching of nitrides. Compared with the conventional planar structure, structures based on GaN nanowire arrays have a number of advantages. A nanowire size of less than a few hundred nm can help completely eliminate the threading dislocations formed during homoepitaxial growth. Therefore, the crystal quality of GaN nanowires can be improved much higher than that of the conventional planar structure. Also, because of the small dimensions of nanowires, the lateral strain relaxation in nanowires on either the top or sidewall plane can lead to a higher level of indium incorporation during InGaN/GaN MQW growth. In addition, the growth of c-axis-oriented GaN nanowires can lead to nonpolar or semipolar planes on either the sidewall or slanted plane. The commonly used conventional planar c-plane InGaN/GaN microLEDs on sapphire substrates suffer from acute piezoelectric polarization due to the large lattice mismatch between GaN and InGaN, which leads to the QCSE and results in decreased radiative recombination efficiency, as is widely known. However, the exposed nonpolar planes (m-planes) of GaN nanowire arrays are known to eliminate piezoelectric polarization, which can dramatically reduce the QCSE in the quantum well.

GaN nanowire arrays are typically grown by MOCVD and MBE. In many previous studies on catalyst-free MOCVD with SAG, Ga-polar GaN nanowire arrays were successfully grown on a GaN template. N-polar GaN nanowires also have recently been successfully grown on a GaN template by constant-mode MOCVD growth. The pulsed-mode MOCVD growth technique was first introduced by Hersee et al. in 2006 [57]. Since then, many research groups have used this technique to successfully to form GaN nanostructures in hexagonal rod shape with six $\{1\bar{1}00\}$ m-planes forming the vertical sidewalls of the structures on a GaN template. For example, successful selective growth of vertically well-aligned Ga-polar GaN nanowire arrays on c-plane GaN templates by a pulsed-mode MOCVD technique was reported and the growth mechanism was explained [58]. Because elemental Ga is more reactive with most mask surfaces, it took longer to develop selective epitaxy processes for MBE. Initial attempts with $SiO_2$ masks and Al pedestal regions produced differences in nucleation density but not true selectivity. Better results have been obtained with titanium (Ti) masks that are intentionally converted to titanium nitride (TiNx) in situ, and this method was found critical in obtaining consistent diameters in nanowires [59–61]. It has also been shown that through varying the size and spacing of nanowires that the incorporation of indium can be tuned in a single growth step, potentially enabling the monolithic growth of multicolor devices [62–65]. Aledia reported the growth of blue-emitting core-shell nanowire LEDs on silicon wafers (8" and 12" diameters) using MOCVD growth technology [66]. For axial nanowire LEDs, MBE is used to grow InGaN/GaN MQW and p-type GaN on c-plane of template n-type GaN nanowire [67, 68].

The two different commonly reported structure for nanowire LEDs are shown in Figure 10.8. The core-shell (coaxial) nanowire structures can be fully grown using MOCVD. So far, the axial nanowire structure has been demonstrated using only MBE. Since axial nanowires can provide a solution for augmented reality/mixed reality display solutions with its monolithic RGB, directional emission, and high brightness, developing a process based on the MOCVD technique will be of great value.

A number of startup companies have publicly discussed their nanowire LED technologies including Glo [69–71], Aledia [66, 72], and NS Nanotech [73–76].

### 10.4.1 Growth of Core-Shell Nanowire LED

A core-shell nanowire LED is typically based on a p-n- or a p-i-n-junction. The difference between a p-n junction and a p-i-n-junction is that the latter has a wider active region. The wider active region allows for a higher probability of recombination in the i-region. Each nanowire comprises a first conductivity type (e.g., n-type) nanowire core and an enclosing second conductivity type (e.g., p-type) shell for forming a p-n or pin junction that in operation provides an active region for light generation. While the first conductivity type of the core is described herein as an n-type semiconductor core and the second conductivity type shell is described herein as a p-type semiconductor shell, it should be understood that their conductivity types may be reversed.

In principle, one single nanowire is enough for forming a nanowire LED, but due to the small size, nanowires are preferably arranged in arrays comprising hundreds, thousands, or tens of thousands or more of nanowires side by side to form the LED structure. For illustrative purposes the individual nanowire LED devices will be described herein as being made up from nanowire LEDs having an n-type nanowire core and a p-type shell at least partly enclosing the nanowire core and an intermediate active region, which may comprise a single intrinsic or lightly doped (e.g., doping level below $10^{16}$ $cm^{-3}$) semiconductor

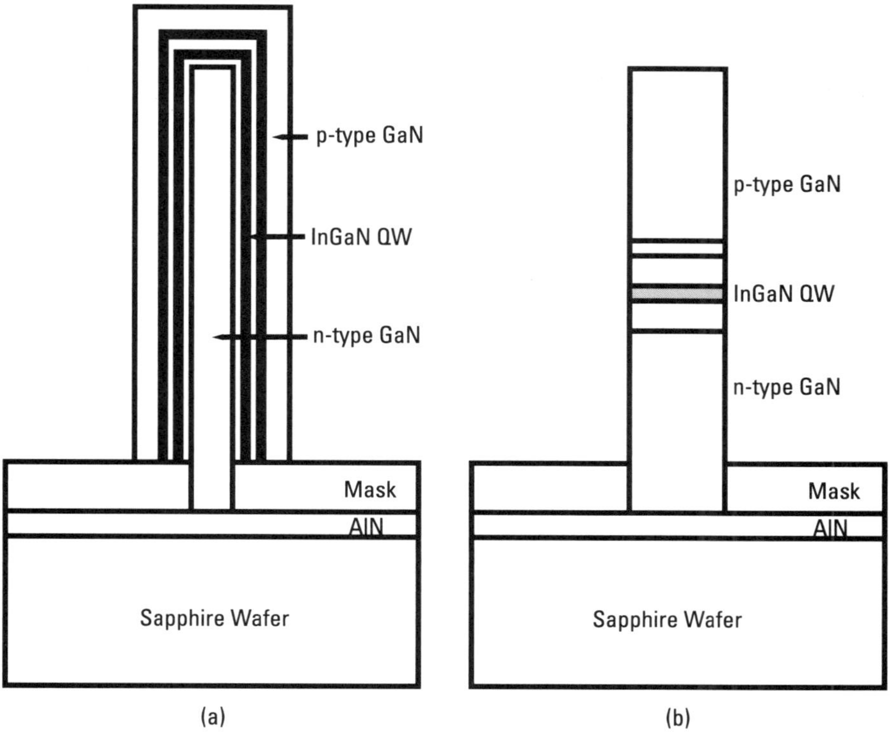


**Figure 10.8** (a) Schematic illustration of a single core-shell nanowire structure. The core–shell configurations are practically impossible to realize with MBE due to the shadowing problem inherent in this high-vacuum deposition. The MOCVD technology does not suffer from this limitation and is therefore the preferred choice for development of NW-LEDs on an industrial scale. (b) Schematic illustration of a single axial nanowire structure. The axial nanowire configurations are practically difficult to realize with MOCVD. The MBE is the preferred choice for growing axial nanowire LEDs.

layer or one or more quantum wells, such as 3–10 quantum wells comprising a plurality of semiconductor layers of different thicknesses and gaps.

Preferably, the substrate is adapted to function as a current transport layer connecting to the die n-side of each nanowire LED. This can be accomplished by having a substrate that comprises a semiconductor buffer layer arranged on the surface of the substrate facing the nanowire LEDs, as shown Figure 10.8 by way of example, a III-nitride laver, such as a GaN and/or AlGaN buffer layer on a Si substrate. The buffer layer is usually matched to the desired nanowire material and thus functions as a growth template in the fabrication process. For an n-type core, the buffer layer is preferably also doped n-type. The buffer layer may comprise a single layer (e.g., GaN), several sublayers (e.g., GaN and AlGaN) or a graded layer that is graded from high Al content AlGaN to a lower Al content AlGaN or GaN.

The method for growing catalyst-free nanowire core involves the growth mask on the buffer layer. Openings are then formed in the growth mask to expose the buffer layer. The openings are preferably well controlled, both in regard to their diameter and their relative positioning. Several techniques known in the art can be used for the procedure, including, but not limited to, electron beam lithography, nanoimprint lithography, optical lithography, and reactive ion etching (RIE) or wet chemical etching methods. The openings are about 100–400 nm and pitched 500–5000 nm apart. The openings define the position and the diameter of the nanowire cores to be produced. Then, the nanowire cores are grown by a MOCVD or MBE. The theory of catalyst-free nanowire growth is discussed in the literature [77–79]. In the MOCVD-based process, the precursor source flows are continuous or pulsed. The precursor source flow rates are adjusted to achieve a low supersaturation in the growth zone. The V/III-ratio should be 100 or less. It should be noted that this V/III-ratio is considerably lower than the ratios used for bulk film growth. In other words, the nanowire core is grown at a low V/III ratio at a relatively low temperature (e.g., below 800°C). Then, one or more shells shown in Figure 10.8 are grown on the core by increasing the temperature above 800°C, such as 900°C–1200°C, increasing the V/III ratio to a higher amount than that used for the core growth (e.g., a V/III ratio higher than 100, such as 200–1,000). For example, the n-GaN nanowire core may be grown by MOCVD using $NH_3$ and TMG gas sources and an optional doping source gas (e.g., a Si containing source gas). The $NH_3$ flow rate may be 0.2 to 3.0 sccm during core growth and 50 to 100 sccm during shell growth. TMG flow rate may be between 0.12 and 1.2 $\mu$mol/min, for example.

If desired, an intermediate n-GaN shell may be formed on the n-GaN core before forming the active region shell. The n-GaN shell may be formed at the high temperature (above 800°C, such as 900°C–1200°C) and high V/III ratio higher than 100, such as 200–1,000. This shell is shown in Figure 10.8(a) and has a smooth (i.e., straight) outer sidewall (i.e., the m-plane radial sidewall). When the quantum well active region shell is formed on a smooth radial surface of the intermediate n-GaN shell, a low number of defects result, which helps improve the quality of the active layer shells grown on the n-GaN shell and the internal quantum efficiency. Finally, an EBL made of AlGaN and a p-type GaN shell are grown to finish the p-i-n structure shown in Figure 10.8(a).

Different additional layers may be deposited on the p-electrode. For example, layers that improve electrical conductivity or coupling of light out from/into the nanowire may be deposited on the nanowire.

For a top emitting device, the p-electrode needs to be transparent (i.e., it should transmit the majority of light emitted by the LED). ITO is a suitable material for the p-electrode, in particular for the top emitting nanowire LED. The ITO preferably has a thickness of 500 nm. ITO has also been extensively used for planar components where LED devices are formed by layer-by-layer techniques. In such components the thickness of the ITO layer is preferably about 150 nm since this is enough to obtain an acceptable current spreading. One drawback with increased thickness is that the ITO has a comparatively high absorption of light. Therefore, the ITO thickness is kept as low as possible. Another reason for keeping the ITO thickness low is that the ITO cannot readily be wet etched if too thick (i.e., more than 150 nm). Other suitable materials for a p-electrode on a top emitting device are ZnO, doped ZnO, and other TCOs. Important parameters for this material are good transparency, electrical conductivity, and the ability to make low resistive contact to the shell. High thermal conductivity is also desirable, together with a matching refractive index (depending on configuration).

### 10.4.2 Growth of Axial Nanowire LED

An axial nanowire LED is typically based on a p-n- or a p-i-n-junction, the same as for a core-shell nanowire LED. However, instead of forming the p-n or p-i-n junction along the m-plane as in core-shell nanowire LED, the junction is formed along the c-plane, as shown in Figure 10.8(b).

The method for growing catalyst-free nanowire template involves the growth mask on the buffer layer. Openings are then formed in the growth mask to expose the buffer layer. The openings are preferably well controlled, both in regard to their diameter and their relative positioning. Several techniques known in the art can be used for the procedure including, but not limited, to electron beam lithography, nanoimprint lithography, optical lithography, and reactive ion etching (RIE) or wet chemical etching methods. The openings are about 50-300 nm, and pitched 500–5000 nm apart. The openings define the position and the diameter of the nanowire template to be produced. Then, the nanowire template is grown by a MOCVD or MBE. In the MOCVD based process, the precursor source flows are continuous or pulsed. The precursor source flow rates are adjusted to achieve a low supersaturation in the growth zone. The V/III-ratio should be 100 or less. It should be noted that this V/III-ratio is considerably lower than the ratios used for bulk film growth. In other words, the nanowire template is grown at a low V/III ratio at a relatively low temperature (e.g., below 800°C). For example, the n-GaN nanowire template may be grown by MOCVD using ammonia ($NH_3$) and TMG (trimethylgallium) gas sources and an optional doping source gas (e.g., Silicon containing source gas). If desired, an intermediate n-GaN layer may be formed on the n-GaN template before forming the active region. The n-GaN layer may be formed at a relatively higher temperature (above 800°C) using MBE. This layer should have a smooth top surface (i.e., the c-plane) with low number of defects. When the quantum well active region is formed on a smooth top surface of the intermediate n-GaN layer, less defects and less nonradiative recombination result, which helps achieve higher internal quantum efficiency. Finally, an electron barrier shell layer (EBL) made of AlGaN and a p-type GaN shell are grown to finish the p-i-n structure using MBE technique, as shown in Figure 10.8(b) [68, 80, 82–84].

Much reduced polarization field has been predicted by theory and realized by experiments using axial nanowire architecture [80-85]. When the diameter of the nanowire is less than a critical value, strain is relaxed, which is the root cause for the piezoelectric field in conventional c-plane light-emitting diode structures.

## References


[1] Pohl, U., "Methods of Epitaxy," in *Epitaxy of Semiconductors: Physics and Fabrication of Heterostructures,* Second Edition, Cham, Switzerland: Springer, 2020, pp. 427–467.

[2] Lundin, W., and R. Talalaev, "Epitaxial Systems for III-V and III-Nitride MOVPE," in *Metalorganic Vapor Phase Epitaxy (MOVPE) Growth, Materials Properties, and Applications* (S. Irvine and P. Capper, eds.), Wiley, 2019, pp. 423–466.

[3] Irvine, S., and P. Capper (eds.), *Metalorganic Vapor Phase Epitaxy (MOVPE): Growth, Materials Properties, and Applications,* Wiley, 2019.

[4] O'Steen, M., E. Readinger, S. Farrell, M. Marek, M. Doran, and D. Hanser, "Systems and Technology for Production-Scale Molecular Beam Epitaxy," in *Molecular Beam Epitaxy,* Elsevier, 2018, pp. 649–675.

[5] Mohammad, S., W. Kim, A. Salvador, and H. Morkoç, "Reactive Molecular-Beam Epitaxy for Wurtzite GaN," *MRS Bulletin,* Vol. 22, No. 2, 1997, pp. 22–28.

[6] Torvik, J., M. Leksono, J. Pankove, B. Van Zeghbroeck, H. Ng, and T. Moustakas, "Electrical Characterization of GaN/SiC NP Heterojunction Diodes," *Applied Physics Letters,* Vol. 72, No. 11, 1998, pp. 1371–1373.

[7] Haus, E., I. Smorchkova, B. Heying, et al., "The Role of Growth Conditions on the p-doping of GaN by Plasma-Assisted Molecular Beam Epitaxy," *Journal of Crystal Growth,* Vol. 246, 2002, pp. 55–63.

[8] Heinke, H., V. Kirchner, S. Einfeldt, and D. Hommel, "X-Ray Diffraction Analysis of the Defect Structure in Epitaxial GaN," *Applied Physics Letters,* Vol. 77, No. 14, 2000, pp. 2145–2147.

[9] Lebedev, V., B. Schröter, G. Kipshidze, and W. Richter, "The Polarity of AlN Films Grown on Si (111)," *Journal of Crystal Growth,* Vol. 207, No. 4, 1999, pp. 266–272.

[10] Lu, L., H. Yan, C. Yang, et al., "Study of GaN Thin Films Grown on Vicinal SiC (0001) Substrates by Molecular Beam Epitaxy," *Semiconductor Science and Technology,* Vol. 17, No. 9, 2002, p. 957.

[11] Wang, X., and A. Yoshikawa, "Molecular Beam Epitaxy Growth of GaN, AlN and InN," *Progress in Crystal Growth and Characterization of Materials,* Vol. 48, 2004, pp. 42–103.

[12] Wu, J., and W. Walukiewicz, "Band Gaps of InN and Group III Nitride Alloys," *Superlattices and Microstructures*, Vol. 34, 2003, pp. 63–75.

[13] Bhuiyan, A., A. Hashimoto, and A. Yamamoto, "Indium Nitride (InN): A Review on Growth, Characterization, and Properties," *Journal of Applied Physics*, Vol. 94, No. 5, 2003, pp. 2779–2808.

[14] Nanishi, Y., Y. Saito, and T. Yamaguchi, "RF-Molecular Beam Epitaxy Growth and Properties of InN and Related Alloys," *Japanese Journal of Applied Physics*, Vol. 42, No. 5R, 2003, p. 2549.

[15] Shen, X., T. Ide, M. Shimizu, and H. Okumura, "Growth and Characterizations of InGaN on N-and Ga-Polarity GaN Grown by Plasma-Assisted Molecular-Beam Epitaxy," *Journal of Crystal Growth*, Vol. 237, 2002, pp. 1148–1152.

[16] Amano, H., N. Sawaki, I. Akasaki, and Y. Toyoda, "Metalorganic Vapor Phase Epitaxial Growth of a High Quality GaN Film Using an AlN Buffer Layer," *Applied Physics Letters*, Vol. 48, No. 5, 1986, pp. 353–355.

[17] Amano, H., I. Akasaki, T. Kozawa, et al., "Electron Beam Effects on Blue Luminescence of Zinc-Doped GaN," *Journal of Luminescence*, Vol. 40, 1988, pp. 121–122.

[18] Nakamura, S., N. Iwasa, M. Senoh, and T. Mukai, "Hole Compensation Mechanism of P-Type GaN Films," *Japanese Journal of Applied Physics*, Vol. 31, No. 5R, 1992, p. 1258.

[19] Nakamura, S., T. Mukai, M. Senoh, and N. Iwasa, "Thermal Annealing Effects on P-Type Mg-Doped GaN Films," *Japanese Journal of Applied Physics*, Vol. 31, No. 2B, 1992, p. L139.

[20] Kim, W., A. Botchkarev, A. Salvador, G. Popovici, H. Tang, and H. Morkoc, "On the Incorporation of Mg and the Role of Oxygen, Silicon, and Hydrogen in GaN Prepared by Reactive Molecular Beam Epitaxy," *Journal of Applied Physics*, Vol. 82, No. 1, 1997, pp. 219–226.

[21] Berishev, I., E. Kim, A. Fartassi, M. Sayhi, and A. Bensaoula, "Mg Doping Studies of Electron Cyclotron Resonance Molecular Beam Epitaxy of GaN Thin Films," *Journal of Vacuum Science & Technology A: Vacuum, Surfaces, and Films*, Vol. 17, No. 4, 1999, pp. 2166–2169.

[22] Ptak, A., T. Myers, L. Romano, C. Van de Walle, and J. Northrup, "Magnesium Incorporation in GaN Grown by Molecular-Beam Epitaxy," *Applied Physics Letters*, Vol. 78, No. 3, 2001, pp. 285–287.

[23] Namkoong, G., W. Doolittle, and A. Brown, "Incorporation of Mg in GaN Grown by Plasma-Assisted Molecular Beam Epitaxy," *Applied Physics Letters*, Vol. 77, No. 26, 2000, pp. 4386–4388.

[24] Kim, W., A. Salvador, A. Botchkarev, O. Aktas, S. Mohammad, and H. Morcoç, "Mg-Doped P-Type GaN Grown by Reactive Molecular Beam Epitaxy," *Applied Physics Letters*, Vol. 69, No. 4, 1996, pp. 559–561.

[25] Nakayama, H., P. Hacke, M. Khan, T. Detchprohm, K. Hiramatsu, and N. Sawaki, "Electrical Transport Properties of P-GaN," *Japanese Journal of Applied Physics*, Vol. 35, No. 3A, 1996, p. L282.

[26] T. Tanaka, A. Watanabe, H. Amano, et al., "P-Type Conduction in Mg-Doped GaN and Al0. 08Ga0. 92N Grown by Metalorganic Vapor Phase Epitaxy," *Applied Physics Letters*, Vol. 65, No. 5, 1994, pp. 593–594.

[27] Bernardini, F., V. Fiorentini, and A. Bosin, "Theoretical Evidence for Efficient P-Type Doping of GaN Using Beryllium," *Applied Physics Letters*, Vol. 70, No. 22, 1997, pp. 2990–2992.

[28] Neugebauer, J., and C. Van de Walle, "Chemical Trends for Acceptor Impurities in GaN," *Journal of Applied Physics*, Vol. 85, No. 5, 1999, pp. 3003–3005.

[29] Green, D., U. Mishra, and J. Speck, "Carbon Doping of GaN with CBr4 in Radio-Frequency Plasma-Assisted Molecular Beam Epitaxy," *Journal of Applied Physics*, Vol. 95, No. 12, 2004, pp. 8456–8462.

[30] Duchemin, J., "Low-Pressure MOVPE: The Time of the Pioneers," *Journal of Crystal Growth*, Vol. 601, 2023, p. 126939.

[31] Koleske, D., A. Wickenden, R. Henry, W. DeSisto, and R. Gorman, "Growth Model for GaN with Comparison to Structural, Optical, and Electrical Properties," *Journal of Applied Physics*, Vol. 84, No. 4, 1998, pp. 1998–2010.

[32] Uchida, Y., K. Ito, S. Tsukimoto, Y. Ikemoto, et al., "Epitaxial Growth of GaN Layers on Metallic TiN Buffer Layers," *Journal of Electronic Materials*, Vol. 35, 2006, pp. 1806–1811.

[33] Ito, K., Y. Uchida, S. Lee, et al., "Effects of TiN Buffer Layer Thickness on GaN Growth," *Journal of Electronic Materials*, Vol. 38, 2009, pp. 511–517.

[34] Watanabe, T., K. Ito, S. Tsukimoto, et al., "Growth of GaN on Nitriding TiN Buffer Layers," *Materials Transactions*, Vol. 46, No. 9, 2005, pp. 1975–1978.

[35] Chen, N., W. Lien, C. Shih, P. Chang, T. Wang, and M. Wu, "Nitride Light-Emitting Diodes Grown on Si (111) using a TiN Template," *Applied Physics Letters*, Vol. 88, No. 19, 2006.

[36] Shinkai, S., and K. Sasaki, "Influence of Sputtering Parameters on the Formation Process of High-Quality and Low-Resistivity HfN Thin Film," *Japanese Journal Applied Physics*, Vol. 38, 1999, p. 2097.

[37] Yang, B., A. Trampert, O. Brandt, B. Jenichen, and K. Ploog, "Structural Properties of GaN Layers on Si (001) Grown by Plasma-Assisted Molecular Beam Epitaxy," *Journal of Applied Physics*, Vol. 83, No. 7, 1998, pp. 3800–3806.

[38] Akasaka, T., Y. Kobayashi, S. Ando, and N. Kobayashi, "GaN Hexagonal Microprisms with Smooth Vertical Facets Fabricated by Selective Metalorganic Vapor Phase Epitaxy," *Applied Physics Letters*, Vol. 71, No. 15, 1997, pp. 2196–2198.

[39] Hersee, S., X. Sun, and X. Wang, "The Controlled Growth of GaN Nanowires," *Nano Letters*, Vol. 6, No. 8, 2006, pp. 1808–1811.

[40] Seifert, W., D. Asoli, and Z. Bi, Nitride Nanowires and Method of Producing Such, US Patent 7,829,443, 2010.

[41] Ahmed, K., High Performance Light Emitting Diode and Monolithic Multi-Color Pixel, US Patent 10,957,818, 2021.

[42] Fujieda, S., M. Mizuta, and Y. Matsumoto, "Growth Characterization of Low-Temperature MOCVD GaN–Comparison between N2H4 and NH3," *Japanese Journal of Applied Physics*, Vol. 26, No. 12R, 1987, p. 2067.

[43] Koukitu, A., Y. Kumagai, N. Kubota, and H. Seki, "Thermodynamic Analysis on the MOVPE Growth of Nitride Semiconductors Using Hydrazine," *physica status solidi (b)*, Vol. 216, No. 1, 1999, pp. 707–712.

[44] An, Q., A. Jaramillo-Botero, W. Liu, and W. Goddard III, "Reaction Pathways of GaN (0001) Growth from Trimethylgallium and Ammonia versus Triethylgallium and Hydrazine Using First Principles Calculations," *The Journal of Physical Chemistry C*, Vol. 119, No. 8, 2015, pp. 4095–4103.

[45] Reilly, C., N. Hatui, T. Mates, et al., "Properties of AlN/GaN Heterostructures Grown at Low Growth Temperatures with Ammonia and Dimethylhydrazine," *Crystals*, Vol. 11, No. 11, 2021, p. 1412.

[46] Sartel, C., S. Gautier, S. Hamady, et al., "Low Temperature Homoepitaxy of GaN by LP-MOVPE Using Dimethylhydrazine and Nitrogen," *Superlattices and Microstructures*, Vol. 40, No. 4–6, 2006, pp. 476–482.

[47] Gautier, S., C. Sartel, S. Ould-Saad, J. Martin, A. Sirenko, and A. Ougazzaden, "GaN Materials Growth by MOVPE in a New-Design Reactor Using DMHy and NH3," *Journal of Crystal Growth*, Vol. 298, 2007, pp. 428–432.

[48] Sato, H., H. Takahashi, A. Watanabe, and H. Ota, "Preparation of GaN Films on Sapphire by Metalorganic Chemical Vapor Deposition using Dimethylhydrazine as Nitrogen Source," *Applied Physics Letters*, Vol. 68, No. 25, 1996, pp. 3617–3619.

[49] Muthuraj, V., C. Reilly, T. Mates, S. Nakamura, S. DenBaars, and S. Keller, "Properties of High to Ultrahigh Si-doped GaN Grown at 550°C by Flow Modulated Metalorganic Chemical Vapor Deposition," *Applied Physics Letters*, Vol. 122, No. 14, 2023, p. 142103.

[50] Keller, S., U. Mishra, and S. DenBaars, "Flow Modulation Epitaxy of Indium Gallium Nitride," *Journal of Electronic Materials*, Vol. 26, 1997, pp. 1118–1122.

[51] Lee, B., Thin-Film III-V Devices for Low-Cost Detection and Energy Conversion, Doctoral Dissertation, University of Michigan, https://dx.doi.org/10.7302/3882, 2021.

[52] Christiansen, K., M. Luenenbuerger, B. Schineller, M. Heuken, and H. Juergensen, "Advances in MOCVD Technology for Research, Development and Mass Production of Compound Semiconductor Devices," *Optoelectronics Review*, Vol. 4, 2002, pp. 237–242.

[53] Pedersen, H., S. Barry, and J. Sundqvist, "Green CVD—Toward a Sustainable Philosophy for Thin Film Deposition by Chemical Vapor Deposition," *Journal of Vacuum Science & Technology A*, Vol. 39, No. 5, 2021.

[54] Ahmed, K., "Micro LEDs Efficiency Targets for Displays," *SID Symposium Digest of Technical Papers*, Vol. 50, No. 1, 2019, pp. 125–128.

[55] Pelzel, R., "A Comparison of MOVPE and MBE Growth Technologies for III-V Epitaxial Structures," in *CS MANTECH Conference*, 2013, pp. 105–108.

[56] P. Dapkus, "A Critical Comparison of MOCVD and MBE for Heterojunction Devices," *Journal of Crystal Growth*, Vol. 68, No. 1, 1984, pp. 345–355.

[57] Hersee, S., X. Sun, and X. Wang, "The Controlled Growth of GaN Nanowires," *Nano Letters*, Vol. 6, No. 8, 2006, pp. 1808–1811.

[58] Jung, B., S. Bae, Y. Kato, et al., "Morphology Development of GaN Nanowires using a Pulsed-Mode MOCVD Growth Technique," *CrystEngComm*, Vol. 16, No. 11, 2014, pp. 2273–2282.

[59] Bertness, K., N. Sanford, and A. Davydov, "GaN Nanowires Grown by Molecular Beam Epitaxy," *IEEE Journal of Selected Topics in Quantum Electronics*, Vol. 17, No. 4, 2010, pp. 847–858.

[60] Sekiguchi, H., K. Kishino, and A. Kikuchi, "Ti-Mask Selective-Area Growth of GaN by RF-Plasma-Assisted Molecular-Beam Epitaxy for Fabricating Regularly Arranged InGaN/GaN Nanocolumns," *Applied Physics Express*, Vol. 1, 2008, p. 124002.

[61] Kishino, K., T. Hoshino, S. Ishizawa, and A. Kikuchi, "Selective-Area Growth of GaN Nanocolumns on Titanium-Mask-Patterned Silicon (111) Substrates by RF-Plasma-Assisted Molecular-Beam Epitaxy," *Electronics Letters*, Vol. 44, 2008, p. 819–821.

[62] Sekiguchi, H., K. Kishino, and A. Kikuchi, "Emission Color Control from Blue to Red with Nanocolumn Diameter of InGaN/GaN Nanocolumn Arrays Grown on Same Substrate," *Applied Physics Letters*, Vol. 96, 2010, p. 231104.

[63] Kishino, K., A. Yanagihara, K. Ikeda, and K. Yamano, "Monolithic Integration of Four-Colour InGaN-Based Nanocolumn LEDs," *Electronics Letters*, Vol. 51, 2015, p. 852–854.

[64] Kishino, K., K. Nagashima, and K. Yamano, "Monolithic Integration of InGaN-Based Nanocolumn Light-Emitting Diodes with Different Emission Colors," *Applied Physics Express*, Vol. 6, 2012, p. 012101.

[65] Ra, Y.- H. R. Wang, S. Y. Woo, et al., "Full-Color Single Nanowire Pixels for Projection Displays," *Nano Letters*, Vol. 16, 2016, p. 4608–4615.

[66] Tchoulfian, P., U. Steegmueller, B. Amstatt, M. Broell, and P. Gilet, "GaN-on-Silicon Nanowire Technology for MicroLED Devices," *In Proceedings of SPIE*, Vol. 12441, 2023, pp. 49–52.

[67] Pandey, A., Y. Malhotra, P. Wang, K. Sun, X. Liu, and Z. Mi, "N-Polar InGaN/GaN Nanowires: Overcoming the Efficiency Cliff of Red-Emitting Micro-LEDs," *Photonics Research*, Vol. 10, No. 4, 2022, pp. 1107–1116.

[68] Pandey, A., Y. Xiao, M. Reddeppa, et al., "A Red-Emitting Micrometer Scale LED with External Quantum Efficiency > 8%," *Applied Physics Letters*, Vol. 122, No. 15, 2023.

[69] Monemar, B., B. Ohlsson, N. Gardner, and L. Samuelson, "Nanowire-Based Visible Light Emitters, Present Status and Outlook," in *Semiconductors and Semimetals*, Vol. 94, 2016, pp. 227–271.

[70] Bi, Z., Z. Chen, F. Danesh, and L. Samuelson, "From NanoLEDs to the Realization of RGB-Emitting MicroLEDs," in *Semiconductors and Semimetals*, Vol. 106, 2021, pp. 223–251.

[71] Gardner, N., P. Svensson, Y. Chang, O. Kryliouk, L. Romano, and L. Samuelson, "III-Nitride Nanowire LEDs," in *CLEO: Science and Innovations*, 2013, pp. CF2E-3.

[72] Gilet, P., and I. Robin, "Nanostructures on Silicon to Solve the Active Display Paradigms," in *SID Symposium Digest of Technical Papers*, Vol. 49, No. 1, 2018, pp. 684–687.

[73] Ra, Y., R. Wang, M. Stevenson, S. Coe-Sullivan, and Z. Mi, "Sub-Micron Full-Color LED Pixels for Micro-Displays and Micro-LED Main Displays," in *SID Symposium Digest of Technical Papers*, Vol. 51, No. 1, 2020, pp. 432–435.

[74] Liu, X., Y. Wu, Y. Malhotra, et al., "Submicron Full-Color LED Pixels for Microdisplays and Micro-LED Main Displays," *Journal of the Society for Information Display*, Vol. 28, No. 5, 2020, pp. 410–417.

[75] Stevenson, M., D. Laleyan, Z. Mi, and S. Coe-Sullivan, "Display Technology Responds to COVID-19 Challenges," in *SID Symposium Digest of Technical Papers*, Vol. 52, No. 1, 2021, pp. 863–863.

[76] Pandey, A., Y. Malhotra, M. Reddeppa, et al., "Nanowire Micro-LEDs for Augmented Reality and Virtual Reality (AR/VR) Displays,"in *SID Symposium Digest of Technical Papers*, Vol. 54, No. 1, 2023, pp. 148–150.

[77] Dubrovskii, V., "Modeling Catalyst-Free Growth of III-V Nanowires: Empirical and Rigorous Approaches," *Nanomaterials*, Vol. 13, No. 7, 2023, p. 1253.

[78] Gibson, S., and R. LaPierre, "Model of Patterned Self-Assisted Nanowire Growth," *Nanotechnology*, Vol. 25, No. 41, 2014, p. 415304.

[79] Dubrovskii, V., "Theory of MBE Growth of Nanowires on Reflecting Substrates," *Nanomaterials*, Vol. 12, No. 2, 2022, p. 253.

[80] Park, B., J. Lee, C. Koch, M. Wölz, L. Geelhaar, and S. Oh, "High-Resolution Mapping of Strain Partitioning and Relaxation in InGaN/GaN Nanowire Heterostructures," *Advanced Science*, Vol. 9, No. 22, 2022, p. 2200323.

[81] Pandey, A., J. Min, M. Reddeppa, et al., "An Ultrahigh Efficiency Excitonic Micro-LED," *Nano Letters*, Vol. 23, No. 5, 2023, pp. 1680–1687.

[82] Guo, W., M. Zhang, A. Banerjee, and P. Bhattacharya, "Catalyst-Free InGaN/GaN Nanowire Light Emitting Diodes Grown on (001) Silicon by Molecular Beam Epitaxy," *Nano Letters*, Vol. 10, No. 9, 2010, pp. 3355–3359.

[83] Pandey, A., J. Min, Y. Malhotra, et al., "Strain-Engineered N-Polar InGaN Nanowires: Towards High-Efficiency Red LEDs on the Micrometer Scale," *Photonics Research*, Vol. 10, No. 12, 2022, pp. 2809–2815.

[84] Glas, F., "Critical Dimensions for the Plastic Relaxation of Strained Axial Heterostructures in Free-Standing Nanowires," *Physical Review B*, Vol. 74, No. 12, 2006, p. 121302.

# About the Author

**Khaled Ahmed** received BS and MS degrees in electrical engineering from Ain Shams University, Egypt, in 1991 and 1994, respectively, and a PhD degree in electrical engineering in 1998 from North Carolina State University. Dr. Ahmed joined Intel Corporation in 2015 where he is currently a senior principal engineer and chief technology officer of the Systems Supply Chain group. Dr. Ahmed architected the MicroLED Display program at Intel, inventing key patents in the area of microscopic devices assembly technology and equipment, nanowire and nanopyramid light-emitting diode structures, microLED driving circuits, thin-film transistors, light management technologies including metasurface devices, quantum dot patterning technologies, and display architectures.

Before joining Intel, Dr. Ahmed was with Advanced Micro Devices, Inc., Conexant Systems Inc., Applied Materials, Inc., and Intermolecular, Inc., all in California, from 1997 to 2015. Dr. Ahmed has served as a technical program committee member for the Display Week Conference since 2016 and has won the Semiconductor Research Corporation Best Industry Liaison in 2008. Dr. Ahmed sponsored multiple research programs at Purdue University, Penn State University, University of California San Diego, University of Southern California, and the Indian Institute of Technology Bombay.

Dr. Ahmed has authored over 150 patents (granted and pending) covering technologies such as semiconductor devices, semiconductors manufacturing equipment, microLED device architecture, microLED display architecture, metasurface optical elements for display and photonics applications, and optical interconnects technology. Dr. Ahmed was awarded Intel Top Inventor Awards in 2021, 2022, and 2023.

Dr. Ahmed has authored more than 50 peer-reviewed papers on semiconductor devices, metrology, semiconductor manufacturing equipment, and display technologies.

Dr. Ahmed is known for his strategic thinking and entrepreneurial spirit. He cofounded a company along with others working at JPL/NASA and University of Southern California targeting the manufacturing of III-V photodetectors on 300-mm silicon wafers for lidar and optical interconnect applications.

# Index

## Artech House Applied Photonics Library

Brian Culshaw and Marc Wuilpart, Series Editors

*The ABCs of Fiber Optic Communication,* Sudhir Warier

*Acousto-Optic Signal Processing: Fundamentals and Applications,* Pankaj K. Das and Casimer De Cusatis

*Advanced Optical Communication Systems and Networks*, Milorad Cvijetic and Ivan B. Djordjevic

*Applications of Modern RF Photonics,* Preetpaul Singh Devgan

*Bistabilities and Nonlinearities in Laser Diodes,* Hitoshi Kawaguchi

*Chemical and Biochemical Sensing with Optical Fibers and Waveguides,* Gilbert Boisdé and Alan Harmer

*Coherent and Nonlinear Lightwave Communications,* Milorad Cvijetic

*Coherent Doppler Wind Lidars in a Turbulent Atmosphere,* Viktor Banakh and Igor Smalikho

*Coherent Lightwave Communication Systems,* Shiro Ryu

*Digital Optical Measurement Techniques and Applications,* Pramond Rastogi, Editor

*DWDM Fundamentals, Components, and Applications*, Jean-Pierre Laude

*Electromagnetic and Photonic Simulation for the Beginner: Finite-Difference Frequency-Domain in MATLAB®*, Raymond C. Rumpf

*Electro-Optical Systems Performance Modeling,* Gary Waldman

*Elliptical Fiber Waveguides,* R. B. Dyott

*Engineering Optical Networks,* Sudhir Warier

*Fiber Bragg Gratings: Fundamentals and Applications in Telecommunications and Sensing,* Andrea Othonos and Kyriacos Kalli

*Fiber Optics Communications,* Henry F. Taylor

*The Fiber-Optic Gyroscope, Third Edition,* Hervé C. Lefèvre

*Fiber-Optic Sensors for Biomedical Applications,* Daniele Tosi and Guido Perrone

*Field Theory of Acousto-Optic Signal Processing Devices,* Craig R. Scott

*Finite Element Modeling Methods for Photonics,* B. M. Azizur Rahman and Arti Agrawal

*Frequency Stabilization of Semiconductor Laser Diodes,* Tetsuhiko Ikegami, Shoichi Sudo, and Yoshihisa Sakai

*Fundamentals of Multiaccess Optical Fiber Networks,* Dennis Mestdagh

*Germanate Glasses: Structure Spectroscopy and Properties,* Alfred Margaryan and Michael Piliavin

*Handbook of Distributed Feedback Laser Diodes, Second Edition,* Geert Morthier and Patrick Vankwikelberge

*Highly Coherent Semiconductor Lasers,* Motoichi Ohtsu

*High-Power Optically Activated Solid-State Switches,* Arye Rosen, Fred Zutavern

*Integrated Optics: Design and Modeling,* Reinhard Marz

*Introduction to Electro-Optical Imaging and Tracking Systems,* Shaheen A. Hovanessian and Khalil Seyrafi

*Introduction to Glass Integrated Optics*, S. Iraj Najafi

*Introduction to Infrared and Electro-Optical Systems*, Third Edition, Ronald G. Driggers, Melvin H. Friedman, John W. Devitt, Orges Furxhi and Anjali Singh

*Introduction to Radiometry and Photometry, Second Edition,* William Ross McCluney

*Introduction to Semiconductor Integrated Optics,* Hans P. Zappe

*Laser Communications in Space,* Stephen Lambert

*Liquid Crystal Devices: Physics and Applications*, Vladimir G. Chigrinov

*Lithium Niobate Photonics,* James E. Toney

*MicroLED Devices and Systems,* Khaled Ahmed

*Military Laser Technology and Systems,* David H. Titterton

*Natural Photonics and Bioinspiration*, Sébastien R. Mouchet and Olivier Deparis

*New Photonics Technologies for the Information Age: The Dream of Ubiquitous Services,* Shoichi Sudo and Katsunari Okamoto, editors

*Optical Document Security, Third Edition,* Rudolf L. van Renesse

*Optical FDM Network Technologies,* Kiyoshi Nosu

*Optical Fiber Amplifiers: Materials, Devices, and Applications,* Shoichi Sudo, editor

*Optical Fiber Communication Systems,* Leonid Kazovsky, Sergio Benedetto and Alan Willner

*Optical Fiber Sensors, Volume One: Principles and Components,* Brian Culshaw and John P. Dakin

*Optical Fiber Sensors, Volume Two: Systems and Applications,* Brian Culshaw and John P. Dakin

*Optical Fiber Sensors, Volume Three: Components and Subsystems,* John Dakin and Brian Culshaw, editors

*Optical Fiber Sensors, Volume Four: Applications, Analysis, and Future Trends*, John Dakin and Brian Culshaw, editors

*Optical Interconnection: Foundations and Applications,* John Caulfied and Christopher S. Tocci

*Optical Measurement Techniques and Applications,* Pramod Rastogi

*Optical Network Theory,* Yitzhak Weissman

*Optical Transmission for the Subscriber Loop,* Norio Kashima

*Optical Transmission Systems Engineering,* Milorad Cvijetic

*Optoelectronics for Low-Intensity Conflicts and Homeland Security,* Anil K. Maini

*Optoelectronic Techniques for Microwave and Millimeter-Wave Engineering,* William M. Robertson

*Passive Optical Components for Optical Fiber Transmission,* Norio Kashima

*Photonic Applications for Radio Systems and Networks*, Fabio Cavaliere and Antonio D'Errico

*Plasmonic Optical Fiber Biosensors*, Christophe Caucheteur and Médéric Loyez

*Polarization in Optical Fibers,* Alan Rogers

*Principles of Modern Optical Systems, Volume 1,* Deepak Uttamchandani and Ivan Andonovic, editors

*Principles of Modern Optical Systems, Volume 2,* Deepak Uttamchandani and Ivan Andonovic, editors

*Reliability and Degradation of III-V Optical Devices,* Osamu Ueda

*Securing Information and Communications Systems,* Stephen Furnell, Sokratis Katsikas, Javier Lopez, and Ahmed Patel

*Semiconductor Raman Lasers,* Ken Suto and Jun-Ichi Nishizawa

*Semiconductors for Solar Cells,* Hans Joachim Moller

*Semiconductor Quantum Wells and Superlattices for Long-Wavelength Infrared Detectors,* M. Omar Manasreh

*Signal Processing and Performance Analysis for Imaging Systems,* S. Susan Young, Ronald G. Driggers, and Eddie L. Jacobs

*Single-Mode Optical Fiber Measurement: Characterization and Sensing,* Giovanni Cancellieri and Franco Chiaraluce

*Smart Structures and Materials,* Brian Culshaw

*Substrate Surface Preparation Handbook*, Max Robertson

*Surveillance and Reconnaissance Imaging Systems: Modeling and Performance Prediction*, Jon C. Leachtenauer and Ronald G. Driggers

*Tunable Laser Diodes,* Markus-Christian Amann and Jens Buus

*Ultrafast Diode Lasers: Fundamentals and Applications,* Peter Vasilev

*Understanding Optical Fiber Communications,* Alan Rogers

*Wavelength Division Multiple Access Optical Networks,* Andrea Borella, Giovanni Cancellieri and Franco Chiaraluce

*Wired and Wireless Seamless Access Systems for Public Infrastructure*, Tetsuya Kawanishi

For further information on these and other Artech House titles, including previously considered out-of-print books now available through our In-Print-Forever® (IPF®) program, contact:

Artech House
685 Canton Street
Norwood, MA 02062
Phone: 781-769-9750
Fax: 781-769-6334
e-mail: artech@artechhouse.com

Artech House
16 Sussex Street
London SW1V 4RW UK
Phone: +44 (0)20 7596-8750
Fax: +44 (0)20 7630-0166
e-mail: artech-uk@artechhouse.com

Find us on the World Wide Web at: www.artechhouse.com